ANESTHETIC UPTAKE and ACTION

ANESTHETIC UPTAKE and ACTION

Edmond I. Eger, II, M.D.

Professor of Anesthesia
The University of
California, San Francisco

To Michael
For a good time in Washington
Ted Eger
5 Dec 07

The Williams & Wilkins Company
Baltimore, Maryland

Made in the United States of America

Library of Congress Catalog Card Number 73-6904
SBN 683-02771-9

Reprinted 1975
Reprinted 1976

Composed and printed at the
Waverly Press, Inc.
Mt. Royal and Guilford Aves.
Baltimore, Md. 21202, U.S.A.

Special Contributors

Special chapters have been contributed to this volume by the following:

Ralph A. Epstein, M.D., Assistant Professor of Anesthesiology, Columbia Presbyterian Medical Center, New York, New York. (*Chapter 18*)

Michael J. Halsey, M.A., D. Phil., Member of Scientific Staff, Medical Research Council, Division of Anaesthesia, Clinical Research Centre, Harrow, Middlesex, England. (*Chapter 3*)

René H. Levy, Ph.D., Assistant Professor of Biopharmaceutics, Department of Pharmaceutical Sciences, School of Pharmacy, University of Washington, Seattle, Washington. (*Chapter 20*)

Malcolm Rowland, Ph.D., Associate Professor of Pharmacy and Pharmaceutical Chemistry, University of California, San Francisco, California. (*Chapter 21*)

Lawrence J. Saidman, M.D., Associate Professor of Anesthesia, Department of Anesthesia, University of California, San Diego, California. (*Chapters 16 & 17*)

Preface

Our understanding of how drugs used in the practice of anesthesia reach, act at and are removed from their sites of action has gone well beyond the qualitative descriptions available only a few years ago. This understanding has played a fundamental role in changing anesthesiology from an art to a science, from a specialty that advanced by trial and error to one in which results could be anticipated and predicted. As would be expected, our knowledge of anesthetic uptake and action is scattered through hundreds of reports, and the newest knowledge sometimes conflicts with that obtained earlier. It is the purpose of this book to reduce volume, establish coherency and referee differences of opinion. To accomplish these purposes, I have deliberately followed two policies. First, where conflict exists, I have emphasized the data most apt to be correct. Second, where no data or concepts (or insubstantial amounts of either) exist I have not hestitated to speculate. Thus, the reader must beware of thoughts preceded by "if" or "perhaps" or "possibly."

The first section of the book is devoted to the inhaled anesthetics while subsequent sections cover barbiturates, muscle relaxants and local anesthetics. Each section considers first how the agent acts and second what factors influence the concentration and movement of the agent within the tissues of the body. All sections approach each principle from several viewpoints with the thought that if a reader fails to grasp an idea in one guise, he may be helped by another. Thus, each major concept is described by text, by illustrations and by mathematics. Usually, it is not necessary to follow more than one of these descriptions to follow the book's course—although understanding from one viewpoint strengthens the understanding from another. The mathematical proofs will appeal to only a minority of readers and therefore they exist mainly as footnotes which can be read or passed over.

The questions at the end of each chapter have two aims. One group of questions (the larger group) allows the reader to test his comprehension of the material covered. The second group hopefully will stimulate the reader to consider the implications of the chapter material. There may be no answer, or at least no unambiguous answer, to the latter group of questions.

I owe a great deal to Drs. R. A. Epstein, M. J. Halsey, R. H. Levy, M. Rowland and L. J. Saidman who not only contributed their own chapters, but also suggested revisions of other chapters. I wish to thank several friends who have critiqued portions of the manuscript. These included Drs. E. N. Cohen, R. H. deJong, W. K. Hamilton, T. F. Hornbein, A. S. Keats, E. S. Munson, B. E. Waud and D. R. Waud. A number of anesthesia residents including B. E. Filner, D. Gura and D. W. Kent also have given me the benefit of their criticism. Since this book is directed to the resident and practitioner, their viewpoint was especially pertinent. I am particularly appreciative of the advice and encouragement given by Dr. H. H. Bendixen. Without his support, this book might not exist. Finally, I am indebted to Mrs. Thayer Taft for her editing and untiring retyping of the manuscript.

Contents

Chapter 1

MAC

"Ether contributes other benefits besides preventing . . . pain. It keeps patients still, who otherwise would not be."

John Snow

MAC is the minimum alveolar concentration of anesthetic at 1 atmosphere that produces immobility in 50 percent of those patients or animals exposed to a noxious stimulus. It is a measure of anesthetic potency (potency equals the reciprocal of the partial pressure of an agent required to achieve a given anesthetic effect) which, as indicated by the above quotation from John Snow, has been used clinically since the discovery of anesthesia. Because MAC will be particularly useful to us in future chapters, this chapter will discuss the measurement of MAC and the factors which influence MAC.

Before beginning that discussion I would like to explain my selection of MAC as opposed to some other index of potency. Apart from a modest element of personal bias, there are several objective reasons for that choice. First, as indicated by the Snow quotation and by our own experience, the end-point of abolition of movement is an important element of clinical anesthesia. Obviously, paralysis produced by curare would achieve the same end—but without the achievement of two other essential properties of anesthesia: amnesia and analgesia. It appears that both of these properties are obtained at an alveolar concentration of anesthetic which by itself suppresses movement in response to a noxious stimulus. In fact, amnesia results from doses of an agent which often are too small to abolish volitional movement (1). Although remembrance of intraoperative events has been reported to occur during anesthesia, for these cases "anesthesia" almost invariably included paralysis by muscle relaxants (2, 3).

A second reason for the choice of MAC is that it is equally applicable to all inhaled anesthetics. The same cannot be said for Guedel's signs (4) or the characteristics noted by Woodbridge (5) in his description of "nothria." Many of these signs or characteristics result from anesthetic side effects and vary from agent to agent. For example, ether, cyclopropane and fluroxene increase sympathetic activity and thereby cause a dose-related pupillary dilation, whereas halothane fails to enlarge the pupil (6). Halothane (7), but not ether (8), may depress respiration during anesthesia sufficiently for surgery. Surely then, respiratory changes (or circulatory changes for that matter) cannot be used to characterize all anesthetics. Even reflex responses (laryngeal, carinal, vagal) vary between the anesthetic states produced by anesthetics. Such side effects of anesthesia are useful to the clinician who must administer neither too much nor too little of a particular anesthetic. But these signs of "depth" of anesthesia vary from agent to agent and therefore cannot provide a universal definition of anesthetic potency. This is in contrast to MAC which can be applied to all anesthetics.

A third reason for the choice of MAC is that it equals the partial pressure of anesthetic (in percent of 1 atmosphere pressure) at the anesthetic site of action. This assumes that the alveolar partial pressure is transmitted without change to arterial blood (9) and that, given sufficient time for equilibration, the partial pressure at the site of action equals the partial pressure in arterial blood. We shall demonstrate later that these are reasonable assumptions under normal circumstances. The use of alveolar concentrations (the "AC" in MAC) contrasts with the use of inspired concentrations or concentrations of anesthetic in arterial or venous blood. Neither the inspired nor the blood concentrations may bear a constant relation to the concentration or partial pressure at the anesthetic site of action. An appreciation of this point requires that we define the term "partial pressure" and the relations between partial pressure and concentration. In a gaseous phase, partial pressure equals the fractional concentration of the gas in question times total pressure. In any phase the partial pressure is a measure of the tendency of an anesthetic to leave or escape from that phase. It is synonomous with "activity." As we shall see in Chapter 4, a given partial pressure may produce different concentrations in different phases (blood, alveolar gas or tissues). Thus, at equilibrium, although the partial pressure in all phases may be equal the concentrations may vary, and the concentration in one phase, such as blood, is not necessarily representative of the concentration in brain.

Determination of MAC

In animals MAC is determined as follows (10). The animal is anesthetized with the agent to be studied. The alveolar concentration is measured and held constant at a predetermined level for at least 15 minutes to insure equilibration between alveoli and the central nervous system. The animal is then stimulated (usually for a full minute) and observed for movement or lack of movement. The stimulus normally is produced by application of a large hemostat to the tail (tail clamp) or by passage of electrical current through subcutaneous electrodes. Movement of the head, torso or legs may follow. We arbitrarily do not consider stiffening, coughing or hyperventilation as movement. If movement fails to occur then the alveolar concentration is lowered to 80 percent of the previous value and the process of equilibration and stimulus-response is repeated. Eventually this process derives the anesthetic concentrations permitting and preventing movement. The concentration midway between these brackets is MAC. For example, if 1.0 percent alveolar halothane prevents movement while 0.8 percent permits movement then the halothane MAC equals 0.9 percent. Note that in fact MAC might have been slightly above 0.8 or below 1.0 or about 10 percent different from the calculated 0.9 figure. A smaller error results if smaller differences are used for the bracketing concentrations. This, however, greatly increases the time required to determine MAC. Usually the bracketing of MAC is repeated 1 or 2 times in the same animal. A group of animals studied in this manner provide an average MAC for this agent in this species and an estimate of the variability of MAC.

Determination of MAC in man differs from the determination in animals in that the stimulus is the surgical skin incision and, in practice, only one observation can be obtained for each patient. Several patients are anesthetized with the agent to be studied and the alveolar concentration held constant for at least 15 minutes at one of several predetermined levels. The levels chosen are both above and below the one estimated to permit movement in response to surgical incision. The results are plotted as percentage of patients moving at each concentration. From a visual line of best fit drawn through these points the concentration (MAC) preventing 50 percent of patients from responding can be estimated (fig. 1,1) (11). This technique fails to give an estimate of MAC variability unless many groups of patients are studied or unless the data are analyzed by Probit analysis (12). Probit analysis allows an objective estimate of both MAC and its variability.

Factors Not Affecting MAC

One of the surprising aspects of MAC is its constancy. When we began our studies of MAC we anticipated a large biological variability, and the need for many determinations to give meaning to an average MAC value especially if it were to be compared with MAC values of other anesthetics. To our delight, MAC proved to be remarkably constant.

Effect of Variable Stimulus, Species, Sex and Duration of Anesthesia

The value obtained for MAC is not critically dependent on the choice or intensity of the noxious stimulus. Different stimuli, such as electrical

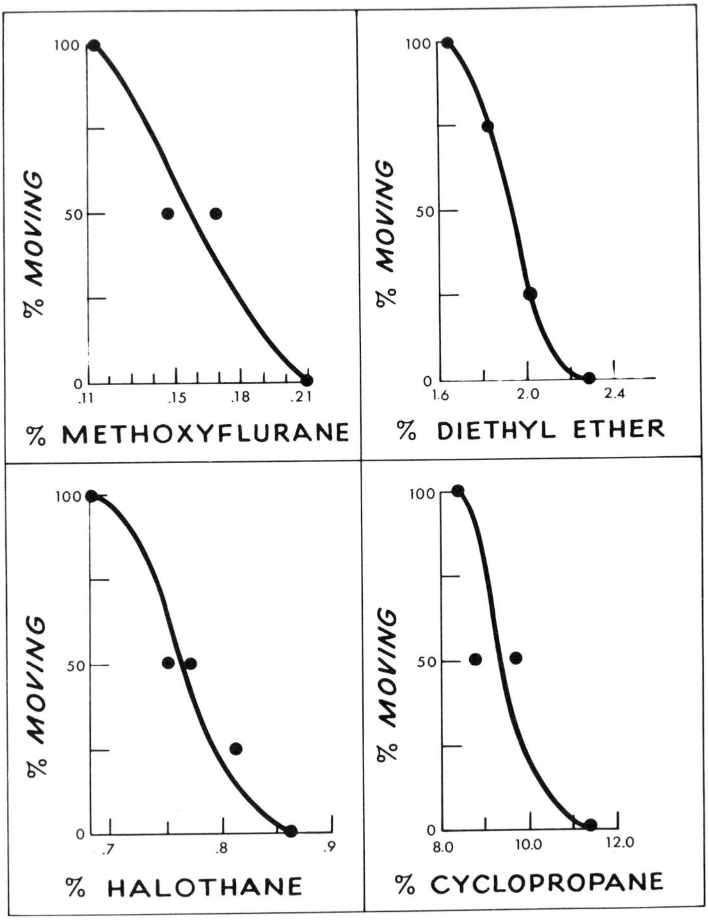

FIG. 1,1. The percent of patients moving in response to surgical incision decreases from 100 percent to zero over a narrow range of alveolar concentrations. Note that zero concentration is far to the left of each curve. This is true for all anesthetics tested as illustrated by the 4 agents in this figure. MAC is the concentration preventing movement in 50 percent of patients. In these examples, MAC is 0.16 for methoxyflurane, 1.9 for ether, 0.76 for halothane and 9.2 for cyclopropane, all expressed as percent of anesthetic in alveolar air. (Reproduced with permission from Saidman, L. J., Eger, E. I., II, Munson, E. S., Babad, A. A., and Muallem, M.: Minimum alveolar concentration of methoxyflurane, halothane, ether and cyclopropane in man: Correlation with theories of anesthetia. Anesthesiology 28: 994–1002, 1967.)

current passed through needle electrodes in the skin, the tail clamp or skin incision all require the same alveolar concentration to suppress movement (10). Increasing the intensity of stimulus beyond a certain strength fails to alter MAC. The halothane MAC determined by application of 30 volts to subcutaneous electrodes does not differ from the MAC determined with 50 volts. Concomitant application of 40 volts and tail clamp led to the same MAC determined by individual application of either stimulus (10).

Variability of MAC in a given species is small. In the dog the standard deviation from the average MAC equals 10 to 20 percent of the MAC value (13). Anesthetic requirement as indicated by MAC shows still less variation in a given animal (10). Perhaps more remarkable is the smallness of the variability of the average MAC from species to species or even from one class of animals to another (table 1,1).

Time does not seem to affect MAC. Halothane MAC determined on the same dog on successive weeks varies an average of 8 percent. Similar constancy of MAC has been obtained with cyclopropane in rat (32). In the same dog on a given day, the variation between successive determinations is also 8 percent (fig. 1,2) (10). MAC after 10 hours of halothane anesthesia was not significantly different from that measured during the first 1 to 2 hours. Similar results were obtained with fluroxene and cyclopropane. Thus, duration of anesthesia does not affect MAC in dogs. The same is true in man when subjected to two incisions (usually bilateral herniorrhaphies) at different times during the same anesthetic. The dose required to suppress movement in response to second incision did not differ from that required for the first incision (Gregory, G. A., unpublished data).

The sexes are equally affected by anesthesia. Munson (unpublished data) found no difference in cyclopropane MAC in male compared to

TABLE 1,1

*MAC values for anesthetics in different species**

Agent	Dog	Man	Cat	Rat or Mouse	Goldfish	Toad
Methoxyflurane	0.23 ± 0.03 (14)	0.16 (11)	0.23 ± 0.02 (15)	0.22 (16)	0.13 (17)	0.22 (18)
Chloroform	0.77 ± 0.10 (13)			0.8 (19)	0.63 (17)	
Halothane	0.87 ± 0.12 (14)	0.75 (11, 20, 21)	0.82 ± 0.10 (15)	0.95 to 1.1 (22)	0.76 (17)	0.67 (18)
Isoflurane	1.5 (23)	1.15 (24)				
Enflurane	2.2 ± 0.26 (13)	1.68 (25)	1.2 ± 0.1 (15)			
Ether	3.04 ± 0.53 (14)	1.92 (11)	2.1 ± 0.1 (15)	3.2 (19)	2.2 (17)	1.63 (18)
Fluroxene	6.0 ± 1.1 (14)	3.4 (26)				
C_3H_6	17.5 ± 3.8 (14)	9.2 (11)	19.7 ± 1.0 (15)	17 (27)		9.0 (18)
C_2H_4		67 (20)		130 (28)		
Xe	119 ± 8 (14)	71 (29)		95 (30)		
N_2O	188 ± 35 (14)	105 (31)		150 (30)		81.5 (18)
SF_6	490 ± 40 (13)			610 (30)		
CF_4	2600 ± 800 (13)			1900 (30)		

* This table demonstrates the low variability of MAC among species or even classes of animals. All values are given as a percent of 1 atmosphere. Some of the variation results from differences in technique used to demonstrate MAC. Dog values were obtained with either tail clamp or electrical stimuli, whereas the stimulus in man was surgical incision or an electrical pulse (nitrous oxide). Perhaps this partly explains the consistently lower figures for man. Age may also explain this difference since human values were obtained in 30 to 55 year old patients (except for nitrous oxide where the age was 20 to 30 years). Cats and rats were tested with a tail clamp; for mice the inspired dose abolishing the righting reflex was measured. Goldfish were electrically stimulated. Mammal temperatures ranged from 36 to 39°C. Goldfish temperatures were 25° and toads 20 to 22°C.

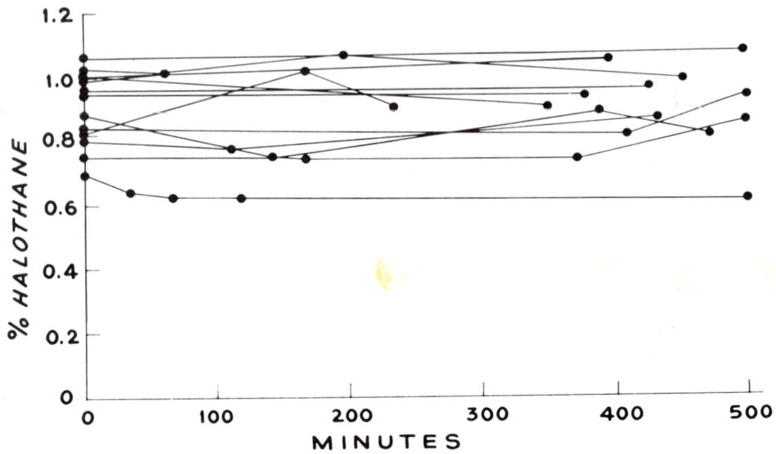

FIG. 1,2. The halothane MAC of 7 dogs was determined on 12 occasions during 5 to 10 hours of anesthesia. Changes occurring with time are illustrated. No difference was found between the first determination (0 minutes) and the last. It should be noted that anesthesia had been induced 1 to 2 hours prior to the first determination. (Reproduced with permission from Eger, E. I., II, Saidman, L. J., and Brandstater, B.: Minimum alveolar anesthetic concentration: a standard of anesthetic potency. Anesthesiology 26: 756–763, 1965.)

female rats. We found no differences between MAC in human males and females (unpublished data).

Effect of Acid-Base Changes

Changes in metabolic acid-base status fail to alter anesthetic requirements (33). MAC was unchanged by infusion of sufficient sodium bicarbonate to induce a base excess of 7 mEq or by intravenous hydrochloric acid to induce a 20 mEq base deficit. Similarly, arterial pH values from 7.6 to 6.9 induced by changes in arterial PCO_2 failed to alter MAC.

A $PaCO_2$ as low as 10 torr and as high as 90 torr produces no measurable change in MAC for halothane (33) (fig. 1,3). In a study over a narrower range of partial pressures (22 to 38 torr) (34) we confirmed this lack of effect of $PaCO_2$ on MAC in man. Andersen and Shim (18) similarly found no change in toad MAC from hyperventilation sufficient to elevate pH to 7.6.

The failure of $PaCO_2$ to alter MAC appears to conflict with the clinical impression that either hyperventilation or administration of CO_2 augments the depth of anesthesia. The conflict is more apparent than real. Although no effect is apparent below a $PaCO_2$ of 90 torr, above this level CO_2 increases the anesthetic effect of halothane (fig. 1,3). CO_2 alone is anesthetic in normal dogs at 245 torr (33). In contrast, imposition of a central (cerebrospinal fluid) acidosis by infusion of hydrochloric acid permits a $PaCO_2$ of 145 torr to be anesthetic alone. The evidence in dogs suggests that the effect of CO_2 is best related to its effect on cerebrospinal fluid hydrogen ion rather than to CO_2 partial pressure or arterial pH (fig. 1,4). No effect is seen above a cerebrospinal fluid pH of 7.1, whereas complete CO_2 narcosis results at a pH of 6.8 to 6.9.

Hyperventilation may have three effects which would appear to increase depth of anesthesia. As we shall see in Chapter 7, an increase in ventilation increases the alveolar anesthetic concentration and thereby may increase the anesthetic effect of any given inspired concentration. The clinician correctly perceives an increase in anesthetic depth but should not conclude that this resulted from a fall in $PaCO_2$. Secondly, the fall in CO_2 acts to augment one of the *secondary* effects of anesthesia; a lowered $PaCO_2$ decreases or abolishes ventilatory drive. The clinician obtains greater abdominal muscle relaxation through the inactivity of the accessory muscles of respiration. Lastly, a reduction in $PaCO_2$ causes cerebral blood flow to fall. The consequent reduction in oxygen delivery to the brain may augment the effect of anesthesia. Our initial studies failed to support this notion. However, Cullen (35) suggested that this failure might have come from our use of halothane in 100 percent oxygen, with dissolved oxygen countering hypoxia secondary to reduced blood flow. The clinician usually administers halothane in a mixture of nitrous oxide and oxygen rather than oxygen alone. In this case there would be less dissolved oxygen to compensate for the reduction in cerebral blood flow. Some studies of patients after surgery do suggest that cerebral injury under anesthesia may be wrought by hyperventilation. In these studies showing postoperative abnormalities in flicker fusion (36) or reaction time (37), air or nitrous oxide-oxygen was the respired gas. On the other hand, Blenkarn *et al.* (38) found no difference due to hypocapnia (versus eucapnia) in 5 tests of cognitive and perceptual-motor function in humans subjected to thiopental-nitrous oxide-curare anesthesias without operation.

To test the role of inspired oxygen concentration, Cullen (35) examined MAC in dogs during hypocapnia with halothane administered in oxygen compared with halothane in air. Hyperventilation failed to change MAC when oxygen was inspired but caused a decrease of 11 percent of the eucapnic MAC when air formed the background gas. Whether such a slight change could be clinically detectable might be debated.

Effect of Changes in Arterial Oxygen

Changes in arterial oxygen partial pressure (PaO_2) over a wide range fail to affect MAC in dogs except for the small reduction with concomitant hyperventilation noted above. Halothane MAC at PaO_2 of 40 torr equals that at 500 torr (fig. 1,5) (39). However, if PaO_2 is reduced

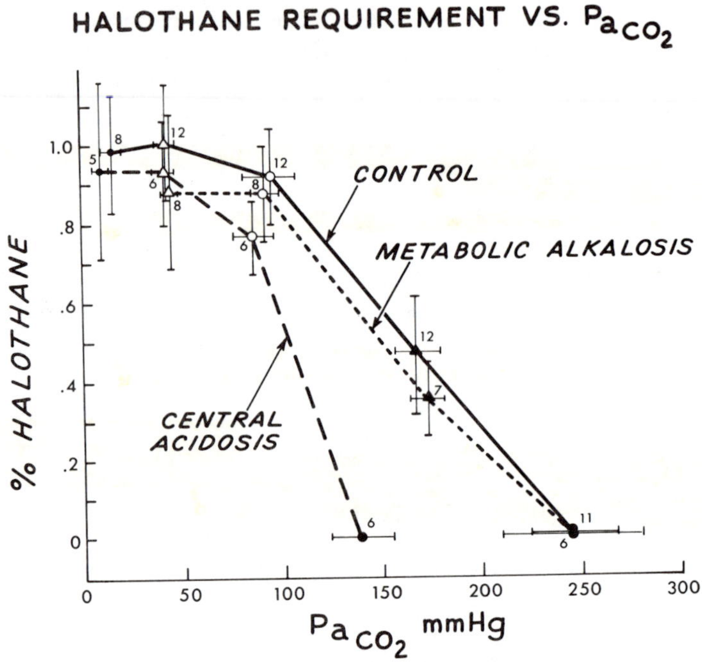
HALOTHANE REQUIREMENT VS. Pa_{CO_2}
CONTROL
METABOLIC ALKALOSIS
CENTRAL ACIDOSIS
% HALOTHANE
1.0
.8
.6
.4
.2
0
0
50
100
150
200
250
300
Pa_{CO_2} mmHg

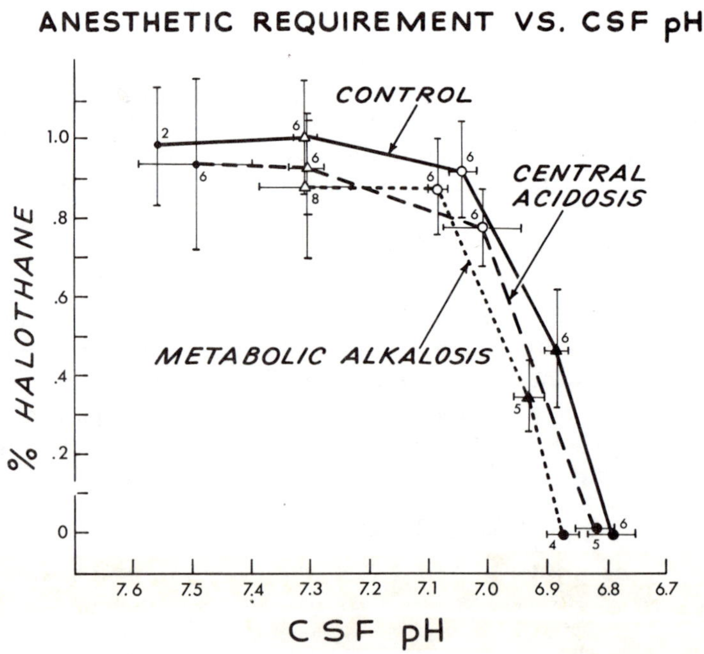
ANESTHETIC REQUIREMENT VS. CSF pH
CONTROL
CENTRAL ACIDOSIS
METABOLIC ALKALOSIS
% HALOTHANE
1.0
.8
.6
.4
.2
0
7.6
7.5
7.4
7.3
7.2
7.1
7.0
6.9
6.8
6.7
CSF pH

below 40 torr, MAC decreases. The reduction is particularly steep below 30 torr (fig. 1,5).

The excellent correlation between MAC and arterial oxygen content during hypoxia does not apply to induced isovolemic anemia (fig. 1,6) (40). In 6 dogs we progressively reduced the hematocrit by phlebotomy and by concomitant infusion of dextran or autologous plasma. Arterial blood pressure was unaffected by the exchange. The resulting anemia failed to alter MAC until the oxygen content fell below 5 volumes percent. Further decreases in hemoglobin reduced MAC. In contrast to the lack of an effect from anemia, when content was reduced to 5 volumes percent by low inspired oxygen, MAC fell to one-third of its original value (fig. 1,6). The difference is not surprising, since cerebral tissues require a minimum venous oxygen tension of 20 torr or more to prevent lactic acidosis (41, 42). The demand of brain tissue for oxygen may be met during anemia by increasing cerebral blood flow. For example, a 4 fold increase in flow would completely compensate for an anemia which reduced oxygen content to one-fourth normal. But no increase in flow could sustain brain oxygen tension above 20 torr during hypoxia which produced a reduction in arterial oxygen content to one-fourth normal. Such a content exists at a PaO_2 of only 17 torr (normal pH).

Neither hypoxia nor isovolemic anemia influence MAC until they attain levels which produce decompensation of the body defenses against oxygen deprivation. Levels of hypoxia and anemia sufficient to affect MAC cause a progressive metabolic acidosis and are only slightly higher then levels causing cardiovascular or respiratory arrest. For example, 2 of the 6 animals died following reduction of their hematocrit from 10 to 8 percent. At 10 percent, MAC had not been significantly altered.

Effect of Changes in Arterial Pressure

Hypertension induced by phenylephrine fails to affect MAC though the blood pressure may be twice normal (10, 43). Similarly MAC remains unaffected by the slight fall in blood pressure induced by guanethidine

FIG. 1,3. Halothane MAC decreases when $PaCO_2$ exceeds 90 mm Hg. The CO_2 MAC is that $PaCO_2$ at which no halothane is required (i.e., 245 mm Hg). MAC of CO_2 is little affected by metabolic alkalosis induced by sodium bicarbonate infusion. When cerebrospinal fluid acidosis was induced prior to the study by hyperventilation and intravenous hydrochloric acid infusion, CO_2 MAC decreased from 245 mm Hg to 145 mm Hg. The *numbers* at each point indicate the number of dogs in each sample. *Bars* indicate standard deviation. (Reproduced by permission from Eisele, J. H., Eger, E. I., II, and Muallem, M.: Narcotic properties of carbon dioxide in the dog. Anesthesiology 28: 856–865, 1967.)

FIG. 1,4. This figure is identical to 1,3 except that the changes in halothane MAC are related to changes in cerebrospinal fluid (CSF) pH. Unlike the previous figure, halothane requirement approaches zero at a consistant point regardless of the treatment. (Reproduced with permission from Eisele, J. H., Eger, E. I., II, and Muallem, M.: Narcotic properties of carbon dioxide in the dog. Anesthesiology 8: 856–865, 1967.)

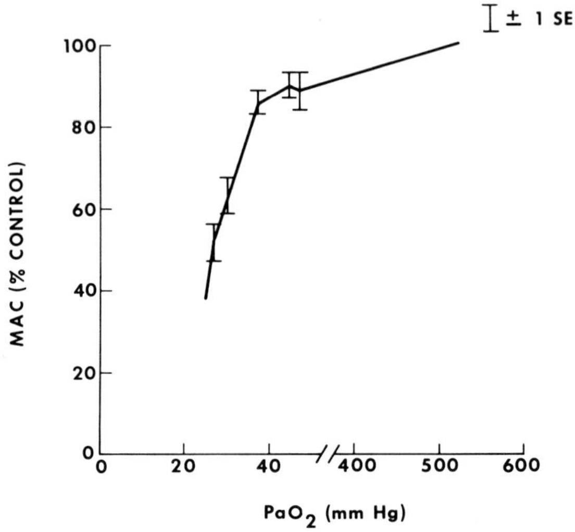

FIG. 1,5. Halothane MAC in dogs shows no significant change over a range of PaO_2 values extending from 40 to 500 torr. Below a PaO_2 of 30 to 40 torr, MAC shows a sharp decrease. (Reproduced with permission from Cullen, D. J., and Eger, E. I., II: The effects of hypoxia and isovolemic anemia on the halothane requirement (MAC) of dogs. I. The effect of hypoxia. Anesthesiology 32: 28–34, 1970.)

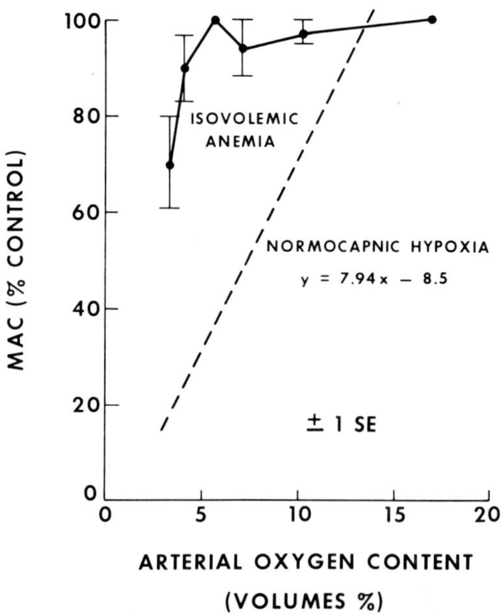

FIG. 1,6. A progressive reduction in MAC accompanies a fall in arterial oxygen content due to a lower inspired oxygen (*dashed line*) but no fall in MAC results from a fall in content due to anemia until the content falls below 5 volumes percent (*continuous line* and *points*). (Reproduced with permission from Cullen, D. J., and Eger, E. I., II: The effects of hypoxia and isovolemic anemia on the halothane requirement (MAC) of dogs: III. The effects of acute isovolemic anemia. Anesthesiology 32: 46–50, 1970.)

(Miller, R. D., unpublished data). Reduction in blood pressure to one-third to one-half of control by hemorrhage reduces halothane MAC to 80 percent of control (10). Such hypovolemia induces a base deficit of 2 to 6 mEq—perhaps indicating that as in hypoxia and anemia this change in MAC requires the imposition of a life-threatening stress.

Physiological Factors Which Alter Anesthetic Requirement

The previous section suggested that only the application of extreme stress changes MAC. Such changes in MAC are not immediately reversed by removal of the stress, implying a residual structural or biochemical change in the brain.

Circadian Rhythms and MAC

However, some natural causes can change MAC without apparent brain damage. Small changes are related to circadian rhythms. In rats subjected to a 12 hour alternating cycle of light and dark, halothane or cyclopropane MAC increases 5 to 10 percent above average if anesthesia is induced in the dark portion of the cycle; that is, the time of greatest rat activity. Conversely, the lowest values are obtained during the light portion of the cycle (27). Such variations might explain the small variability in MAC in a given animal on a given day or among patients.

Effect of Changes in Body Temperature

Clinicians have long recognized that very little anesthetic is required for hypothermic patients. Several investigations of MAC confirm this clinical impression (17, 44–47). Although hypothermia reduces MAC for all agents, the reduction per degree decrease in body temperature varies from agent to agent. In dogs halothane or methoxyflurane requirement falls 5 percent with each degree centigrade from 37°C (45). However, cyclopropane MAC falls by only 2 percent per degree. The relationship for ether and fluroxene, 4 percent per degree, lies between these extremes (table 1,2). Qualitatively similar but greater changes occur in rats (fig. 1,7) (46). The ascent of MAC with temperature follows the same path as descent indicating neither hysteresis nor structural damage (fig. 1,7) (46). The implications of temperature dependent changes in MAC relate both to theories of narcosis and to uptake and distribution of inhaled anesthetics—subjects discussed in succeeding chapters. The implications for clinical anesthesia are obvious: most patients lose heat during operation both because anesthesia reduces metabolism and because anesthesia increases skin blood flow. By transferring heat from the body core to the skin, increased skin blood flow caused by anesthesia may reduce esophageal temperature 0.5 to 1.0°C within 15 minutes following induction of anesthesia (48). Body heat also is lost during operation from open pleural or peritoneal cavities and by administration

TABLE 1,2*

Agent	Number of Dogs	MAC at 37°C	Change in MAC/10°C	Decrease in MAC/10°C
				%
Cyclopropane	6	15.9 ± 3.6	3.0 ± 1.5	20 ± 9
Diethyl ether	5	3.3 ± 0.7	1.2 ± 0.5	38 ± 11
Fluroxene	8	6.6 ± 0.8	2.8 ± 1.2	42 ± 15
Methoxyflurane	7	0.24 ± 0.03	0.13 ± 0.03	52 ± 11
Halothane	6	0.87 ± 0.11	0.44 ± 0.88	53 ± 8

* The MAC values in this table represent means of small groups of animals. The values therefore vary slightly from the much larger group represented in table 1,1. The change in MAC/10°C indicates the decrease in absolute percent gas concentration required to prevent movement in response to tail clamp per 10°C lowering of body temperature from 37°C. Values are the average ±1 standard deviation. (Regan, M. J., and Eger, E. I., II: Effect of hypothermia in dogs on anesthetizing and apneic doses of inhalation agents. Anesthesiology 28: 689, 1967.)

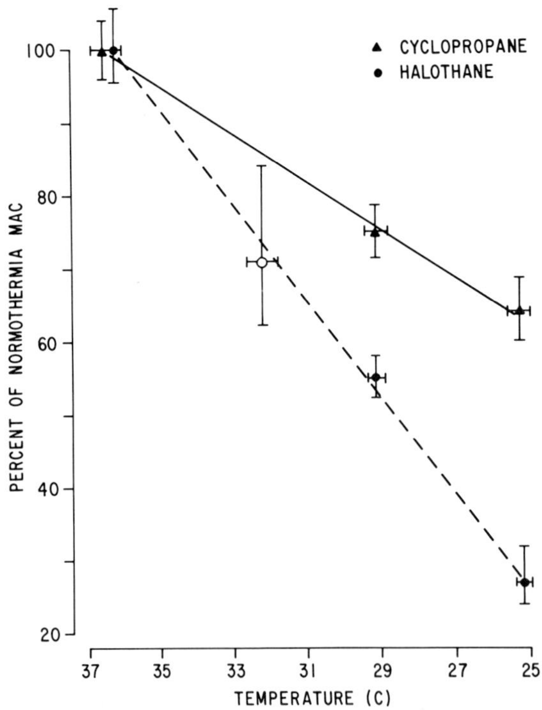

FIG. 1,7. Although a decrease in body temperature lowers both cyclopropane (*triangles*) and halothane (*circles*) MAC, the change is twice as great with halothane. In both cases the relationship follows a straight line. The *unfilled circle* for halothane was obtained during rewarming while all other points were obtained during cooling. (Reproduced with permission from Munson, E. S.: Effect of hypothermia on anesthetic requirement in rats. Lab. Anim. Sci. 20: 1109–1113, 1970.)

of cold intravenous fluids. Normothermic preoperative patients often cool inadvertently to 31 to 35°C during surgery. The reduction in anesthetic requirement associated with cooling must be considered by the anesthetist who may otherwise overdose the patient by using a concentration optimal only at 37°C.

As anticipated, an increase in body temperature increases MAC. The quantitative changes indicated above for hypothermia probably also apply to hyperthermia, but data in mammals are limited to studies of halothane in dogs at 39 to 40°C (44). These data support the long held clinical impression of an increased anesthetic requirement for febrile patients. The use of greater anesthetic doses in these patients, however, should be tempered by the decreased physiological reserve imposed by the disease causing the fever as well as the increased metabolic demands levied by hyperthermia itself.

Effect of Changes in Thyroid Function

The MAC changes induced by elevating or lowering body temperature probably are not related to changes in oxygen consumption since large changes in oxygen consumption induced by hyper- or hypothyroidism in normothermic dogs cause relatively small changes in halothane MAC. For example, hypothyroidism reduces oxygen consumption by 36 percent without significantly lowering MAC. Conversely, hyperthyroidism raises MAC only 15 percent whereas uptake of oxygen increases by 32 percent (49). Similarly, 2 fold variations in whole body oxygen consumption induced by thyroid or antithyroid medications do not affect cyclopropane MAC in rats. However, oxygen consumption in rat brain slices is not affected by prior thyroid medication, and thus, the changes in whole body oxygen consumption cited above may be misleading (50).

Age and MAC

The anesthetist has long known to reduce anesthetic dose in older patients. Until recently the quantitative aspects of this relationship were unknown (12, 51). We found that halothane MAC descends from a high of 1.1 percent in the neonate to a low of 0.63 in the 70 year old (fig. 1,8) (51). The changes with age may be correlated with many aspects of the aging process. For example, neuronal density decreases with age and cerebral metabolic rate decreases with age. These, however, may be mere associations and not have a cause and effect relationship. Regardless of cause, the anesthetist must temper his ministrations to avoid overdosing the elderly.

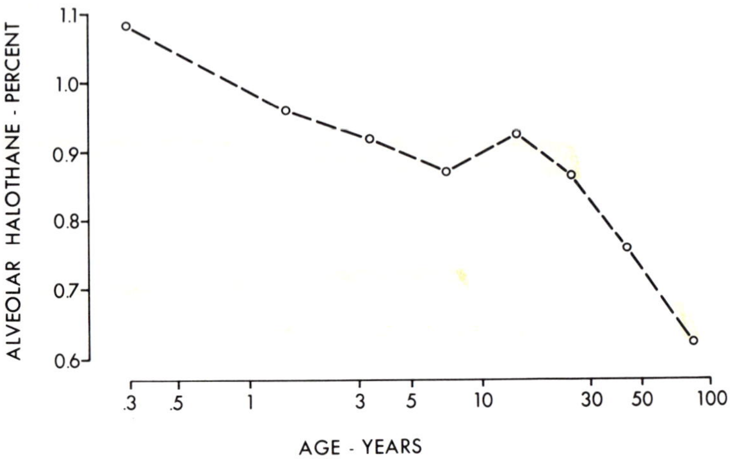

FIG. 1,8. Halothane MAC (*vertical axis*) constantly decreases with age, with the possible exception of a slight increase at puberty. (Reproduced with permission from Gregory, G. A., Eger, E. I., II, and Munson, E. S.: The relationship between age and halothane requirement in man. Anesthesiology. 30: 488–491, 1969.)

Effect of Adjuvants and Other Drugs on MAC

Narcotics and Diazepam

Two drugs given concomitantly each may modify the action of the other. The effects of some interactions are obvious. It is not surprising that narcotics reduce MAC. In humans premedication with 8 to 15 mg of morphine decreases halothane MAC by 7 percent (fig. 1,9) (21) and fluroxene MAC by 20 percent (26). Similarly, pentazocine, morphine and meperidine reduce cyclopropane MAC in rats (fig. 1,10) (47). The effect of morphine and meperidine is dose-related. Each logarithmic increase in narcotic dose produces a proportional reduction in cyclopropane MAC. Although pentazocine also reduces MAC, the reduction appears to reach an upper limit or ceiling effect at 20 mg/kg.

Another common premedicant, diazepam, also reduces halothane MAC in man. In 17 patients given 0.2 mg/kg of diazepam intravenously 15 to 30 minutes prior to incision, halothane MAC was 0.48 percent (52), as compared to a MAC of 0.73 percent in unmedicated patients. Diazepam may have a ceiling effect. In 5 patients, administration of 0.4 mg/kg of diazepam reduced MAC to 0.4 percent (52), a figure only slightly less than that produced by 0.2 mg/kg.

Atropine and Scopolamine

Intraperitoneal atropine, 0.015 mg/kg does not alter cyclopropane MAC in rats (Munson, E. S., DiFazio, C. A. and Coker, W., unpublished data). Small doses of scopolamine also have no effect on MAC in rats. A large dose of scopolamine (0.48 mg/kg) causes a maximum decrease in MAC of 14 percent in MAC 1 hour after administration. The small effect of scopolamine and absent effect of atropine may relate to the limited passage of atropine and possible scopolamine into rat brain. Atropine passes more readily into the cat and dog central nervous system (53). If atropine passes into human brain as easily as into the dog brain, then a reduction in MAC by scopolamine may occur in man.

Interactions between Inhaled Agents

The interaction between anesthetics in their effect on MAC appears to be additive. The simultaneous use of 70 to 75 percent nitrous oxide produces a striking reduction in fluroxene or halothane MAC (fig. 1,9). Our work with xenon-halothane and ethylene-halothane combinations suggests additive effects. Half a MAC of ethylene or xenon plus half a MAC of halothane produces the same effect as one MAC of either alone (20, 29) (fig. 1,11). Assuming all anesthetic effects are simply additive then the 70 percent reduction in halothane or fluroxene MAC produced by the addition of 70 to 75 percent nitrous oxide allows us to predict a nitrous oxide MAC of about 100 percent. A similar MAC was predicted from combinations of isoflurane and nitrous oxide (Dolan, W. M. *et al.*,

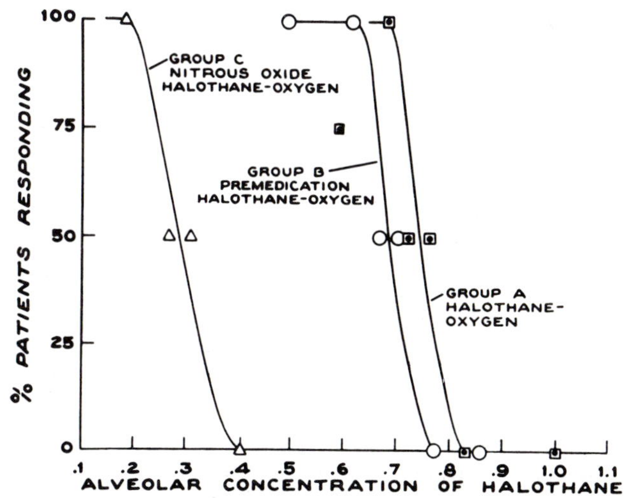

FIG. 1,9. Both premedication with 8 to 15 mg of morphine (*group B*) or addition of 70 percent nitrous oxide (*group C*) reduce the alveolar concentration of halothane required to eliminate movement in response to surgical incision. (Reproduced with permission from Saidman, L. J., and Eger, E. I., II: Effect of nitrous oxide and of narcotic premedication on the alveolar concentration of halothane required for anesthesia. Anesthesiology 25: 302–306, 1964.)

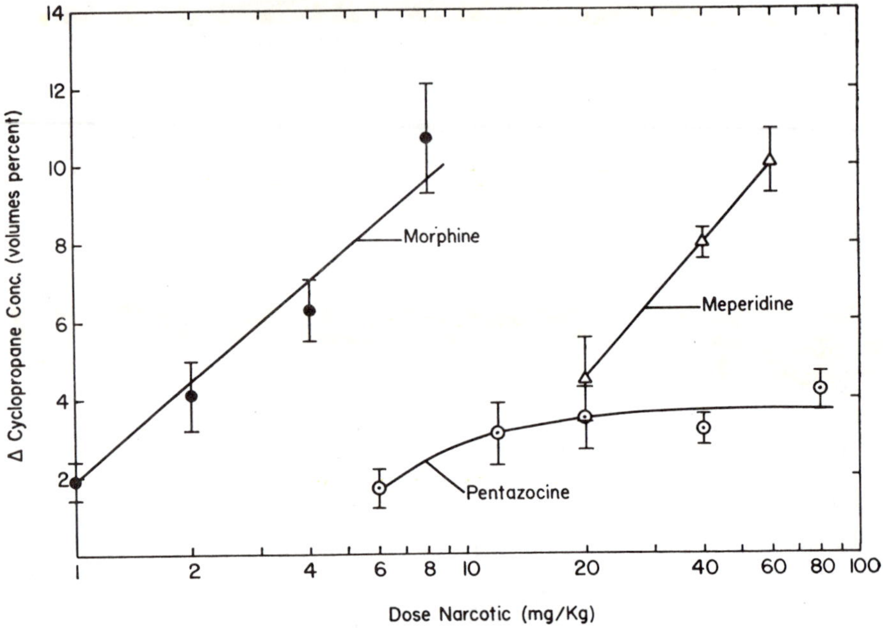

FIG. 1,10. A larger dose of morphine or meperidine causes a greater change (Δ) in cyclopropane MAC (*vertical axis*). The effect with pentazocine is limited. Note that the "change" is a reduction in MAC and not an increase as the illustration might suggest from the positive slope of the graphs. (Reproduced with permission from Hoffman, J. C., and DiFazio, C. A.: The anesthesia-sparing effect of pentazocine, meperidine, and morphine. Arch. Int. Pharmacodyn. Thèr. 186: 261–268, 1970.)

unpublished data). This estimate for man accords well with the study by Paul Bert (54) who reported 16 operations in humans conducted under nitrous oxide alone at partial pressures of 1.0 to 1.1 atmospheres, plus 0.2 atmospheres of oxygen. Finally, the estimate of 100 percent also agrees with the results of the study by Winter *et al.* (31). They determined the nitrous oxide MAC in human volunteers anesthetized with nitrous oxide in oxygen and subjected to electrical stimulation.

DeFazio *et al.* (28) have found additive effects for halothane-fluroxene, cyclopropane-teflurane and cyclopropane-halothane combinations in rats. They also, however, found a slight but significant antagonism between cyclopropane and ethylene or cyclopropane and nitrous oxide as evidenced by the failure of 15 to 20 percent nitrous oxide or ethylene to reduce the cyclopropane MAC. Concentrations of nitrous oxide or ethylene above 15 to 20 percent were additive with cyclopropane.

Effect of Alcoholism

In his studies of nitrous oxide, Bert (54) noted that 1 patient, a chronic alcoholic, was only paritally anesthetized by 1.15 atmospheres of nitrous oxide. "Resistance" of these patients to anesthetics is a long-established clinical impression. Han (55) reported a dramatic increase in halothane MAC in chronic alcoholics. However, Munson found no response to incision in 3 chronic alcoholics anesthetized with 0.8 percent halothane (Munson, E. A., unpublished data).

MAC and Central Nervous System Catecholamines

Drugs which alter central nervous system catecholamines or their release also alter anesthetic requirement. Drugs such as alpha methyl dopa (Aldomet) or reserpine deplete cerebral catecholamines and decrease MAC (fig. 1,12) (43, 56). Guanethidine depletes peripheral but not central catecholamine stores and interestingly does not alter MAC (56) (fig. 1,12). The maximum effect of drugs which reduce central catecholamines is limited, reducing MAC roughly 30 percent regardless of further increases in dose. This observation implies that a portion of anesthetic effect may be achieved through the inhibition of sympathetic pathways. It also implies that other pathways must be blocked to achieve anesthesia.

The opposite effect, an increase in MAC, results from the intravenous

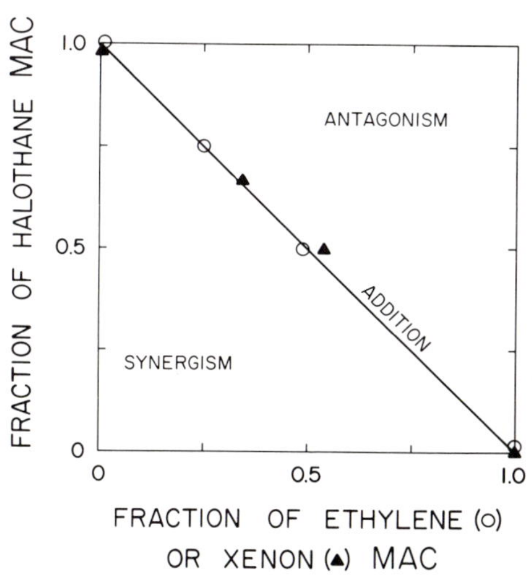

FIG. 1,11. In man, the sum of the fraction of the ethylene or xenon MAC which must be added to the halothane MAC in order to produce unresponsiveness to surgical incision equals 1 for all combinations tested. That is, all results lie on the line marked "addition." (Adapted with permission from Miller, R. D., Wahrenbrock, E. A., Schroeder, C. F., Knipstein, T. W., Eger, E. I., II, and Buechel, D. R.: Ethylene-halothane anesthesia: Addition or synergism? Anesthesiology 31: 301–304, 1969 and Cullen, S. C., Eger, E. I., II, Cullen, B. F., and Gregory, G. P.: Observations on the anesthetic effect of the combination of xenon and halothane. Anesthesiology 31: 305–309, 1969.)

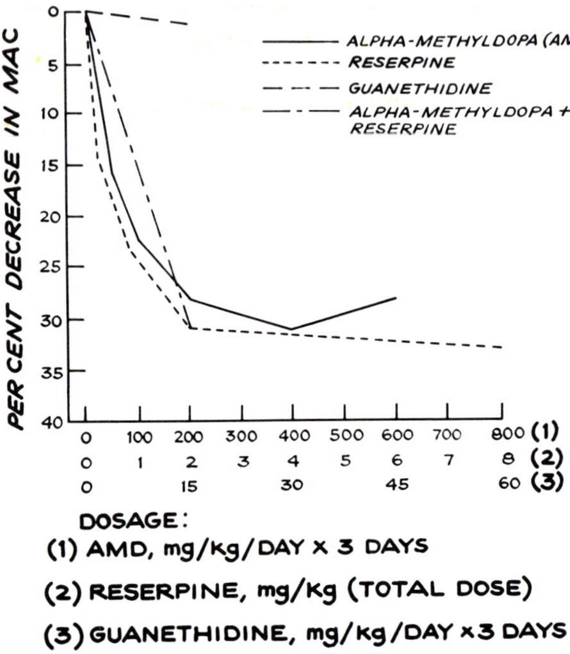

FIG. 1,12. Alpha-methyl dopa, reserpine or the combination of these two drugs cause a reduction in halothane MAC in dogs. Guanethidine, although causing the same depletion of peripheral catecholamines as the other drugs, alters neither central catecholamines nor MAC. (Reproduced with permission from Miller, R. D., Way, W. L., and Eger, E. I., II: The effects of alpha-methyl-dopa, reserpine, guanethidine, and iproniazid on minimum alveolar anesthetic requirement (MAC). Anesthesiology 29: 1153–1158, 1968.)

administration of d-amphetamine (43), a drug which releases catecholamines. The increase in MAC is dose-related and may be very large (fig. 1,13). Prior administration of drugs which deplete or block the synthesis of central catecholamines partially or completely blocks the stimulatory effect of d-amphetamine. Alkalosis induced by hyperventilation diminishes or abolishes the effect. The basis for the effect of hyperventilation is unknown, but it is not due to a pH dependent increase in nonionized amphetamine nor to an increase in amphetamine blood levels (43). Chronic administration of amphetamine to dogs (2.5 mg/kg/day for 7 days) results in a 22 ± 3 (SE) percent *decrease* rather than an increase in MAC (43). Chronic administration depletes central catecholamines as evidenced by lack of a pressor response to tyramine. Thus, chronically administered amphetamine acts like reserpine and alpha methyl dopa.

These observations have implications for the anesthetist in his management of the patient who abuses amphetamine or similar stimulants (dextroamphetamine and possible cocaine). The acute abuser may require larger anesthetic doses, while the chronic abuser or the patient who has recently ceased ingestion of stimulants may have decreased anesthetic requirements. Another potential hazard is that the acute administration of amphetamine may cause hyperthermia (43), probably through an increase in metabolism but possibly also by decreasing skin blood flow.

The above evidence suggests an important role for catecholamines as modifiers of anesthetic effect. We also know that many anesthetics themselves modify sympathetic activity and catecholamine release. Do these agents increase their own MAC by causing the release of central catecholamines? As yet, we have no answer.

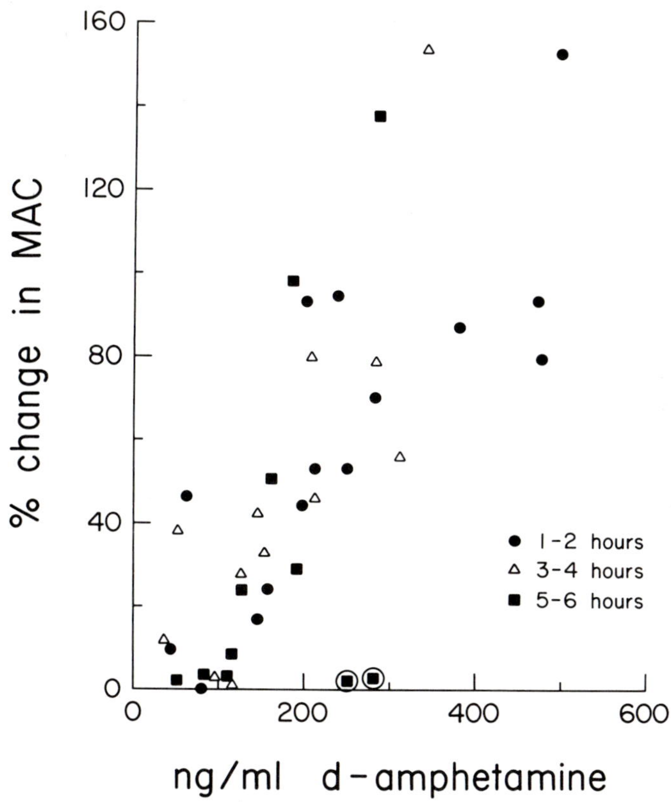

FIG. 1,13. Dextro-amphetamine administration to dogs produces an increase in halothane MAC (*vertical axis*) which is directly related to the serum level of amphetamine (*horizontal axis*). Two exceptions to this relationship (*circles, filled boxes*) appeared 5 to 6 hours after administration of amphetamine and may have resulted from the depletion of cathecholamine stores. (Reproduced with permission from unpublished data of Johnston, R. R., Way, W. L., and Miller, R. D.)

MAC as the Measure of Anesthetic Dose

Since MAC is a yardstick of anesthetic requirement which applies to all inhaled anesthetics it may be used as a comparative measure of anesthetic dose. It may be used to test the correlation of anesthetic dose with various physical properties supporting this or that theory of anesthesia (see Chapter 3). It also is useful as a yardstick by which the pharmacological effects of anesthetics may be compared. Thus, we may look at the effect of multiples of MAC of halothane or cyclopropane or other anesthetics on respiration (8), or circulation (48) or on the effectiveness of muscle relaxants (57). The use of MAC for this purpose has been criticized on the grounds that an increase in concentration to twice, 3 times or 4 times MAC for one anesthetic may not produce an effect equivalent to an identical increase with another agent. In at least one sense this is not a criticism. If we choose one anesthetic over another for its respiratory, circulatory, neuromuscular or other action, this implies that we recognize a quantitative difference between the effect of comparable doses of each anesthetic. Although MAC may not be the perfect yardstick for such a comparison, as noted earlier in this chapter,

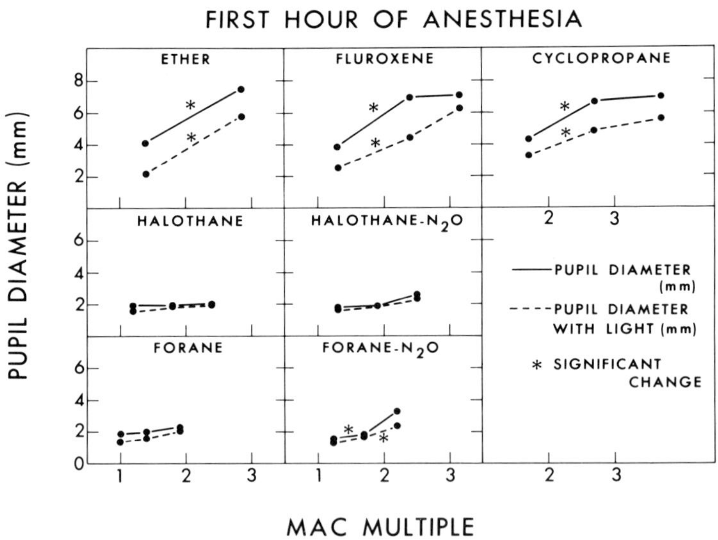

FIG. 1,14. Pupil diameter (*vertical axis*) in unstimulated young human volunteers is increased by ether, fluroxene or cyclopropane and further increased by higher doses of these agents (MAC, *horizontal axis*). The pupil is not dilated by halothane or isoflurane (Forane). Shining a light into the eye caused the pupil to constrict (*dashed lines* connect the resulting pupillary diameters) but constriction became increasingly sluggish (not shown in figure) as anesthetic dose increased. (Reproduced with permission from Cullen, D. J., Eger, E. I., II, Stevens, W. C., *et al.*: Clinical signs of anesthesia. Anesthesiology. 36: 21–36, 1972.)

there is no alternative standard which is equally applicable to all anesthetics.

Finally, we can relate multiples of MAC to the clinically used manifestations of anesthetic depth such as eye signs or pulse and blood pressure (6). Ether, fluroxene and cyclopropane stimulate sympathetic activity and tend to cause a dose-related pupillary dilation which is absent with halothane or isoflurane, a beta-sympathetic stimulating anesthetic (fig. 1,14). On the other hand, no particular relationship between depth and blood pressure or heart rate is apparent for ether, cyclopropane or fluroxene except that at the deepest level of fluroxene, tachycardia and hypertension appear. Conversely, halothane and isoflurane produce a dose-related depression of blood pressure without affecting pulse rate (except for an increase in rate at the deepest levels of isoflurane when combined with nitrous oxide). These data illustrate the nature of the "signs" of anesthesia which, though useful as guides to the conduct of clinical anesthesia with individual agents, are too diverse to provide a basis for a universal definition of anesthesia depth.

The practical application of the clinical "signs" noted above is limited by the situation in which the observations were made: these data came from young, healthy unmedicated volunteers not subjected to surgical stress. These "signs" may be modified by narcotic and atropine premedication, the stimulus of operation, or blood loss. Such modifications, of course, may bear no relation to anesthetic depth and great care must be taken to distinguish between change in signs owing to changes in anesthetic depth and changes in signs secondary to responses to physiological or pharmacological stress.

Summary

The older definitions of anesthetic depth lack a description of dose and effect which can be applied equally to all inhalation anesthetics. In contrast, MAC precisely defines anesthetic dose and its relationship to an all-or-none response (movement). Abolition of movement is one of the prime criteria of general anesthesia. Moreover, MAC is applicable to all inhaled anesthetics.

MAC may be used to evaluate factors which influence anesthetic requirement. A number of these have little effect on MAC. These include duration of anesthesia, circadian rhythms, hyper- or hypothyroidism, $PaCO_2$ up to 90 torr, hyperventilation to 10 torr, severe metabolic acidosis or alkalosis, PaO_2 from 40 to 500 torr, anemia to a hematocrit of 10 percent or phenylephrine induced hypertension. Some extreme stresses produce irreversible or slowly reversible reductions in MAC. These include $PaCO_2$ greater than 90 torr, PaO_2 less than 40 torr and a hematocrit less than 10. Aging also reduces MAC. Body temperature reduction lowers MAC reversibly and elevation of temperature increases MAC. Reserpine or alpha methyl dopa which deplete central catecholamines reduce MAC, while iproniazide and dextroamphetamine which release central catecholamines raise MAC. Depressants such as narcotics or other anesthetics lower MAC, the latter in a simple, additive fashion. The clinician must allow for changes in anesthetic requirement induced by these factors lest he give too much or too little anesthetic.

Besides its value in quantifying factors influencing anesthetic requirement, MAC may be helpful in testing theories of narcosis. It also may be used as a yardstick by which the pharmacological effects of anesthetics can be compared. Such comparisons are indispensable to the evaluation of new anesthetics. Finally, by providing a standard expression of anesthetic dose, MAC may be helpful in redefining clinical signs of anesthetic depth.

QUESTIONS

1. What other alternatives are there to the use of MAC to define anesthetic dose? Where are such alternatives superior and inferior?
2. What factors have little or no influence on anesthetic dose as defined by MAC? Which of these will alter MAC if carried to a sufficient extreme? What factors may alter MAC reversibly?
3. Should a mentally retarded child have a reduced MAC?
4. What does the constancy of MAC with time imply to clinical practice?
5. How do you reconcile the clinical impression that hyperventilation causes deepening of anesthesia with the finding that MAC is unchanged by lowering $PaCO_2$?
6. If an increase in carbon dioxide stimulates the sypathetic nervous system and causes the central release of catecholamines, why is MAC unaffected by increases in $PaCO_2$ up to 90 torr?
7. How would the addition of hypercapnia affect the reduction in MAC produced by a given, low PaO_2? Why?
8. Both anemia and hypoxia reduce MAC. With hypoxia, this reduction correlates with changes in arterial oxygen content, whereas no such correlation is apparent for anemia (fig. 1,6). Suggest a reason for this difference.
9. If circadian variations occur in man, at what hours of the day would you expect MAC to be greatest in a normal person? In a night watchman?
10. What circumstance surrounding the requirement for and use of blood might alter anesthetic requirement?
11. What implications from the studies with reserpine and amphetamine might be used to explain the changes in MAC seen with hyperthyroidism? With age?
12. Which premedications may alter MAC?

13. Why might the administration of ephedrine during an anesthetic alter anesthetic requirement? Why should methoxamine not change MAC?
14. How might drug abuse alter anesthetic requirement?

REFERENCES

1. Mazzia, V. D. B. and Randt, C. T.: Amnesia and eye movement in first stage anesthesia. Arch. Neurol. 14: 544–525, 1966.
2. Hutchinson, R.: Awareness during surgery. A study of its incidence. Brit. J. Anaesth. 33: 463–469, 1961.
3. Sia, R. L.: Consciousness during general anesthesia. Curr. Res. Anesth. Analg. 48: 363–366, 1969.
4. Guedel, A. E.: *Inhalation Anesthesia*, Ed. 2. The Macmillan Company, New York, 1951.
5. Woodbridge, P. D.: Changing concepts concerning depth of anesthesia. Anesthesiology 18: 536–550, 1957.
6. Cullen, D. J., Eger, E. I., II. Stevens, W. C., et al: Clinical signs of anesthesia. Anesthesiology 36: 21–36, 1972.
7. Munson, E. S., Larson, C. P., Jr., Babad, A. A., Regan, M. J., Buechel, D. R., and Eger, E. I., II: The effects of halothane, fluroxene and cyclopropane on ventilation: a comparative study in man. Anesthesiology 27: 716–728, 1966.
8. Larson, C. P., Eger, E. I., II. Muallem, M., Buechel, D. R., Munson, E. S., and Eisele, J. H.: The effects of diethyl ether and methoxyflurane on ventilation: II. A comparative study in man. Anesthesiology 30: 174–184, 1969.
9. Eger, E. I., II, and Bahlman, S. H.: Is the end-tidal anesthetic partial pressure on accurate measure of the arterial anesthetic partial pressure? Anesthesiology 35: 301–303, 1971.
10. Eger, E. I., II, Saidman, L. J., and Brandstater, B.: Minimum alveolar anesthetic concentration: a standard of anesthetic potency. Anesthesiology 26: 756–763, 1965.
11. Saidman, L. J., Eger, E. I., II, Munson, E. S., Babad, A. A., and Muallem, M.,: Minimum alveolar concentration of methoxyflurane, halothane, ether and cyclopropane in man: Correlation with theories of anesthesia. Anesthesiology 28: 994–1002, 1967.
12. Nicodemus, H. F., Nassiri-Rahimi, C., Bachman, L., and Smith, T. C.: Median effective doses (ED50) of halothane in adults and children. Anesthesiology 31: 344–348, 1969.
13. Eger, E. I., II, Lundgren, C., Miller, S. L., and Stevens W. C.: Anesthetic potencies of sulfur hexafluoride, carbon tetrafluoride, chloroform and Ethrane in dogs; Correlation with the hydrate and lipid theories of anesthetic action. Anesthesiology 30: 129–135, 1969.
14. Eger, E. I., II, Brandstater, B., Saidman, L. J., Regan, M. J., Severinghaus, J. W., and Munson, E. S.: Equipotent alveolar concentrations of methoxyflurane, halothane, diethyl ether, fluroxene, cyclopropane, xenon and nitrous oxide in the dog. Anesthesiology 26: 771–777, 1965.
15. Brown, B. R., Jr., and Crout, R. J.: A comparative study of the effect of five general anesthetics on myocardial contractibility. I. Isometric conditions. Anesthesiology 34: 236–245, 1971.
16. Waizer, P. R., Baez, S., and Orkin, L. R.: A method for the determination of minimum alveolar concentration of anesthetic in the rat. Unpublished data.
17. Cherkin, and Catchpool, J. F.: Temperature dependence of anesthesia in goldfish. Science 144: 1460–1462, 1964.

18. Shim, C. U., and Andersen, N. B.: The effect of oxygen on minimal anesthetic requirements in the toad. Anesthesiology 34: 333–337, 1971.

19. Robbins, B. H.: Preliminary studies of the anesthetic activity of fluorinated hydrocarbons. J. Pharmacol. Exp. Ther. 86: 197–204, 1946.

20. Miller, R. D., Wahrenbrock, E. A., Schroeder, C. F., Knipstein, T. W., Eger, E. I., II, and Buechel, D. R.: Ethylene-halothane anesthesia. Anesthesiology 31: 301–304, 1969.

21. Saidman, L. J., and Eger, E. I., II: Effect of nitrous oxide and of narcotic premedication on the alveolar concentration of halothane required for anesthesia. Anesthesiology 25: 302–306, 1964.

22. White, P., Johnston, R. R., and Eger, E. I., II: Unpublished data.

23. Joas, T., and Stevens, W. C.: Unpublished data.

24. Stevens, W. C., *et al.*: Unpublished data.

25. Gion, H., and Saidman, L. J.: The minimum alveolar concentration of enflurane in man. Anesthesiology 35: 361–364, 1971.

26. Munson, E. S., Saidman, L. J., and Eger, E. I., II: Effect of nitrous oxide and morphine on the minimum anesthetic concentration of fluroxene. Anesthesiology 26: 134–139, 1965.

27. Munson, E. S., Martucci, R. W., and Smith, R. E.: Circadian variations in anesthetic requirement and toxicity in rats. Anesthesiology. 32: 507–514, 1970.

28. DiFazio, C. A., Brown, R. E., Ball, C. G., *et al.*: Additive effects of anesthetics and theories of anesthesia. Anesthesiology 36: 57–63, 1972.

29. Cullen, S. C., Eger, E. I., II, Cullen B. F., and Gregory, P.: Observations on the anesthetic effect of the combination of xenon and halothane. Anesthesiology 31: 305–309, 1969.

30. Miller, K. W., Paton, W. D. M., Smith, E. B., and Smith, R. A.: Physico-chemical approaches to the mode of action of general anesthetics. Anesthesiology 36: 339–351, 1972.

31. Winter, P. M., Hornbein, T. F., Smith, G., *et al.*: *Hyperbaric Nitrous Oxide Anesthesia in Man: Determination of Anesthetic Potency (MAC) and Cardiorespiratory Effects*, pp. 103–104. Abstracts, American Society of Anesthesiologists Meeting, October, 1972.

32. Hoffman, J. C., and DiFazio, C. A.: The anesthesia sparing effect of pentazocine, meperidine and morphine. Arch. Int. Pharmacodyn. Thèr. 186: 261–268, 1970.

33. Eisele, J. H., Eger, E. I., II, and Muallem, M.: Narcotic properties of carbon dioxide in the dog. Anesthesiology 28: 856–865, 1967.

34. Bridges, B. E., Jr., and Eger, E. I., II: The effect of hypocapnia on the level of halothane anesthesia in man. Anesthesiology 27: 634–637, 1966.

35. Cullen, D. J., and Eger, E. I., II: The effect of extreme hypocapnia on the anesthetic requirement (MAC) of dogs. Brit. J. Anaesth. 43: 339–343, 1971.

36. Allen, G. D., and Morris, L. E.: Central nervous system effects of hyperventilation during anesthesia. Brit. J. Anaesth. 34: 296–305, 1962.

37. Wollman, S. B., and Orkin, L. R.: Postoperative human reaction time and hypocarbia during anaesthesia. Brit. J. Anaesth. 40: 920–926, 1968.

38. Blenkarn, G. D., Briggs, G., Bell, J., and Sugioka, K,: *Cognitive Function after Hypocapnia Hypoventilation* pp. 41–42. Abstracts of Scientific Papers, American Society Anesthesiologists, 1971.

39. Cullen, D. J., and Eger, E. I., II: The effects of hypoxia and isovolemic anemia on the halothane requirement (MAC) of dogs. I. The effect of hypoxia. Anesthesiology 32: 28–34, 1970.

40. Cullen, D. J., and Eger, E. I., II: The effects of hypoxia and isovolemic anemia on the

halothane requirement (MAC) of dogs: III. The effects of acute isovolemic anemia. Anesthesiology 32: 46–50, 1970.
41. Cohen, P. J., Alexander, S. C., Smith, T. C., Reivach, N., and Wollman, H: The effects of hypoxia and normocarbia on cerebral blood flow and metabolism in conscious man. J. Appl. Physiol. 23: 183–189, 1967.
42. Alexander, S. C., Smith, T. C. Strobel, G., Steven, G. W., and Wollman, H.: Cerebral carbohydrate metabolism of man during respiratory and metabolic alkalosis. J. Appl. Physiol. 24: 66–72, 1968.
43. Johnston, R. R., Way, W. L., and Miller, R. D.: Alterations of anesthetic requirement by amphetamine. Anesthesiology 36: 357–363, 1972.
44. Eger, E. I., II, Saidman, L. J., and Brandstater, B.: Temperature dependence of halothane and cyclopropane anesthesia in dogs: Correlation with some theories of anesthetic action. Anesthesiology 26: 764–770, 1965.
45. Regan, M. J., and Eger, E. I., II: The effect of hypothermia in dogs on anesthetizing and apneic doses of inhalation agents. Anesthesiology. 28: 689–699, 1967.
46. Munson, E. S.: Effect of hypothermia on anesthetic requirement in rats. Lab. Anim. Sci. 20: 1109–1113, 1970.
47. Hoffman, J. C., and DiFazio, C. A.: The anesthesia sparing effect of pentazocine, meperidine, and morphine. Arch. Int. Pharmacodyn. Ther. 186: 261–268, 1970.
48. Eger, E. I., II, Smith, N. T., Cullen, D. J., Cullen, B. F., and Gregory, G. A.: A comparison of the cardiovascular effects of halothane, fluroxene, ether and cyclopropane in man: A resumé. Anesthesiology 34: 25–41, 1971.
49. Babad, A. A., and Eger, E. I., II: The effects of hyperthyroidism and hypothyroidism on halothane and oxygen requirements in dogs. Anesthesiology 29: 1087–1093, 1968.
50. Munson, E. S., Hoffman, J. C., and DiFazio, C. A.: The effects of acute hypothyroidism and hyperthyroidism on cyclopropane requirement (MAC) in rats. Anesthesiology 29: 1094–1098, 1968.
51. Gregory, G. A., Eger, E. I., II, and Munson, E. S.: The relationship between age and halothane requirement in man. Anesthesiology 30: 488–491, 1969.
52. Perisho, J. A., Buechel, D. R., and Miller, R. D.: The effect of diazepam (Valium) on minimum alveolar anaesthetic requirement in man. Canad. Anaesth. Soc. J. 18: 536–540, 1971.
53. Kalser, S. C., Wills, J. H., Gabourel, J. D., Gosselin, R. E., and Epes, C. F.: Further studies of the excretion of atropine-alpha-C 14. J. Pharmacol. Exp. Ther. 121: 449–456, 1957.
54. Bert, P.: Anesthesie par le protoxyde d'azote melange-d'oxygene et employ sous prission. C. R. Acad. Sci. (Paris) 89: 132–135, 1879.
55. Han, Y. H.: Why do chronic alcoholics require more anesthesia? Anesthesiology 30: 341–342, 1969.
56. Miller, R. D., Way, W. L., and Eger, E. I., II: The effects of alpha-methyl dopa, reserpine, guanelthidine, and iproniazid on minimum alveolar anesthetic requirement (MAC). Anesthesiology 29: 1153–1158, 1968.
57. Miller, R.D., Way, W. L., Dolan, W. M., *et al.*: Comparative neuromuscular effects of pancuronium, gallamine, and succinylcholine during Forane and halothane anesthesia in man. Anesthesiology 35: 509–514, 1971.

Chapter 2

Transmission of Messages by the Nervous System

In future chapters, we will speculate on the mode of action of inhaled anesthetics, of barbiturates, of muscle relaxants, and of local anesthetics. Each of these drugs shares one property: all impair the transmission of messages by the nervous system. To understand how they act requires that we understand the process of transmission itself. A description of this process is the aim of this chapter.

The picture to be given is only a sketch. It is drawn without a discussion of opinions at conflict with current views. Those who wish to pursue these important avenues, plus detailed but very readable accounts of current concepts in neurophysiology, should consult the books by Katz (1) and Eccles (2) or the reviews by Hille (3) and Hubbard (4). With few exceptions this chapter is based on their expositions.

The Anatomy of Nervous Pathways

Sensation usually begins at the surface of the body. The energy from an incision, or from touch, warmth or cold is converted to electrical impulses (transduced) by superficial sensors. These electrical impulses (nerve action potentials or NAP) pass to the central nervous system where the impulse is interpreted and a response generated. The response may lead to muscle contraction, to hormonal secretion or to an alteration in the pathways within the nervous system itself.

The drugs which concern us act at one or more of these points: Local anesthetics may interrupt the transduction of a painful stimulus to an electrical impulse or may block the transmission of the impulses leading to the central nervous system. In sufficient concentration local anesthetics may decrease the central perception of these impulses. Inhaled anesthetics and barbiturates may inhibit transmission or central interpretation. Neuromuscular blocking agents mainly confine their attention to the neuromuscular junction, that is, the response part of the pathway.

The processes of transduction, transmission, interpretation and response are carried out by billions of cells whose functions are interrelated in ways which, at best, we dimly understand. We know a good bit more about the basic unit of this complex system, the nerve cell or neuron. The neuron itself is a miniature nervous system which receives, integrates and transmits messages. Let us see how it functions.

Axonal Transmission of Impulses

The peripheral sensory neuron consists of a transducer apparatus which converts a stimulus to an electrical impulse (the NAP), an axon which conducts the NAP over a considerable distance, and a system (the synapses) for communicating this impulse to other neurons. The axon conducts the NAP without diminution, at a high speed, and is ready to conduct subsequent impulses at extremely short intervals. A unique combination of structure and chemistry permits the efficient achievement of these ends.

Anatomy of the Axon Membrane

The axon is a long tube whose wall is composed of lipoprotein. The actual structure of the wall is still uncertain. The classic suggestion that it consists of two layers of lipid sandwiched between two layers of protein (5, 6) has been challenged (7, 8). One of the newer proposals also suggests a lipoprotein structure but one in which the protein molecules form a latticework rather than a continuous layer. The lipid molecules fill and thereby plug the holes between the protein lattice (fig. 2,1). Both the classic and more recent models suggest that the midlayer of the wall is hydrophobic while the outer layers facing the intracellular and extracellular fluids are hydrophilic. The hydrophobic layer forms an electrical barrier to the passage of ions between the intracellular and extracellular fluids. In contrast to the high resistance of the unstimulated axon wall, the intracellular fluid contains several hundred milliequivalents per liter of ions and thus conducts electrical currents with relative ease.

Electrotonic or Cable Transmission

It would seem that little more should be required to conduct the NAP: a pulse generated at one end of an axon should travel unimpeded down its core of ionic fluid to the other end (electrotonic or saltatory transmission). Such would be the case if the resistance to current flow within the axon were small and if little of the current were lost through the axon wall. However, neither of these requirements is met. Resistance to current flow is significant. A significant resistance results from the limited conductivity of the intracellular fluid and from the small cross-section of the nerve fiber. Moreover, the insulation of the axon wall is not perfect. Ions can and do leak through it. Furthermore, by its action as a capacitor the wall may diminish the NAP without the direct passage of ions (i.e., a current may be used up in charging a capacitor).

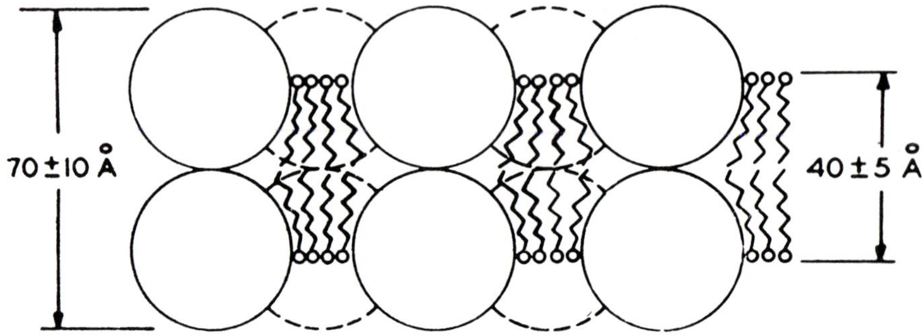

FIG. 2,1. The protein lattice making up the axon wall is formed from globular proteins (*large round circles;* the *dashed line circles* indicate more distant proteins in the lattice). Between these are lipid molecules whose hydrophilic heads face outward at both surfaces of the wall while the hydrophobic tails (the *wavy lines*) dip into the hydrophobic center. Similarly, the protein is hydrophilic at the surfaces of the wall and hydrophobic within. (Reproduced with permission from Vanderkooi, B., and Green, D. E.: Biological membrane structure. I. The protein crystal model for membranes. Proc. Nat. Acad. Sci. U.S.A. 66: 615–621, 1970.)

What Keeps the Impulse Going?

In the absence of some compensatory mechanism, current losses would limit nerve conduction to a few millimeters or less. But built into the axon are relay stations which rejuvenate the faltering impulse and thereby permit its conduction undiminished over the long distances it must travel. Rejuvenation at these relay stations is dependent on three conditions: 1) a difference in ionic composition between the fluid within the axon and that bathing the axon; 2) a difference in potential between these fluids; and 3) a variable and selective permeability of the axon wall to the passage of different ions.

The Development of the Membrane Potential

The ionic composition within the axon differs considerably from that without. The intracellular sodium and chloride concentrations are low, while the concentration of potassium is high. Conversely, the sodium and chloride concentrations bathing the axon are high and the potassium low. The difference in sodium and potassium concentrations is a consequence of the active extrusion of sodium by a "sodium pump" probably with a concomitant coupled injection of potassium (fig. 2,2*A*). The asymmetry of intracellular and extracellular ionic concentrations is sustained by the poor permeability of the resting membrane to both sodium and potassium. However, this small permeability allows both ions to leak down their concentration gradients (figure 2,2*B*). Small though it is, the potassium permeability far exceeds that for sodium, and thus the leakage of potassium is much greater than that of sodium. As a consequence there is an asymmetrical transfer of charges with more positive charges leaving (K^+) the axon than entering (Na^+). An intracellular negativity results and hinders the further transfer of the positive potassium ions. At equilibrium the intracellular negativity prevents any net loss of potassium which is not balanced by a gain of sodium. The intracellular negativity or membrane potential (really a transmembrane potential) thus results from the higher intracellular potassium ion concentration plus a greater membrane permeability to potassium. A secondary effect of the intracellular negativity is the expulsion of negative ions such as chloride. The final equilibrium relationship is illustrated in figure 2,2*C*. As we shall see, the resting negative membrane potential is of fundamental importance to the transmission of nervous impulses.

The sodium pump is essential to the development of the ionic asymmetry which makes the membrane potential possible. But once the potential is developed, the pump is unnecessary to the immediate existence of that potential: the greater membrane permeability to potassium combined with the greater internal potassium concentration

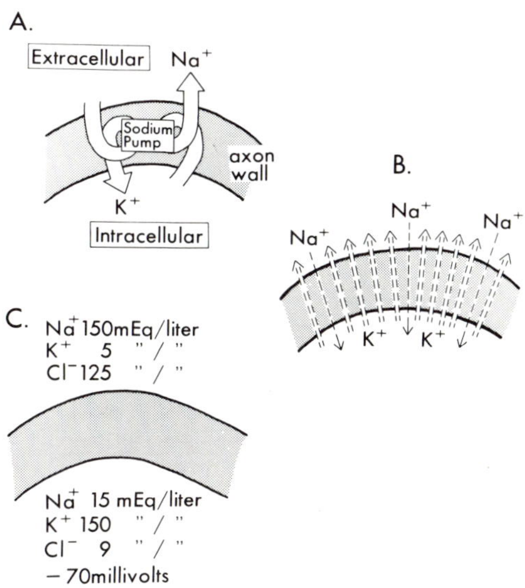

FIG. 2.2. The development of the resting ionic and voltage relationships across the axon membrane (*C*) may be thought of as reflecting two processes (*A* and *B*). First, sodium is ejected from the axon while potassium is injected by the "sodium pump" (*A*) to produce concentration gradients for both ions. Second, a greater membrane permeability for potassium allows potassium to more readily escape from the axon (*B*) with a resulting intracellular negativity. Chloride ions are passively expelled from the cell's interior by this negativity. Note that although these processes are displayed as sequential, they actually proceed concomitantly.

is all that is required. Of course, the membrane potential cannot be maintained indefinitely without the sodium pump. But the ions which are lost through leakage constitute only a very small fraction of those contained within the nerve and therefore the negativity can be sustained for minutes to hours without the pump.

These relationships provide the setting for the propagation of an NAP. An NAP consists of a wave of depolarization and transient reversal of the resting potential which traverses the length of the axon. That is, the negative charge within the axon decreases to a neutral or positive charge which subsequently reverts to its original negativity.

Regeneration of the Nerve Action Potential

The mechanism by which the impulse is propagated may be appreciated from the following experiment. Through a very small electrode inserted into the axon we may deliver brief pulses of current which increase (hyperpolarize) or decrease (depolarize) the internal negativity (fig. 2,3). If we increase the negativity (Fig. 2,3*A*) then when the pulse is turned off, the membrane potential promptly returns to its original value of −70 mV. Similarly if we slightly lower the membrane potential (i.e., make the potential less negative) (B) when the pulse is turned off the membrane potential quickly returns to −70 mV. If we deliver a slightly

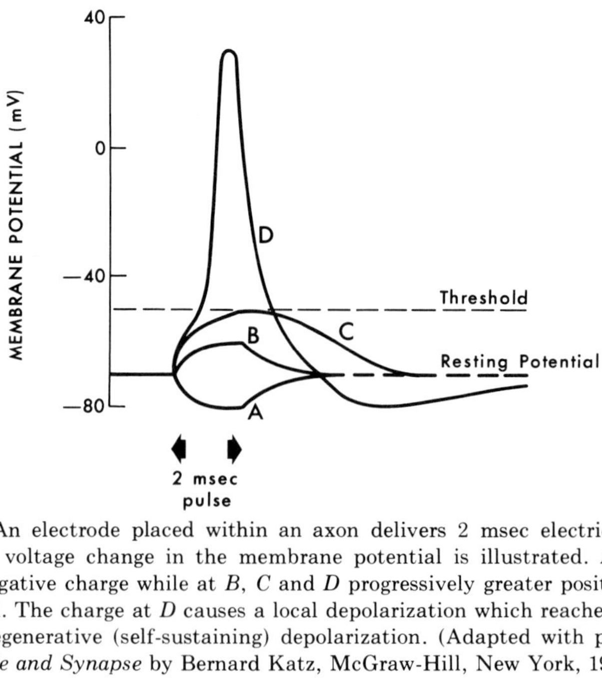

FIG. 2,3. An electrode placed within an axon delivers 2 msec electrical pulses. The concomitant voltage change in the membrane potential is illustrated. At *A* the pulse delivers a negative charge while at *B*, *C* and *D* progressively greater positive charges are administered. The charge at *D* causes a local depolarization which reaches threshold and leads to a regenerative (self-sustaining) depolarization. (Adapted with permission from *Nerve Muscle and Synapse* by Bernard Katz, McGraw-Hill, New York, 1966.)

stronger pulse and lower the potential still further (C) then there may be a delay in the return to the original value. And if we deliver a still stronger pulse (D) then we may trigger an explosive change in the membrane potential. Instead of returning to −70 mV when the pulse is turned off, the membrane potential reaches a threshold value then rapidly decreases to zero, becomes positive and only then returns to and even (transiently) below the original negative value to a hyperpolarized level.

Membrane Potential and Permeability to Sodium and Potassium

What caused this amplification of the delivered pulse through the electrode? Why were pulses A, B and C not amplified? The answer lies in the increase in sodium permeability of the axon membrane that results from a decrease (depolarization) in membrane potential. No change in permeability results from hyperpolarization of the membrane (A). When the pulse is turned off, the inflow leak of sodium (or outflow of chloride) restores the potential to its normal, less negative value. A modest depolarization (B) causes only a small increase in permeability, and when the pulse is abolished the normal efflux of potassium returns the membrane potential to −70 mV. But a slightly greater depolarization (C) increases the permeability to sodium well above the small resting leak. The increased sodium permeability allows an influx of sodium ions from the far higher concentration which surrounds the axon. This influx adds to the positive charges within the cell and thereby sustains the depolarizing effect of our delivered electrical pulse. A brief period follows where the depolarizing influx of sodium balances the effect of the potassium efflux. However, the efflux of potassium eventually predominates, restores the membrane potential to normal and concomitantly reduces the sodium permeability to the normal resting leak. A slightly stronger pulse (D) causes a greater depolarization. As the membrane potential is lowered to −50 mV (threshold), the permeability to sodium increases to a point where the change in voltage induced by the sodium influx becomes self-sustaining or *regenerative* (fig. 2,4). That is, the electrical pulse we delivered is no longer necessary to the continued depolarization of the membrane. The normal efflux of potassium no longer overwhelms or even balances the influx of sodium. With further decreases in potential, the discrepancy becomes still greater because of a continued rise in sodium permeability. However, the permeability soon reaches a maximum and then rapidly decreases to normal. The return to normal occurs even if the membrane potential is artificially held at a depolarized level. That is, the increased sodium permeability cannot be sustained.

These changes involving sodium now give way to changes which govern

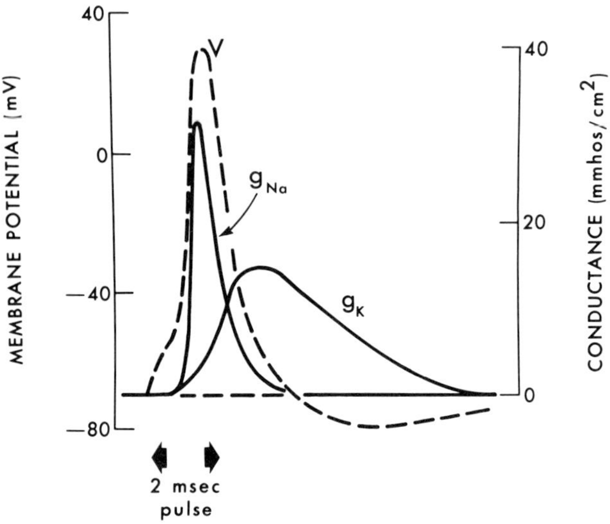

FIG. 2,4. The membrane depolarization illustrated in figure 2,3*D* is reproduced here (*V*, *dashed line*) with the associated changes in the conductance of sodium (g_{Na}) and potassium (g_K). We may consider that conductance changes usually reflect similar changes in permeability. Thus, an increase in g_{Na} results in an increased flow of sodium ions down their concentration gradient into the axon. Notice that the membrane depolarization is closely associated with the unopposed early increase in g_{Na}. Restoration of the membrane potential results from the fall in g_{Na} and rise in g_K. (Adapted with permission from Hodgkin, A. L., and Huxley, A. F.: A quantitative description of membrane current and its application to conduction and excitation in nerve. J. Physiol. 117: 500–544, 1952.)

potassium permeability. As the sodium permeability wanes the permeability to potassium waxes (well beyond the normal resting value). The result is an augmentation of the potassium efflux and a rapid rise in the membrane potential which overshoots the resting −70 mV value. This hyperpolarization results from the increased potassium permeability which allows a greater than normal leak of potassium ions. The negativity approaches the maximum potential which can be produced by the unopposed potassium gradient. The permeability to potassium decreases to normal within milliseconds and the nerve is ready to repeat the process that followed the pulse at D (fig. 2,3).

Transmission of nerve impulses is based on this process. Like the pulse applied in our experiment, depolarization occurring in one segment of membrane lowers the membrane potential in the adjacent segment. Despite current losses through leaks and the capacitative nature of the axon membrane, the potential in the adjacent membrane easily is lowered to the threshold value. The subsequent depolarization amplifies (regenerates) the signal and in turn lowers the membrane potential to the threshold value in the next adjacent segment.

Some Properties of Sodium and Potassium Channels

The increase in sodium permeability which causes the explosive depolarization seen in figure 2,3*D* results from the opening of holes or "pores" in the membrane. It is these pores which are the "relay stations" alluded to earlier. No one has ever seen a sodium pore but indirect evidence allows us to speculate on its appearance (9). It is formed in a thinned portion of the membrane wall so that it looks like a hole rather than a tunnel (fig. 2,5). The individual pore measures at least 3.1 by 5.1 Angstroms in cross-section, a size sufficient to allow the passage of the sodium ion with 3 of its waters of hydration. The pore probably is lined with 8 oxygens of which one pair is an ionized carboxylic acid. Finally, the gate to the pore (which determines whether the pore is open or closed) is held in place by calcium so that a surfeit of calcium hinders the increase in permeability normally produced by a fall in membrane potential.

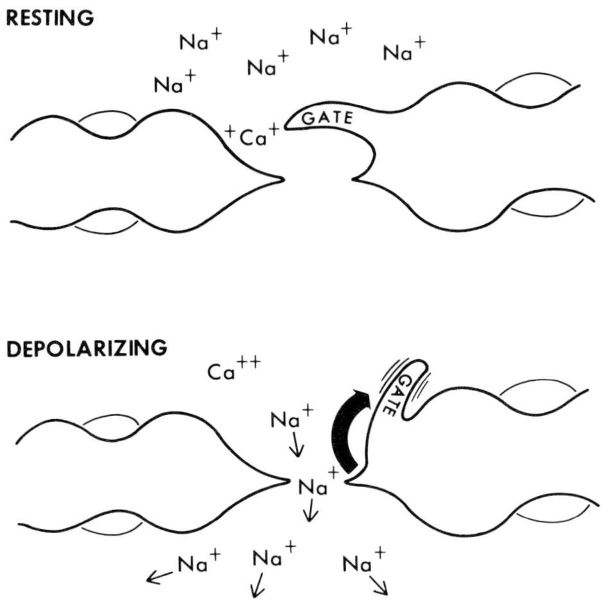

FIG. 2.5. The sodium chanel illustrated here differs from the potassium channel (fig. 2,6) in that it is a pore or hole in the cell membrane rather than a tunnel. At rest, the opening to the pore is covered by a gate and the gate is held in place by calcium. Depolarization to threshold dislodges the calcium and causes the gate to withdraw. Diffusion of sodium ions through the open pore into the axon produces the depolarizing voltage which is electrotonically transmitted (not shown here) to the next sodium pore. The reader should bear in mind that the illustration is imaginary, and that no one has ever seen a sodium pore.

The increase in potassium permeability is similarly caused by the opening of channels through the axon wall. The sodium and potassium channels are independent structures (3). The potassium channels are tunnels (rather than holes or pores) through which 4 or 5 ions might concomitantly diffuse in single file with their shells of hydration (fig. 2,6). The tunnel-like nature of the potassium channel makes its conductance (i.e., the ease with which potassium can pass through) far lower than the conductance of the sodium channel. However, there are about 50 times as many potassium as sodium channels, and thus the difference in the sum of the conductances of the open sodium versus open potassium channels is small.

A number of questions remain. We know that a lowering of membrane potential is associated with the opening of the sodium pores, but how this is accomplished is unclear. The opening may result from a displacement of the calcium which guards the gate to the pore. The reason for the return of sodium permeability to normal (even in the presence of a continued lower membrane potential) also is unclear. Why does the increase in potassium conductance lag the increase in sodium conductance? Is it related to the tunnel-like configuration of the potassium channel as opposed to the hole-like structure of the sodium pore? And

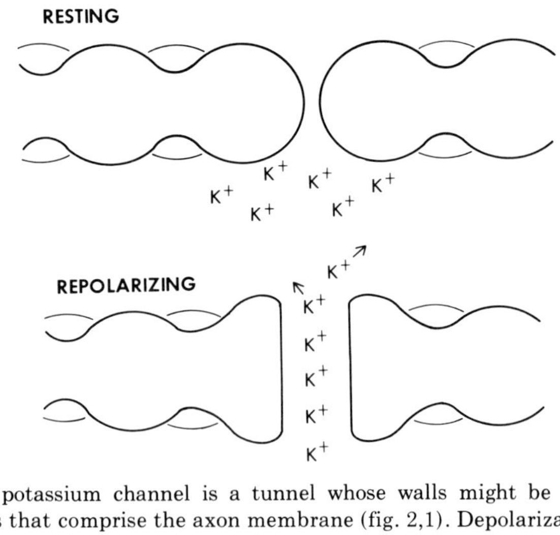

FIG 2,6. The potassium channel is a tunnel whose walls might be composed of the globular proteins that comprise the axon membrane (fig. 2,1). Depolarization may cause a delayed contraction of these proteins which in turn widens the tunnel sufficiently to allow diffusion of potassium out of the axon. The outrush of potassium causes the repolarization which re-establishes the transmembrane potential. As with the sodium pore, no one has ever seen a potassium tunnel, and the reader is cautioned that the illustration may be fanciful.

why is the increased potassium permeability sustained for a far longer period than the increased sodium permeability?

The number of sodium channels is relatively small. Recall that the sodium pore is about 3.1 by 5.1 Angstroms. The nearest pore in an unmyelinated nerve may be several thousand Angstroms distant. Although the potassium pores are more populous, they too, are widely separated. The relative paucity of channels bespeaks the efficiency of nerve conduction. Despite the considerable (albeit brief) fluctuations in voltage that result from the movement of sodium and potassium ions, only a minute fraction of the total intracellular or extracellular ions is transferred with each impulse. Even without the continued action of the sodium pump, the average axon could transmit hundreds to thousands of impulses before the ionic composition would alter sufficiently to halt conduction.

Speeding up the NAP

We have learned that there are two parts to the conduction of a nerve impulse. The first part is a transmission which is analogous to the movement of current through a telephone cable. Were it not for current losses, this "cable transmission" alone would suffice. However, current losses require the second part; something must prevent the cable transmission from petering out. To this end, relay stations (sodium pores) amplify (regenerate) the impulse sufficiently to compensate for current losses. One drawback to these relay stations is that the amplification they supply takes a significant period of time. The imposed delay may be critical to an animal that must fight or flee or simply coordinate rapid movements. Transmission speed may be increased in two ways. Both permit the NAP to travel a greater distance before requiring amplification. One way is to increase the diameter of the axon and thereby reduce the internal resistance to current flow. This may not decrease the absolute loss of current, but does reduce the fraction of the total current lost over any given time and nerve length. Many invertebrates have used this development to insure the rapid transmission of signals. For example, the giant axons of the squid or lobster are large enough to be visable to the naked eye. However, enlargement of the axon is unfeasible where thousands or millions of axons must be employed in parallel—as, for example, in our optic nerves. To meet this need we have developed the myelin sheath. This is a lamellated cylinder of fatty material which surrounds and insulates the axon, and thereby reduces the loss of current through direct and capacitative leakage. The reduced current loss allows the cable transmission of the impulse to extend a great distance (as much as 6 to 8 mm) before requiring amplification. The sheath does not completely cover the nerve. At 0.5 to 3 mm intervals there is a small (less than 1 micron) break in the sheath. This is the node of Ranvier. The sodium and potassium channels are concentrated at this exposed membrane surface; no channels exist (or are needed) in the intervening segments of ensheathed nerve. Obviously, amplification takes place only at the nodes of Ranvier rather than over the entire axon (as occurs in the unsheathed nerve).

Synaptic Transmission

Introduction

We have described how an impulse traverses the length of the neuron. At the end of this neuron it meets and must communicate its message to one or more succeeding cells. The synapse is the connection between this primary and the succeeding neurons. Some other definitions are in order (fig. 2,7). The end of the primary neuron is the nerve terminal: it is "presynaptic." Unlike the axon, the nerve terminal never is sheathed in myelin. The adjacent surface of the succeeding neuron which most immediately perceives the effect of the NAP is "subsynaptic." This would be the end-plate at the neuromuscular junction. The intervening space is the "synaptic cleft." The subsynaptic membrane is a specialized portion of the "postsynaptic" membrane; the postsynaptic membrane forms the surface of the succeeding neuron.

Impulses Require a Chemical Transmitter to Cross the Synapse

The relatively high electrical resistance of the two terminal fiber membranes (as opposed to the low resistance within the axon) prevents the NAP from directly crossing the synaptic cleft. Instead, the NAP of

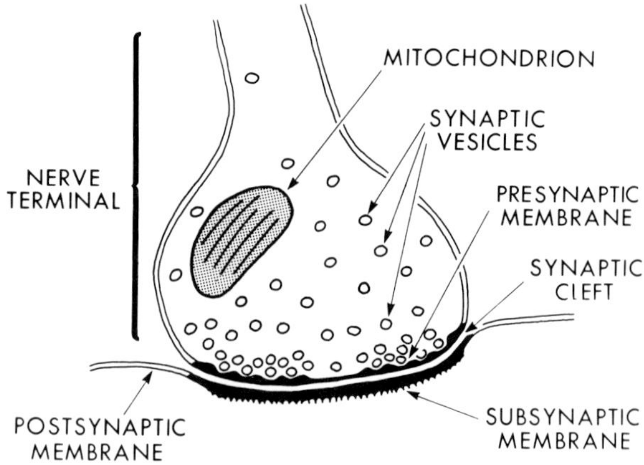

FIG. 2,7. The connection between a primary and succeeding neuron is the synapse illustrated here. Each primary neuron is linked to many succeeding neurons by such synaptic connections.

the primary neuron causes the release of a chemical from the nerve terminal. The chemical diffuses across the synaptic cleft and acts on the subsynaptic membrane. The result may or may not be the generation of a new NAP in the succeeding cell. This uncertainty applies to most neuron-neuron connections, but not to transmission at the neuromuscular junction which almost invariably succeeds in generating a response. The uncertainty also contrasts with the NAP which normally travels the length of the nerve fiber without hindrance. If generated, an impulse in the succeeding neuron would be transmitted in a manner identical to that which supported transmission in the primary neuron.

Several chemicals are capable of affecting the subsynaptic membrane and many of these have been found *in vivo*. However, each nerve terminal contains only one such chemical transmitter. Acetylcholine is known to be capable of initiating a nerve impulse at synaptic ganglia and at neuromuscular junctions, and may be an important chemical transmitter in the central nervous system. Another prominent transmitter is noradrenalin. l-Glutamate, gamma amino butyric acid (GABA), dopamine and glycine also are known to be transmitters. Of these, GABA, dopamine and glycine inhibit rather than cause depolarization. More about inhibition in a moment.

Synaptic Vesicles, the Release of Acetylcholine and Depolarization of the Subsynaptic Membrane

What details surround the release of a chemical transmitter such as acetylcholine from the nerve terminal? Acetylcholine is released in "packets" or "quanta" rather than as individual molecules. A single quantum may consist of as many as 40,000 to 50,000 acetylcholine molecules (4). These quanta probably are released from the synaptic vesicles in the nerve terminal. The synaptic vesicles are spheres of 400 to 600 Angstroms diameter with a limiting membrane of 50 Angstroms thickness. They are concentrated in the portion of the terminal immediately adjacent to the synaptic cleft (fig. 2,7). This portion of the terminal is thickened with dense hillock-like projections. The valleys between hillocks accommodate the vesicles. The vesicles probably attach to and discharge their transmitter through this portion of the terminal membrane. At synapses where noradrenalin is thought to be the transmitter, 400 to 600 Angstrom vesicles also are found in the terminal: their staining characteristics indicate that they hold noradrenalin. Like the acetylcholine containing vesicles, they are concentrated at the terminal membrane bordering the synaptic cleft.

In the absence of a NAP, there is a spontaneous intermittant release of single quanta from the nerve terminal. The released acetylcholine traverses the synaptic cleft and acts on the subsynaptic membrane. To understand the action of acetylcholine we must appreciate that the subsynaptic membrane greatly differs from the adjacent postsynaptic membrane or from the axonal membrane discussed previously. Both the axonal and adjacent postsynaptic membranes contain sodium pores capable of regenerative depolarization; the subsynaptic membrane is not capable of regenerative depolarization. A reduction in membrane potential causes an increase in sodium conductance in the axon or adjacent postsynaptic membranes but has no effect on the subsynaptic membrane. In contrast, acetylcholine causes the depolarization of the subsynaptic membrane but does not depolarize the postsynaptic membrane removed from the subsynaptic area. The subsynaptic depolarization induced by acetylcholine is proportional to the amount of acetylcholine which reaches the membrane. Finally, the subsynaptic depolarization produced by the action of acetylcholine results from the opening of channels which are roughly twice as large as the sodium and potassium channels in the axonal membrane. These larger channels permit the indiscriminate passage of sodium and potassium down their concentration gradients. As a result, the maximum depolarization is of a lesser magnitude than that achievable with the axon membrane where the sodium efflux is not immediately countered by a potassium influx. The subsynaptic potential rises towards −15 mV, a point midway between the potential due to permeability of potassium alone (−90 mV) and sodium alone (+60 mV).

The effect of a single quantum on the subsynaptic membrane is to slightly lower the membrane potential (i.e., make it less negative). Such a slight depolarization is called a miniature end-plate potential (mepp) at a neuromuscular junction and an excitatory postsynaptic potential (EPSP) or inhibitory postsynaptic potential (IPSP) at other synapses. This reduction in potential is too small to cause a NAP in the adjacent postsynaptic membrane. The local alteration in potential is short-lived because the acetylcholine diffuses from the subsynaptic membrane or is quickly hydrolyzed by cholinesterase. The vesicular acetylcholine is restored by reabsorption of the choline by the nerve terminal and recombination with acetate in the nerve terminal cytoplasm. The acetylcholine thus produced may be absorbed by the depleted vesicles. Restoration of vesicular noradrenalin may either be by synthesis or by reabsorption of intact noradrenalin molecules.

The arrival of a NAP at the nerve terminal enormously increases the release of quanta. Many vesicles now become affixed to the presynaptic membrane, and discharge their acetylcholine (or other transmitter) into the synaptic cleft. Except at the neuromuscular junction; the greater subsynaptic depolarization which ensues still is usually insufficient to reach the threshold required for a regenerative depolarization in the adjacent postsynaptic membrane. Unless the effect is augmented, the local depolarization fades and (much as in fig. 2,3 *B* or *C*), no NAP results. The mechanism by which the NAP causes the fixation of vesicles to this membrane and subsequent release of transmitter is unknown, but we do know 1) that the release of quanta is directly related to the magnitude of the NAP (10); and 2) unlike its inhibitory effect on sodium permeability and the NAP, an increase in ionized calcium augments the release of quanta. Magnesium ions exert an opposing (i.e., depressing) effect.

The relationship between the magnitude of the NAP and the release of quanta is of great importance both to synaptic transmission and possibly to the mechanism by which anesthetics act. The release of quanta increases exponentially with each step increase in depolarization (fig. 2,8). For each 15 mV depolarization there is a 10 fold increase in quantal release. From the point of view of both anesthetic mechanisms and of presynaptic inhibitory impulses (see below) the converse effect is of primary concern: failure to depolarize by 15 mV reduces quantal output to one-tenth. For example, in figure 2,8 compare the frequency of mepps

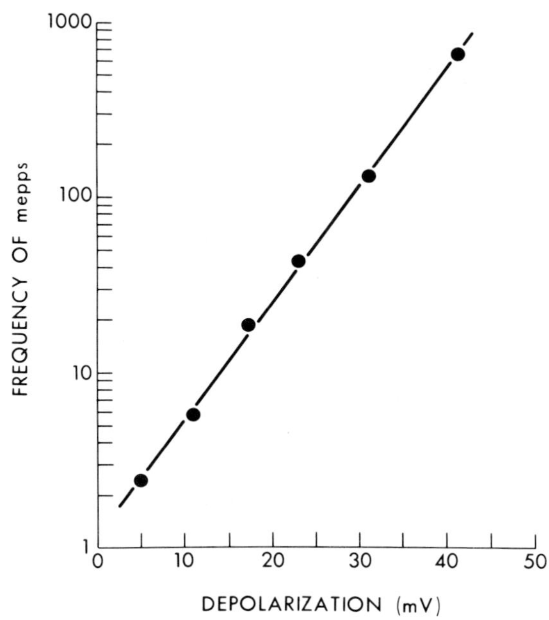

FIG. 2,8. The release of quanta (indicated by the frequency of mepps) is exponentially related to the level of depolarization such that a 15 mV increase in depolarization produces a 10 fold increase in quantal release. (Adapted with permission from Katz, B.: The transmission of impulse from nerve to muscle, and the subcellular unit of synaptic action. Proc. Roy. Soc. Lond. (B) 155: 455–477, 1962.)

(equals quantal release) at 40 and at 25 mV depolarization. The latter is one-tenth the former.

"Readily Releasable" and "Depot" Acetylcholine

Several other factors also influence the number of quanta released by a NAP. The acetylcholine in the nerve terminal exists in two forms: a small "readily releasable" fraction which is immediately available for use as a transmitter and a large "depot" store which serves to replenish the acetylcholine lost from the readily releasable fraction. The readily releasable fraction may be thought of as contained in the vesicles close to or perhaps attached to the portion of nerve terminal membrane bordering the synaptic cleft. The depot store would be contained in the remainder of the vesicles. The readily releasable fraction may become partially exhausted by frequent repeated NAPs such as those produced by tetanic nerve stimulation. This exhaustion is primarily responsible for "fade" during curarization. The transfer rate from the depot store is increased (after a time lag) by tetanic stimulation, but the increase is not sufficient to maintain the resting level of acetylcholine in the readily releasable fraction. Hyperpolarization increases the readily releasable fraction, perhaps by increasing the affinity of vesicles for the presynaptic membrane. The increase in acetylcholine release that occurs following tetany may be due to an exaggeration of the membrane hyperpolarization that follows a NAP. Such an increase in acetylcholine release would explain the facilitation of neuromuscular transmission in partially curarized muscles occurring after tetanic stimulation (posttetanic potentiation). Finally, high demands for the release of acetylcholine increase the synthesis of depot acetylcholine by the choline acetylase system.

Multiple Synapses Affect Each Neuron

To this point we have only noted the contact between one synapse and succeeding neuron (although we noted that one primary neuron innervated several secondary neurons). In fact, multiple synapses from several primary neurons achieve a synaptic connection to *each* secondary neuron. If several adjacent synapses simultaneously depolarize their subsynaptic membranes, a NAP may result from the *summation* of their effects. The postsynaptic membrane threshold for depolarization may vary from one part of the nerve cell to another. The threshold may be high over the dendrites, less over the nerve body and least over the nonmyelinated part of the axon plus the axon hillock from which the axon arises. The latter area is called the "initial segment" (see fig. 2,8). The summation of the excitatory postsynaptic potentials produced by several synapses is most likely to cause a regenerative depolarization at the initial segment—which may be considerably removed from the sites of synaptic contact.

The inability of a single synaptic depolarization alone to initiate a NAP has considerable value (1). It means that a random or inadvertent discharge is unlikely to evoke an unwanted response. The requirement for several depolarizations in adjacent or nearly adjacent areas not only tends to insure that there is good reason for a response but also permits the integration of incoming synaptic information. Particular temporal or spatial combinations predispose to the incitement of a NAP. A few closely juxtaposed synapses which discharge simultaneously are more effective than a larger number of dispersed synapses which discharge chaotically. Thus, the possibility of selective responses can be built into the transmission process.

Inhibitory Synapses

The synaptic release of clinical transmitter may either cause (excitatory synapse) or prevent (inhibitory synapse) a regenerative impulse. A single synapse either excites or inhibits but cannot do both. Both excitatory and inhibitory impulses exert their influence through a release of transmitter which in turn increases the permeability of the subsynaptic membrane. Why then does one cause excitation and the other, inhibition?

Postsynaptic Inhibition

Inhibitory synapses which act at the same level (i.e., on the same postsynaptic membrane) as excitatory synapses are called postsynaptic inhibitory synapses (fig. 2,9). Stimulation of these inhibitory synapses may result in a hyperpolarization of the membrane. Hyperpolarization would occur if potassium conductance were increased (i.e., the potassium channels opened) in the absence of an increase in sodium conductance. This may be seen in the right-hand portion of figure 2,3*D* where the persistent potassium conductance causes the membrane potential to reach nearly −80 mV. The opening of potassium channels would cause inhibition in two ways. First, by causing a postsynaptic hyperpolarization, it increases the depolarization required to produce a regenerative impulse (i.e., it raises the threshold). Second, any current tending to cause depolarization now can be opposed by a far greater than normal outflow of potassium ions. Another postsynaptic mechanism for inhibition would be the opening of additional chloride channels. Although this would not alter the resting potential, it would hinder any tendency to deviate from that potential. The transmitter which causes the opening of potassium or chloride channels may be gamma aminobutyric acid (GABA) or glycine. However, although there is considerable evidence that these compounds are inhibitory transmitters in invertebrates, there is no comparable evidence in mammals.

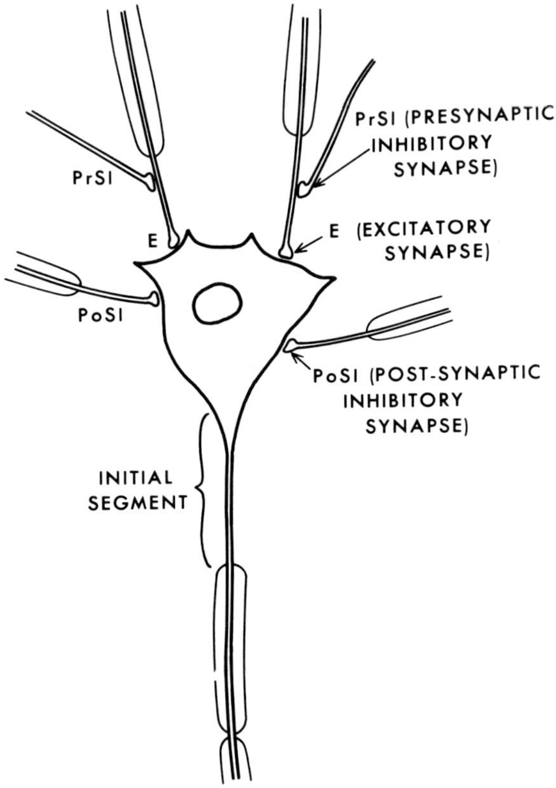

FIG. 2,9. Several synapses may contact any one nerve. Figure 2,6 diagrammatically illustrates two pairs of such synapses: one pair is excitatory (*E*) while the other is inhibitory (*PoSI*). Firing of either excitatory synapse alone is unlikely to produce a regenerative impulse. Simultaneous firing of both (and other excitatory) synapses may cause a regenerative impulse which most likely will originate in the membrane of the initial segment of the axon. The effect of the excitatory synapses may be counteracted by the concomitant or prior firing of the inhibitory (*PoSI*) synapses. Excitation of the presynaptic inhibitory synapses (*PrSI*) may decrease the release of quanta at the excitatory synapses by slightly depolarizing the nerve terminal of the excitatory synapse.

Presynaptic Inhibition

Recall that the number of quanta released from a nerve terminal by the action of a NAP is directly related to the amplitude of the NAP. Anything which reduces the amplitude would decrease the amount of acetylcholine released. Presynaptic inhibitory synapses (fig. 2,9) produce inhibition in precisely this manner. They cause modest depolarization of nerve terminals going to excitatory synapses. The depolarization is insufficient to trigger a regenerative impulse and it does not prevent the transmission of the NAP to the excitatory synapse. But the lower (less negative) membrane potential at that synapse reduces the amplitude of the NAP and thereby decreases the number of quanta released. The reduction in quantal release in turn decreases the subsynaptic depolarization.

Transduction

Less is known about the transduction process than about either axonal or synaptic transmission. The transduction membrane (which is continuous with the afferent axon) resembles the subsynaptic membrane in that it is sensitive to transmitters such as acetylcholine and does not undergo regenerative depolarization (11). The depolarization produced by acetylcholine is converted to a regenerative pulse in the adjacent nerve membrane. It appears that the transduction apparatus is not an important site of action for any of the anesthetic compounds except, perhaps, local anesthetics.

Summary

The transmission of nervous impulses may be divided into the processes of transduction, axonal conduction and transmission at synaptic junctions. Little is known about transduction. Axonal conduction is the result of 1) the "cable transmission" of impulses; and of 2) "relay stations" which sustain the impulse signal. The relay stations depend on an asymmetry of intra-axonal versus extracellular sodium, potassium and chloride ions. They also depend on a selective and variable permeability to sodium and potassium (and chloride?). A decrease in membrane potential (depolarization) at a relay station becomes regenerative because it causes an increase in sodium permeability. The resting membrane potential is subsequently restored by a reduction in sodium permeability and by an increase in potassium permeability. Calcium hinders the relay station action.

Transmission at synapses depends on chemical rather than electrical excitation. The arrival of a NAP at a nerve terminal causes the release of a chemical transmitter (acetylcholine, noradrenalin or other unknown mediators) which crosses the synaptic cleft and acts on the subsynaptic membrane. Calcium is necessary to the release of acetylcholine or noradrenaline. At excitatory synapses the chemical transmitter increases the subsynaptic membrane permeability to both sodium and potassium with a consequent depolarization. Several such depolarizations acting in concert usually are necessary to cause firing in a secondary neuron. At inhibitory postsynaptic synapses, the chemical transmitter increases the subsynaptic permeability to potassium or chloride ions. Both hyperpolarization and an increase in potassium ion efflux or chloride ion influx oppose any tendency to depolarization which might be induced at excitatory synapses. At inhibitory presynaptic synapses, inhibition is accomplished by lowering the membrane potential of the nerve terminal. The resultant reduction in the NAP magnitude decreases the release of quanta and thereby decreases the depolarization of the subsynaptic membrane.

QUESTIONS

1. Why can't a nerve impulse reverse its direction as it travels?
2. How should a reduction in extracellular sodium affect the action potential illustrated in figure 2, *3D*?
3. How would an increase in extracellular potassium affect the resting membrane potential?
4. How would an increase in chloride conductance affect the resting membrane potential?
5. How might strychnine or picrotoxin cause convulsions?
6. Tedrototoxin (poison from the puffer fish) prevents the increase in sodium permeability or depolarization of a nerve membrane. What should this do to an axonal conduction? What should it do to the membrane potential?
7. Suppose we replaced all of the intracellular material of an axon with a high potassium-low sodium solution. What would this do to the axon's ability to generate action potentials?

REFERENCES

1. Katz, B.: *Nerve, Muscle and Synapse*. McGraw-Hill, New York, 1966.
2. Eccles, J. C.: *The Physiology of Synapses*. Academic Press, New York, 1964.
3. Hille, B.: Ionic channels in nerve membranes. Progr. Biophys. 21: 1–32, 1970.
4. Hubbard, J. I.: Mechanism of transmitter release. Progr. Biophys. 21: 33–124, 1970.
5. Danielli, J. F., and Davson, H.: A contribution of the theory of permeability of thin films. J. Cell Physiol. 5: 495, 1935.
6. Robertson, J. D.: The molecular structure and contact relationships of cell membranes. Progr. Biophysics Biophys. Chem. 10: 344, 1960.
7. Green, D. E., and Perdue, J. F.: Membranes as expressions of repeating units. Proc. Nat. Acad. Sci. U.S.A. 55: 1295, 1966.
8. Vanderkooi, G., and Green, D. E.: Biological membrane structure I. The protein crystal model for membranes. Proc. Nat. Acad. Sci. U.S.A. 66: 615, 1970.
9. Hille, B.: The permeability of the sodium channel to organic cations in myelinated nerve. J. Gen. Physiol. 58: 599–619, 1971.
10. Katz, B.: The transmission of impulse from nerve to muscle, and the subcellular unit of synaptic action. Proc. Roy. Soc. Lond. (B) 155: 455–477, 1962.
11. Gray, J. A. B.: Initiation of impulses at receptors. In *Handbook of Physiology*, edited by J. Field, Vol. 1, Sect. 1, Ch. IV, pp. 123–145. American Physiology Society, Washington, 1959.

Chapter 3

Mechanisms of General Anesthesia

M. J. HALSEY

Introduction: Some General Characteristics of Anesthesia

An amazing array of inhaled agents produce general anesthesia in all animals (for example see table 1, 1). These include potent vapors such as methoxyflurane or halothane and also relatively impotent gases such as nitrogen and hydrogen (which cause anesthesia at about 30 and 180 atmospheres, respectively) (1, 2). Theories of general anesthesia must explain how such diverse compounds can produce the same overall effect. It appears that any compound may produce anesthesia if: 1) it can reach the site of anesthetic action; 2) it can attain a certain critical concentration at that site; and 3) its anesthetic effect is not obscured by toxic or other activity at subanesthetic concentrations.

All inhaled agents which produce anesthesia share several characteristics which must affect our thoughts on how they act. First, none form covalent-ionic type bonds with the site of anesthetic action but instead interact through Van der Waal's forces. Van der Waal's forces are weak intermolecular forces (less than 3.5 K joules/mole compared to 50 K joules/mole for some chemical bonds) produced by electrostatic attraction between dipoles. Dipoles are molecules whose electrons are unevenly distributed so that one part of the molecule is more positive and the other part more negative. Dipoles are either permanent (an unequal distribution of electric charge is constantly present), induced (the unequal distribution occurs only when an electric field from another molecule is present) or instantaneous (electron movements within the overall electron cloud cause intermittently uneven distribution). Hydrogen bonds are a special case of Van der Waal's attraction and may be important for some anesthetic interactions.

Second, no "structure-activity" relationship yet can explain the effect of the inhaled agents. That is, they possess no common structure which may be associated with their biological activity. In contrast, structure appears to be very important to the action of intravenous agents, such as the barbiturates and the new steroid induction agents. For example, an experimental steroid, 3 α-hydroxy 5 α-pregnane-10,20 dione has anesthetic activity whereas its 3β-epimer (which has very similar physical properties) is inactive (3). The lack of structure-activity relationships has ruled out the use of model compounds or of specific antagonists in any investigation of anesthetic mode of action.

Third, anesthesia alters the function of almost all systems of the body at both a tissue and cellular level. These effects of anesthesia may relate to a primary process or may be extraneous side effects. It should be remembered that many of these diffuse effects occur at higher concentrations than those required for clinical anesthesia and are therefore unlikely to be involved in a mechanism of narcosis.

Where Do Anesthetics Act?

The following section will examine possible sites of anesthetic action since a knowledge of such a site might suggest a mechanism of action. For example, the demonstration that anesthetics selectively depress transmission through the multineural polysynaptic pathways of the brain stem reticular formation (see below) suggests a critical importance of synaptic transmission to anesthesia. Similarly, if we knew that anesthetics acted in the cell membrane we could ignore changes evoked by anesthetics in plasma (except as they might influence the membrane).

The site of action of anesthesia can be considered at three interrelated levels: the macroscopic (or gross) level; the microscopic (or cellular) level; and the molecular level.

Action at the Macroscopic Level

Reticular Activating System. The brain stem reticular formation is accepted as an important site of anesthetic action. Consciousness requires excitation of the reticular formation, and inhibition of reticular activity produces unconsciousness and anesthesia: stimulation of the reticular formation leads to arousal while destruction of the area causes coma.

Sensory nerve impulses reach the cortex either by a direct quick pathway or by a more slowly conducting central route via the reticular formation (4). The central route is particularly sensitive to anesthetics. Ether anesthesia abolishes the impulse resulting from an auditory stimulus somewhere in its passage through the reticular formation but does not block the direct pathway via the lateral lemniscus. Similarly, nitrous oxide, ethylene and cyclopropane primarily decrease responses evoked from the reticular activating system by stimulation of a radial nerve (5). However, these agents also reduce the direct (rapid) response in the thalamus, although the depression never exceeds 50 percent of control (fig. 3, 1). Reticular stimulation also can cause inhibition of some cortical neurons. However, complex responses such as these may only relate to the excitement state of anesthesia.

Cerebral Cortex. The reticular activating system is not the only central site of interruption of nervous transmission. Electroencephalographic (EEG) evidence suggests that ether may directly affect cortical activity (6), and anesthetic concentrations of halothane, but not methoxyflurane, reduce the sensitivity of cortical neurons to acetylcholine (7). On the other hand, the postsynaptic effects of gamma amino butyric acid are unaffected. As noted in Chapter 2, gamma amino butyric acid may be a transmitter of inhibitory impulses. Similarly, halothane, pentobarbital and ketamine all increase brain glutamine concentration by 40 percent (8). Glutamine or a related amino acid also may be an inhibitory transmitter.

Spinal Cord. General anesthetics may also inhibit transmission of impulses through the spinal cord. For example, electrical stimulation of the tibial nerve in man causes two distinct calf muscle depolarizations. The first (M-response) is due to direct excitation of motor nerve fibers. The second contraction (H-response) is due to the discharge of synapti-

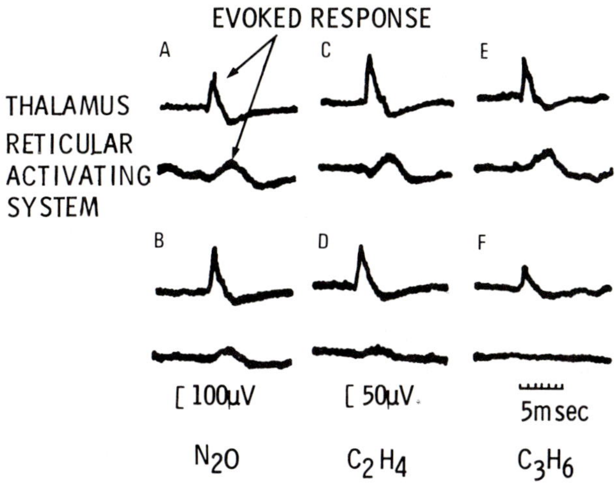

FIG. 3, 1. Stimulation of a cat superficial radial nerve results in two responses in the central nervous system: the upper tracing is the thalamic spike potential while the lower tracing is the midbrain reticular system wave. The upper figures (*A*, *C*, and *E*) are typical control responses. The lower figures illustrate the effects of 77% nitrous oxide (*B*), 77% ethylene (*D*) and 40% cyclopropane (*F*). Note that both evoked responses are affected but the greater effect is on the reticular system. (Reproduced with permission from Davis, H. S., Collins, W. F., Randt, C. T. *et al.:* Effect of anesthetic agents on evoked central nervous system responses: gaseous agents. Anesthesiology 18: 634–642, 1957.)

cally excited spinal motoneurons. That is, stimulation of the tibial nerve causes both an efferent impulse to muscle and also an afferent impulse which discharges spinal motoneurons. Anesthesia depresses the amplitude of the H-response without greatly affecting the M-response. At MAC, about 80 percent of the H-reflex is abolished (9). This depression at the spinal cord is independent of inhibitory influences from higher levels of the nervous system. In animals with transected cervical spinal cords, the depressant effects of halothane and nitrous oxide on dorsal horn cells equals or exceeds the depressant effects found in animals having intact midbrain and hindbrain cord connections. Further support for a direct intraspinal anesthetic action comes from work on cuneate neurons where local perfusion with blood containing halothane causes inhibition of transmission (10).

Polysynaptic versus Monosynaptic Pathways. Polysynaptic pathways are thought to be less resistant than monosynaptic pathways to anesthetic depression. This implies that areas of the brain which contain a multiplicity of synapses (for example, the reticular activating system) may be particularly vulnerable to anesthetics. However, the increasing probability of blockade associated with an increase in the number of synaptic connections (fig. 3, 2) ignores the fact that synapses differ in both sensitivity and transmitter mechanisms, and that they may interact via neuronal loops. Such loops may provide an excitatory or inhibitory action and thereby may produce negative or positive feedback. Any such analysis must be excessively simple and can only begin to describe the human nervous system with its 15/20,000 million neurons each one of which may be directly connected with 10,000 other neurons.

Perhaps little distinction can be made between the relative resistance of monosynaptic and polysynaptic pathways to anesthetic depression. Recall from Chapter 2 that depolarization of a secondary neuron usually requires several synchronous synaptic discharges to that neuron. The chances of depolarization of a secondary neuron increase geometrically with the number of synaptic discharges or the strength of such discharges to that neuron. It is known that the anesthetic depression of the excitatory postsynaptic potentials recorded from one cell is related to the depression of the reflex discharge of the population to which the cell belongs (11). Thus, the characteristics of inhibition of transmission through a single neuron-neuron connection may resemble those described above (fig. 3, 2) for polysynaptic connections. In support of this thesis, inhaled agents depress the transmission of afferent impulses via a single synapse at least as easily as via a synaptic chain (fig. 3, 3) (12).

Peripheral Nerve. It is generally thought that peripheral nerves conduct normally during surgical anesthesia. Anesthetic concentrations of ether and chloroform block synaptic transmission but do not affect axonal conduction in cat sympathetic fibers (fig. 3, 4) (13). Similarly, 3

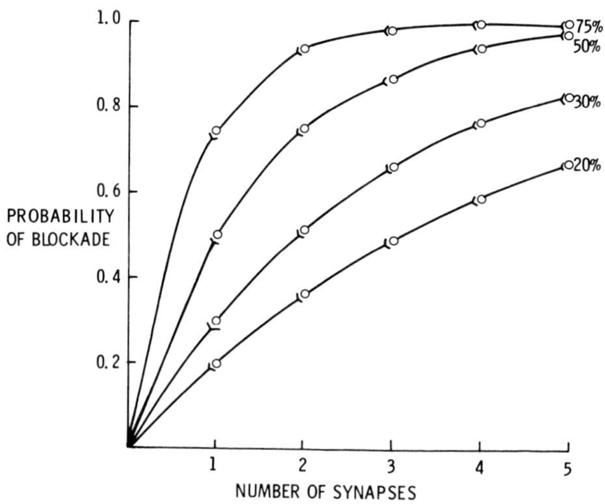

FIG. 3, 2. The probability of blocking a nerve impulse traveling along a synaptic chain is increased with an increase in the number of synaptic links. The different plots are for different probabilities of blocking a single synapse (i.e., 75%, 50%, 30%, 20%). These estimations presume that all synapses are equally sensitive to anesthetics and that probability of blockade equals $1 - (1 - p)^n$ where p is the probability of blocking one synapse and n is the number of synapses.

percent halothane or 80 percent nitrous oxide affects neither impulse generation (transduction) by sensory receptors in feline skin nor impulse conduction via cutaneous nerves (14).

However, one study does suggest a peripheral anesthetic effect at clinically used anesthetic concentrations. Fink and Akamatsu (15) administered nitrous oxide to subjects who had blood flow to one leg occluded by a pneumatic cuff. Sensation of electrical stimuli was lost on the unoccluded side but persisted in the leg with occluded flow. Other evidence also points to a peripheral site of action. Responses to stimulation of pulmonary stretch receptors are augmented at low anesthetic concentrations and depressed by higher concentrations. However, the depression only occurs at concentrations above those used for surgical anesthesia.

Multisites. The problem of certifying one (or more) locus as the primary site of anesthetic action is complicated further by the possibility that one anesthetic may have a dominant effect at one site while the dominant effect of another anesthetic may be located elsewhere. For example, as already noted, halothane reduces the sensitivity of cortical neurons to acetylcholine but methoxyflurane does not alter this sensitivity. Another example is suggested by the electroencephalographic patterns produced by different anesthetics. Although changes in EEG activity can be related to different concentrations of a particular anesthetic, the changes may be very different if another anesthetic is

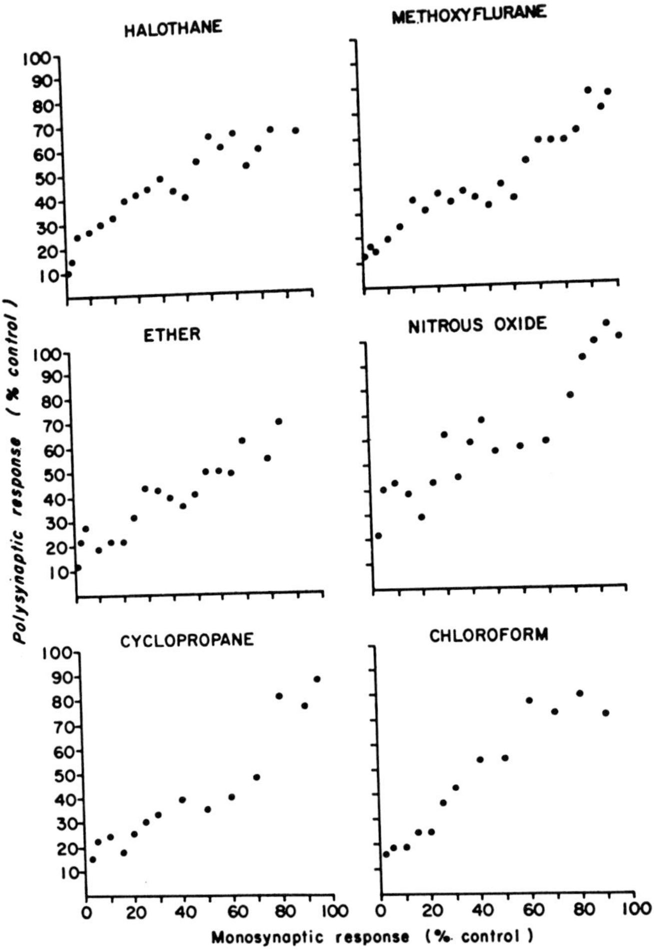

FIG. 3, 3. Concentrations of six different anesthetics depress both monosynaptic and polysynaptic responses to dorsal root stimulation in decerebrate cats. In all cases the anesthetic concentration is increasing from right to left. Note that significant transmission via the polysynaptic pathway remains at concentrations which abolish the monosynaptic response. (Reproduced with permission from DeJong, R. M., Robles, R., Corbin, R. W., *et al.:* Effect of inhalation anesthetics on monosynaptic transmission in the spinal cord. J. Pharmacol. Exp. Ther. 162: 326–330, 1968.)

used. Clark and Rosner (16) have suggested that anesthetics can be classified according to chemical structure and neuroelectric effects in man. There appears to be a relationship between drug structure and regional actions of inhalational agents. For example, the electroencephalographic effects of methoxyflurane, halothane and chloroform are similar to each other but are distinctly different from those of ether, nitrous oxide or cyclopropane.

We conclude that anesthetics act at many sites in the nervous system. We cannot point to one of these sites as the primary site of action, and in fact, anesthesia may result from a concomitant action at many sites.

Action at the Microscopic Level

Does anesthesia result from a failure of the transduction process, of axonal conduction or of synaptic transmission? Concentrations of chloroform or ether causing surgical anesthesia inhibit synaptic transmission, but 3 to 10 times these concentrations are required to inhibit axonal transmission (13). Similarly, a single direct nerve stimulation results in muscular contraction which suggests that axonal conduction and neuromuscular transmission are relatively unaffected. However, the presence of anesthesia causes "fade" in response to stimuli, and the neuromuscular depressant effects of muscle relaxants are directly related to anesthetic depth (17). These effects probably relate to a depression of transmission at the neuromuscular (synaptic) junction rather than any effect on axonal transmission.

If anesthetics act at synapses, which synapses are affected and what part of synaptic transmission is affected? In contrast to barbiturates, it would appear that inhibitory synapses are not preferentially preserved or stimulated during anesthesia with inhaled agents (18). This suggests that blockade at excitatory synapses probably is the major cause of anesthesia. The portion of the neuromuscular junction which appears to be most sensitive to halothane is the postjunctional membrane (19). In the spinal cord, presynaptic endings appear to conduct action potentials

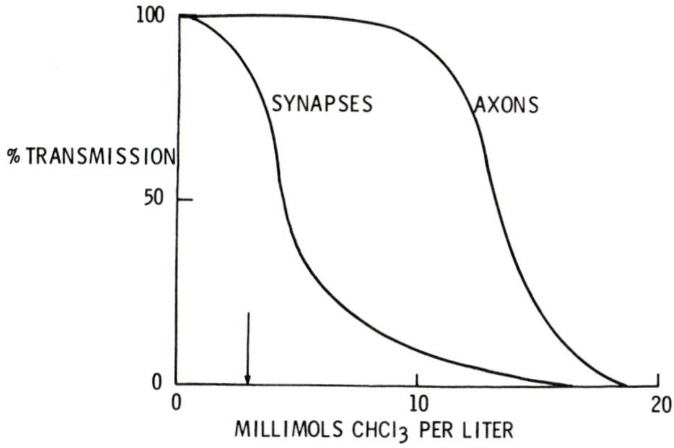

FIG. 3, 4. Chloroform selectively blocks synaptic transmission through the stellate ganglion of the cat at concentrations which are lower than those required to decrease transmission through axons. The concentration of chloroform causing surgical anesthesia is approximately 3 mM/liter (indicated by the *small arrow* on the x-axis). (Adapted with permission from Larrabee, M. G. and Pasternak, J. M.: Selective action of anesthetics on synapses and axons in mammalian sympathetic ganglia. J. Neurophysiol. 15:91–114, 1952.)

normally (11), although the possibility of a small decrease in the terminal nerve action potential cannot be excluded. A small decrease might be sufficient to greatly reduce quantal release of transmitter (see fig. 2, 8). Such reduction has been suggested for barbiturates (20). Anesthesia affects neither synthesis nor storage of transmitter substances. Further, there is no change in the number of synapses participating in transmission (11). Remaining possible causes for failure of synaptic transmission include: 1) impaired release of chemical transmitter; 2) specific antagonism of the transmitter at the postsynaptic membrane; 3) nonspecific stabilization of the subsynaptic membrane. Barbiturates decrease the sensitivity of the subsynaptic membrane to the microiontophoretic application of acetylcholine (21, 22). If this applies to the inhaled anesthetics it would strongly suggest a nonspecific stabilization of the subsynaptic membrane.

Action at the Molecular Level

Correlations of some physical properties of anesthetics with anesthetic potency may implicate a particular subcellular site of action. For example, we may correlate "MAC" with anesthetic lipid solubility or hydrate dissociation pressure (23) (fig. 3, 5). The better correlation with lipids suggests that lipids more closely mimic the site of action. If so, the forces between anesthetics and lipids might indicate the forces between anesthetics and their molecular site of action.

Great care must be taken to select appropriate correlations since an inappropriate selection would not only be useless but misleading (24). The following caricatures describe some of such difficulties (fig. 3, 6). The two anesthetics illustrated by the gentlemen in "A" are considering a liason with a number of possible sites of action such as the two ladies in "B." The lady on the left has nothing to do with an anesthetic effect, while the lady on the right is the true site of anesthetic action. Meanwhile the gentlemen are restrained by their peers (C). These "intrapeer' forces may be related to physical properties which correlate fairly (vapor pressure) to poorly (parachor (25), Van der Waal's constants (26)) with anesthetic potency. One of the best known of the "intrapeer" correlations proposes that equal thermodynamic activities produce equal degrees of anesthesia (27) (table 3, 1 MAC/vapor pressure). This correlates potency with the ideal solubility of a gas or vapor as calculated from Raoult's law with due allowances for the forces between the gas molecules themselves. But, as with any such "intrapeer" relationship, emphasis thus is removed from the interaction of the anesthetic with the true site of action and concentrated on the interaction of the anesthetic with itself. The "intrapeer" forces between similar anesthetic molecules are deficient in that the force contributed by such an imitation site of

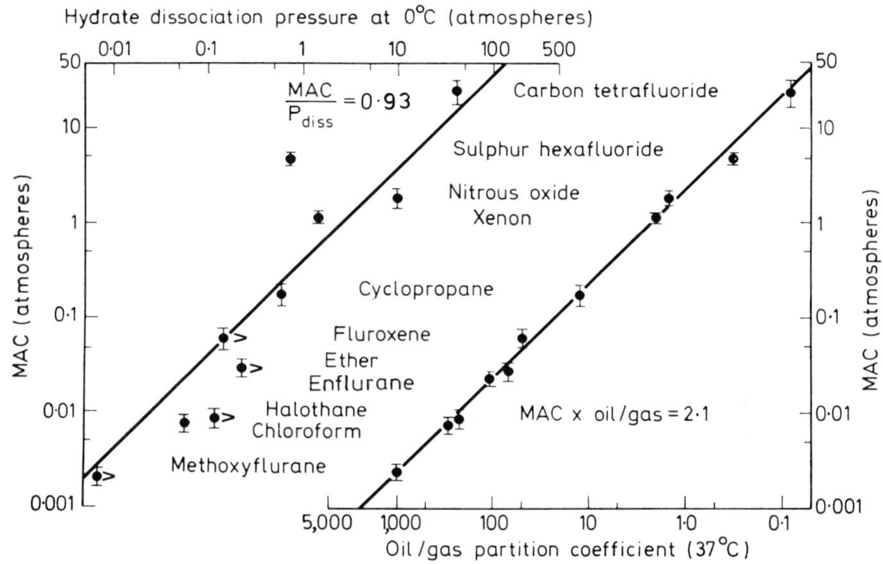

FIG. 3, 5. MAC (in dogs) may be correlated with hydrate dissociation pressure (*left graph, upper scale*) or lipid solubility (*right graph, lower scale*). If the data followed the correlation: MAC/hydrate dissociation pressure equals a constant or MAC × oil/gas partition coefficient equals a constant, the data would lie along the 45°-angle slopes. Similar correlations are obtained using MAC data from humans or mice or other animals. (Adapted with permission from Eger, E. I., Lundgren, C., Miller, S. L. *et al.*: Anesthetic potencies of sulfur hexafluoride, carbon tetrafluoride, chloroform and Ethrane in dogs. Anesthesiology 30: 129–135, 1969.)

action is that of anesthetic with itself and therefore varies from agent to agent.

Choice of a constant imitation site of action reduces the difficulties of interpretation. If the interaction is inconsistent (such as MAC and aqueous solubility or hydrate dissociation pressure) then such a site poorly imitates the force possessed by the true site of anesthetic action (D). But if the interaction is consistent for all anesthetics (such as MAC and lipid solubility) such a site must possess properties similar to those of the site of action (E).

Anesthesia may be produced by the achievement of a certain anesthetic molar concentration at the site of action. If this concentration (K) is the same for all anesthetics, then:

$$P_{An} \times \text{“solubility”} = K \tag{1}$$

where P_{An} is the anesthetizing partial pressure and "solubility" is the solubility at the site of action. The model solvent giving the lowest variability of K would therefore most closely mimic the solvent characteristics of the anesthetic site of action.

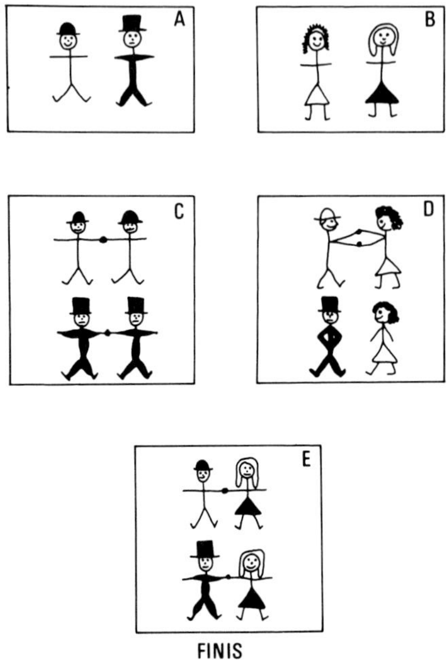

FIG. 3, 6. These caricatures illustrate different types of intermolecular forces between two anesthetic agents (shown in "*A*") and two potential sites of action (shown in "*B*"). "*C*" illustrates the forces between anesthetic molecules themselves. "*D*" illustrates inconsistent forces between anesthetic agents and a false site of action. "*E*" illustrates consistent forces between anesthetic agents and the true site of action. (Adapted from Halsey, M. J., and Kent, D. W.: Molecular mechanisms of anesthesia. Anesthesiology 36: 313–315, 1972.)

A solvent may be characterized by its solubility parameter (δ). The solubility parameter provides a measure of the "cohesive energy density" of the solvent which in turn is an indication of the strength of the forces between the solvent molecules. Solubility parameters may be used to characterize solvents—and hence the site of action—in quantitative terms as opposed to simply saying that the site "resembles" a particular solvent such as benzene or olive oil. The most satisfactory correlation between anesthetic pressure and solubility in pure nonpolar solvents is found for solvents with $\delta = 9 \pm 1$ (cal cm^{-3})$^{1/2}$ (fig. 3, 7) (28). This assumes that anesthesia occurs at a critical molar concentration. If, however, anesthesia occurs at a critical volume concentration of anesthetic, equation 1 must be modified to incorporate the molar volume of the agent at the site of action:

$$P_{An} \times \text{"solubility"} \times \text{molar volume} = K \qquad (2)$$

Inclusion of molar volume raises the most satisfactory correlation to solubility parameters of 10 (cal cm^{-3})$^{1/2}$ or slightly greater (28). By using this analysis it eventually may be possible to ascribe a greater or lesser importance to the inclusion of the molar volume term. That is, if molar volume (as opposed to concentration) is important then the lowest coefficient of variation should be centered at 10 (or greater) rather than 9 (cal cm^{-3})$^{1/2}$. Unfortunately, the available solubility data are insufficient to permit an accurate centering of the lowest point.

TABLE 3, 1

Correlations of anesthetic potencies with three physical properties

Agent	MAC × Oil/Gas Partition Coefficient	MAC/Hydrate Dissociation Pressure	MAC/Vapor Pressure
Methoxyflurane	2.23	<0.32	7.60
Chloroform	2.08	0.12	3.65
Halothane	1.95	<0.073	2.72
Isoflurane	1.48		4.55
Enflurane	2.16		9.29
Ether	1.95	<0.13	5.23
Fluroxene	2.86	<0.39	15.9
Cyclopropane	2.06	0.28	3.42
Xenon	2.26	0.79	
Nitrous oxide	2.63	0.19	3.71
Sulfur hexafluoride	1.44	6.4	23.2
Carbon tetrafluoride	1.90	0.63	
Mean ± SD	2.08 ± 0.41	0.93 ± 1.93	7.93 ± 6.67
Coefficient of variation (%)	20%	210%	84%

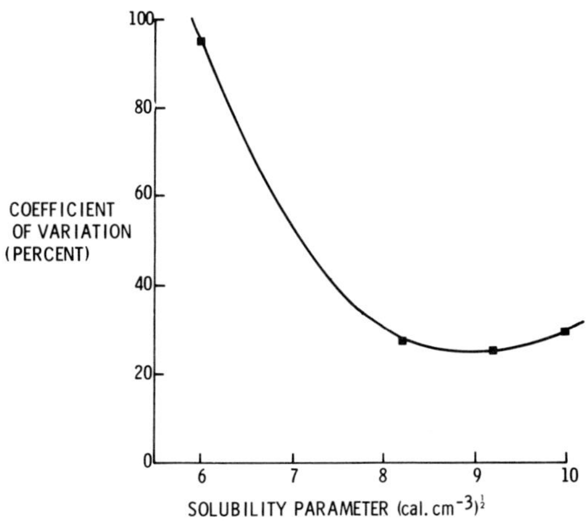

FIG. 3, 7. The coefficient of variation of P_{An} times "solubility" depends on the solvent used and appears to be lowest between 8 and 10 (cal. cm.$^{-3}$)$^{1/2}$. The minimum in the plot indicates the solubility parameter which best mimics that of the site of action. Coefficient of variation equals the standard deviation/mean expressed as a percentage. (Adapted with permission from Miller, K. W., Paton, W. D. M., Smith, E. B. *et al.*: Physiochemical approaches to the mode of action of general anesthesia. Anesthesiology 36: 339–351, 1972.)

These correlation studies indicate that the molecular site of action has hydrophobic properties. This would exclude the aqueous phase ($\delta = 24$) and the overall protein membrane cover ($\delta = 14$) from serious consideration and suggests that the search for a site of anesthesia should concentrate on the lipid regions of the cell membrane or hydrophobic regions within proteins or enzymes ($\delta = 8$ to 10). The increase in anesthetic potency associated with a decrease in body temperature (see fig. 1, 7, Chapter 1) also accords with a hydrophobic site of action. MAC in fish, rats or dogs decreases with hypothermia (i.e., potency increases). For the anesthetics studied, the decline in MAC is proportional to the increase in lipid (but not water) solubility. Thus, the concentration of anesthetic dissolved in a lipid phase at MAC does not vary greatly with temperature. Some variations may result from an anesthetic effect of cold, itself, which becomes dominant at very low temperatures. In homeotherms, a body temperature between 15 and 20°C alone may produce anesthesia. Some interesting experiments remain undone. Carbon tetrafluoride and nitrogen are exceptions to the rule that lipid solubility increases with decreasing temperature. Do their potencies accordingly decrease with hypothermia? Finally, it should be noted that though these data support a lipid site of action they equally support a hydrate (not liquid water) site.

How Do Anesthetics Act?

The previous section discussed the location and properties of the anesthetic sites of action. The following sections will discuss the means by which anesthetics may act at those sites.

The Unitary Hypothesis

It is usually tacitly assumed that all inhalational anesthetics act in the same way. Such a "unitary hypothesis" of anesthesia does not require a single gross site of action. Indeed, as we have seen, there is evidence for several gross sites. The unitary hypothesis *does* require an identity of action at a molecular level. At first glance, the lipid solubility correlation would seem to be good evidence for the unitary hypothesis. However, the correlation might only imply that there are several sites of action which have similar physical characteristics. For example, some anesthetics could inactivate a crucial enzyme, while others could alter the permeability or mobility of protein or lipid areas within the cell membrane.

Several lines of evidence support the unitary hypothesis. For example, multiple sites of action might produce synergism, but in fact, anesthetic effects appear to be additive or antagonistic. Half MAC of one agent plus half MAC of a second agent have the same effect as one MAC of either agent (see fig. 1, 11). Similarly, a study by DiFazio (29) suggested additive effects for one group of anesthetics or a slight antagonism between the effects of cyclopropane and nitrous oxide or ethylene. DiFazio concluded that cyclopropane and nitrous oxide or ethylene may compete at the same site of action, a conclusion which supports the unitary hypothesis.

Further evidence for the unitary hypothesis comes from the parallel nature of the slope of dose-response curves for anesthetics (see also Chapter 1). If dose-response curves are parallel for all anesthetics (i.e., if a proportional increase in concentration produces the same increase in effect for all agents) then the ratio of concentrations for one agent at two given end-points should be the same as the ratio for any other agent. The ratio of "MAC_{awake}" to MAC itself suggests such a constancy (30). MAC_{awake} is the alveolar concentration which just permits a patient to respond to commands. The ratio of MAC_{awake} to MAC produces a narrow range of values for several anesthetics. This is important because different sites of action would likely result in nonparallel dose-response curves. For example, the relationship between MAC and the anesthetic dose causing circulatory depression is inconstant. This is not unexpected since the anesthetic probably acts in different sites in the two cases. The constancy of the ratio of MAC_{awake} to MAC supports but does not prove the anesthetics act on the same site within the nervous system.

A similar line of reasoning also may be used against the unitary hypothesis. Several anesthetics are particularly good analgetics whereas others are not. This implies a variable analgetic/MAC ratio and certainly suggests that these effects result from actions at different sites. Another argument against the unitary hypothesis is that certain anesthetic substances have isomers which are convulsants. For example, Indoklon ($CF_3CH_2OCH_2CF_3$) is a clinically used convulsant agent whereas its geometrical isomer ($(CF_3)_2CHOCH_3$), is an experimental anesthetic. Similarly, enflurane causes convulsions but its isomer isoflurane does not. The argument is marred by the possibility that the same basic process might produce both anesthesia and convulsions. Thus, inhibition of excitatory pathways would produce anesthesia while inhibition of inhibitory pathways (e.g., strychnine) would produce convulsions. In addition, although the anesthetic-convulsant properties of these agents may suggest two sites of action, it is difficult to equate convulsions with the anesthetic state. The fact that anesthetics may affect a convulsant site of action in no way excludes a separate, unitary site. This does not deny that an action at such a convulsant site might influence the anesthetic state.

Another type of dose-response curve has been used to attack the unitary hypothesis. This curve relates the effect of increasing doses of anesthetic to the responses of a number of animals measured at a single end-point such as MAC. Such a curve measures the biological variability of the animals being studied but not the variability of the dose required to achieve different end-points. As such it is not pertinent to this discussion.

Hydrophobic Theories of Anesthesia

An Action on Ionic Channels. The correlation of anesthetic potency and lipid solubility leads to the conclusion that anesthetics act in hydrophobic areas such as those in the cell membrane. If anesthetics act through their effect on the axon membrane, then blockade of the sodium pores is the most likely cause of anesthesia. It is important to realize that although the existence of sodium pores (or other pores) is supported by extensive electrophysiological data, they have not yet been observed in electron micrographs. They may exist either as transient paths, appearing and disappearing, or as permanent structures. They may occur either individually at intervals or in small clusters. The pores blocked must be at the nerve terminal, since all studies suggest that the nerve action potential is not blocked by concentrations of anesthetics sufficient to produce anesthesia. However, as noted previously only a small reduction in the nerve action potential at the nerve terminal is required to reduce markedly the release of transmitter and thereby block synaptic transmission (see fig. 2, 8).

An alternative membrane site of action is the subsynaptic membrane. Recall that this site differs from the axon membrane in several ways. It is depolarized by acetycholine (or other neurotransmitters) but is insensitive to changes in membrane potential. The subsynaptic channels for ionic flux are far larger than the sodium pores of the axon. Both sodium and potassium ions may pass through the channel. Despite these differences, many of the speculations on mechanisms that apply to the sodium pore also apply to this channel.

Sodium pores (fig. 2, 5) may be blocked in several ways. At rest the channels presumably are obstructed by "gates" which may be composed of the polar tails of lecithin molecules. These tails may be held in place by a calcium bridge to proteins surrounding the pore. By weakening the calcium affinity or by causing contraction of the protein, depolarization might rupture the calcium bond and thereby remove the obstructing gates. Anesthetics may act by expanding the protein and thereby reducing the excursion resulting from contraction. The more limited contraction may fail to rupture the calcium bridge. Alternatively, anesthetics might swell or distort the lecithin molecules so that retraction of the obstructing polar tail would be hindered.

Anesthetics may directly block the pore. Mullins (31) suggested that the affinity of anesthetic molecules for the sodium channel walls might hold them in a blocking position (fig. 3, 8*a*). A more complex pore model allows an indirect blocking effect. This model envisions the pore as formed by lipid molecules arranged in spirals stretching lengthwise (closed pore) or flattening sideways (open pore) depending on the transmembrane potential (fig. 3, 8*b*). Anesthetics might prevent the opening of the pore by limiting the freedom of the helix to flatten.

Pore size also may be decreased by the lateral membrane pressure produced by the presence of anesthetics in the membrane (fig. 3, 8*c*). Since the pore size is crucially close to that which would hinder sodium movement, a small reduction in size may be all that is necessary to cause obstruction. The possibility that anesthetics might act by increasing the lateral pressure is supported by the correlation of potency with the changes in lateral pressure produced by anesthetics in artificial lipoprotein films (32).

Contractile proteins may be important to the development of pores in the subsynaptic membrane. Current concepts of membrane structure suggest a far greater mobility of membrane components (including contractile proteins) than traditionally supposed. For example, in the immune response in lymphocytes, protein units within the membrane can come together to form "patches" which then cross-link to form a "cap." Similarly, Allison (33) has speculated that protein migration rearrangements may be necessary to form the subsynaptic receptor sites for transmitter molecules (fig. 3, 9). Further rearrangements resulting from the interaction with transmitter might form the pore necessary for depolarization. By their affinity to hydrophobic portions of the proteins, anesthetics might limit protein mobility and thereby prevent transmitter molecules from activating the subsynaptic membrane.

An Action on Neurotransmitter Release. Anesthetics may act by decreasing the release of neurotransmitters from their vesicles. A failure to release transmitter, or a reduction in the amount of released transmitter may prevent synaptic transmission. The exact mechanism of release is unknown but various models are illustrated in figure 3, 10 (34–36). The release of neurotransmitters by depolarization of the nerve terminal requires a breach of both the vesicle and the nerve terminal membranes. Anesthesia may increase the resistance of either the vesicle or the nerve terminal membrane to rupture. Relevant to such a hypothesis is the demonstration that clinical concentrations of anesthetics protect red cells against hypotonic hemolysis (37). The anesthetic dissolved in the membrane may expand the membrane and permit it to enclose a larger volume without disruption. An alternative explanation would be that the presence of the dissolved anesthetic strengthens the membrane. Either explanation suggests the possibility that anesthetics similarly might act to prevent the rupture of vesicles into the synaptic cleft.

(a)

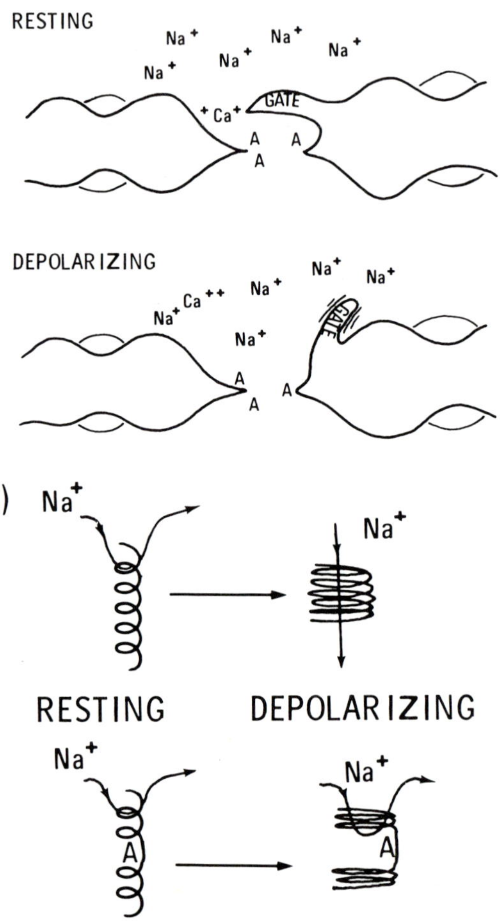

FIG. 3, 8. Anesthetics (A) might block ion pores by: *a*) occupying a site in the pore itself and blocking ion fluxes directly; *b*) interacting with a lipid spiral helix to prevent the opening of the pore; *c*) dissolving in the membrane and thereby exerting a lateral pressure which would narrow the pore.

Experimental Evidence

Pressure Reversal of Anesthesia. An increase in hydrostatic pressure increases anesthetic requirement. Anesthetics lower bacterial luminescence. Luminescence is restored by application of hundreds of atmospheres of pressure. Similarly, tadpoles immobilized by ethyl alcohol revive and swim about if concomitantly pressurized (38). High pressures reverse the anesthesia produced in newts by halothane or pentobarbital.

The above qualitative findings have been assessed quantitatively for the pressure antagonism of nitrous oxide anesthesia in mice (2, 39). An

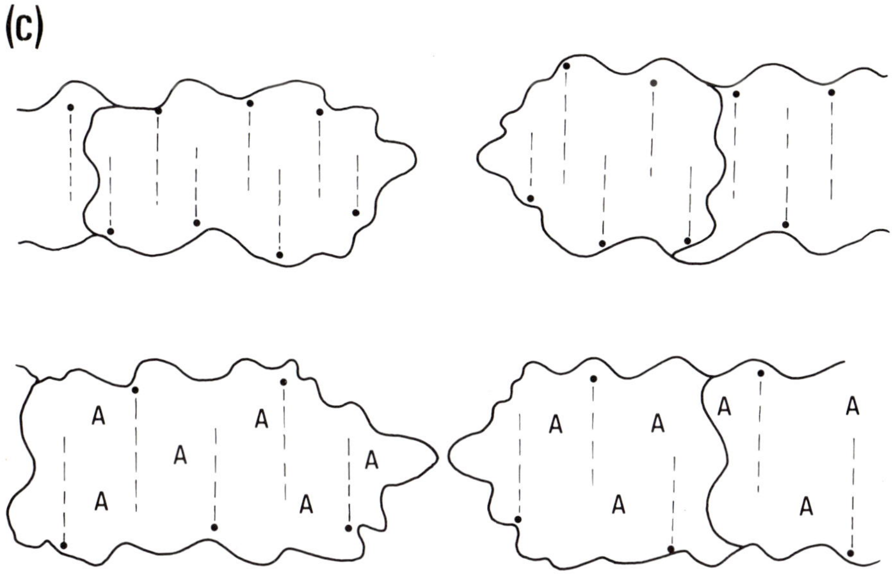

FIG. 3, 8c.

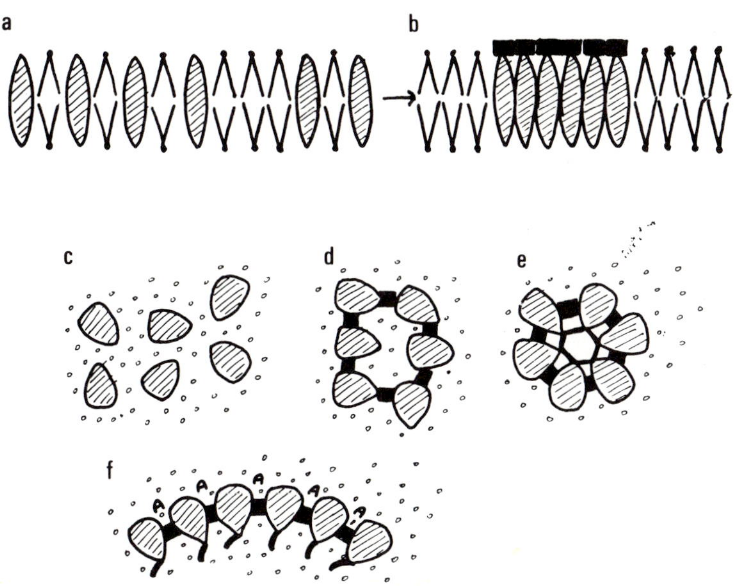

FIG. 3, 9. Proteins (*striped ovals*) may be arranged randomly in the lipid bilayer (*a*) or may move to aggregate together (*b*). The various processes can also be visualized in the subsequent pictures of the surface of the membrane (*c* to *f*). Normally the protein units (now represented as *striped "pear-shaped"* structures) are arranged randomly in a "sea" of lipids (*very small circles*) (*c*). However, in the area of the subsynaptic membrane the protein units are haphazardly linked together by a number of specific products (■) (*d*). Transmitter molecules (—) can further cross-link the proteins, forming an ion-conducting hole with the exclusion of the lipids from the center (*e*). However, if anesthetics (A) also interact with the proteins, the transmitter molecules are unable to induce the formation of the ion-conducting hole (*f*). (Adapted with permission from Allison, A. C.: Analogies between triggering mechanisms in immune and other cellular reactions. In *Cell Interactions*, edited by L. E. Silvestri, pp. 156–161. North Holland, Amsterdam, 1972.)

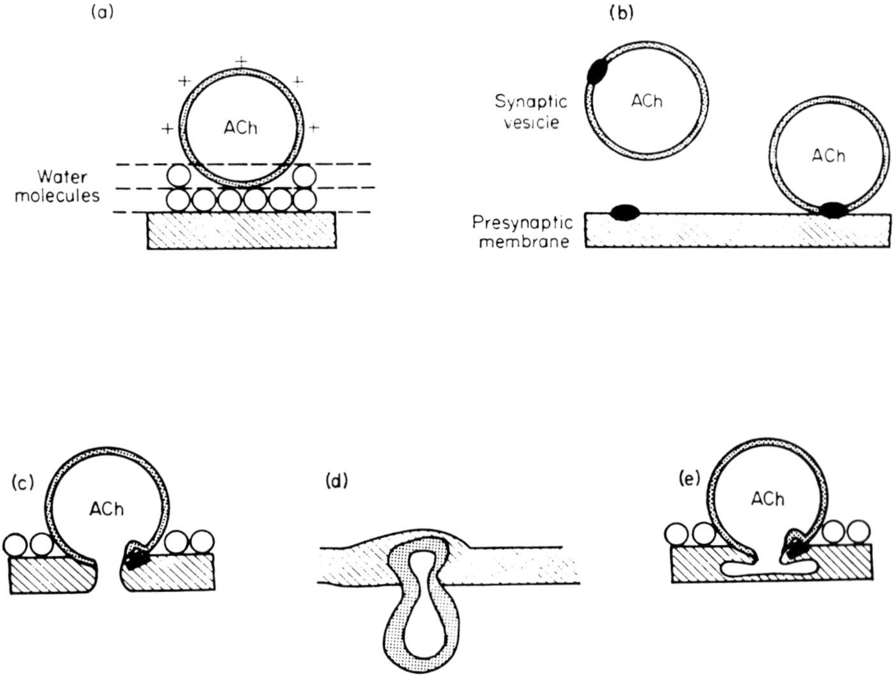

FIG. 3, 10. Possible mechanisms of neurotransmitter release from vesicles are illustrated. Bass and Moore (34) assumed that both vesicle and presynaptic membrane are charged and therefore hydrated (*a*). A nerve impulse reduces the electrical and hydration barrier and allows vesicles to discharge neurotransmitter molecules into the synaptic cleft. Del Castillo and Katz (35) proposed that the vesicles and membrane have complementary receptor sites (*b*). The vesicle therefore can become attached to the membrane and then discharge its contents as shown in (*c*). A nerve impulse might increase the number of active sites in the membrane. Alternative concepts have envisaged the entire vesicle being released (*d*) or the contents of the vesicle being transferred to a membrane store prior to discharge (*e*). (Reproduced with permission from Hubbard, J. I.: Mechanism of transmitter release. Progr. Biophys. 21: 33–124, 1970.)

increase in total pressure achieved by the addition of helium causes a rectilinear increase in the pressure of nitrous oxide required for anesthesia (fig. 3, 11). These relationships bear on some of the preceding speculations on mechanisms. Let us examine the implications of one experiment with the reversal of anesthesia by high pressures of "inert" gases. The effect of increasing helium pressures on nitrous oxide requirement is not equalled by any other gas. Increasing pressures produced by neon do not alter nitrous oxide requirements and increasing pressures produced by hydrogen cause a decrease (fig. 3, 11). These differences may be explained if we assume that the increase in pressure achieved with any gas produces two effects: one is anesthesia and the second is the reversal of anesthesia! The reversal of anesthesia is a

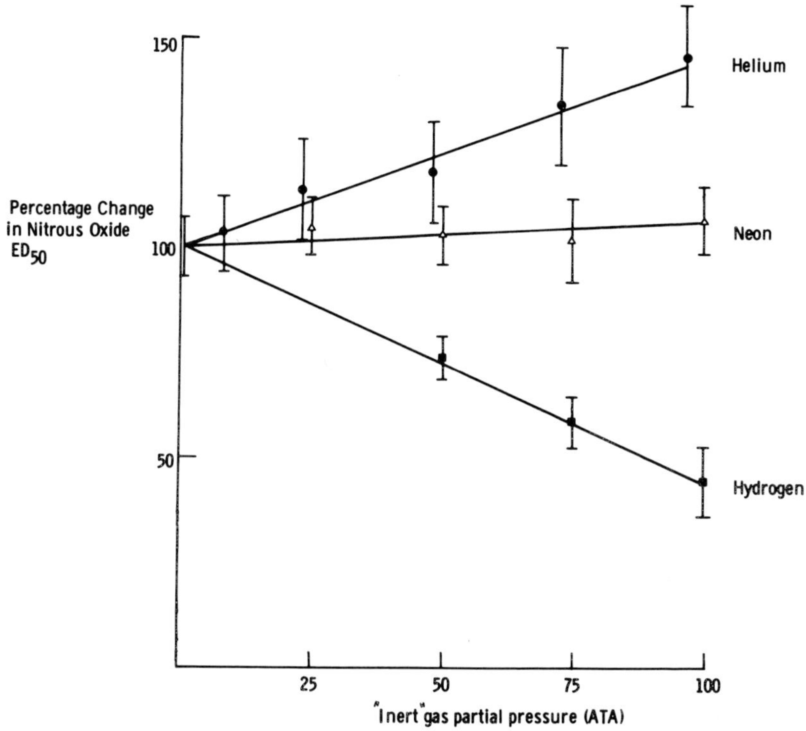

FIG. 3, 11. The partial pressure of nitrous oxide required to produce a loss of righting reflex in mice is plotted against increasing pressures achieved by the addition of helium, neon or hydrogen. Increasing helium pressures increase the nitrous oxide requirement in a linear fashion, indicating that pressure produced with helium antagonizes the effect of anesthesia. Increases in pressure produced with neon do not alter anesthetic requirement. Increases in pressure produced with hydrogen reduce anesthetic requirements as indicated by the decreased partial pressure of nitrous oxide necessary to cause a loss of the righting reflex. (Adapted from Halsey, M. J., and Kent, D. W.: The anesthetic effects of inert gases. In *Abstracts of the American Society of Anesthesiologists Annual Meeting*, p. 105–106, 1972.)

hydrostatic phenomenon and thus common to all gases at a given pressure. That is, 100 atmospheres of hydrogen exerts an anti-anesthetic effect equal to that exerted by 100 atmospheres of helium. But at the same time that each gas exerts its anti-anesthetic effect, it also acts as an anesthetic. Therein lies the difference in the effects of the different gases. If the previously noted correlation of anesthetic potency with lipid solubility can be extended to helium, neon and hydrogen, then we would predict helium to be least potent (it is least lipid soluble), neon intermediate and hydrogen most potent. This, indeed, is what figure 3, 11 suggests. The anesthetic effect of helium is too weak to overcome the anti-anesthetic effect produced by pressure. The two effects are equal in the case of neon and thus cancel each other. With hydrogen, the anesthetic effect predominates, allowing the reduction of nitrous oxide requirement despite an increased pressure.

The hypothesis of a dual anesthetic and anti-anesthetic (hydrostatic) effect of all gases explains why gases such as helium or neon cannot of themselves produce anesthesia. Their potency is less than (helium) or equal to (neon) their antianesthetic effect. The hypothesis also allows the inclusion of helium, neon and hydrogen in the correlation of potency and lipid solubility. To include these gases requires the application of a pressure correction factor of about minus 1.3 MAC for each 100 atmospheres of pressure. Such a correction would allow the inclusion of these gases in table 3, 1 without much alteration in the variance of the MAC times oil/gas partition coefficient ratio.

How might pressure exert its anti-anesthetic effect? The anti-anesthetic effect is probably made up of two parts. An increase in hydrostatic pressure may reduce gas solubility (40). That is, hydrostatic pressure may decrease the number of anesthetic molecules which can be present at the site of action at a given partial pressure. For example, suppose that 1 atmosphere of gas X causes anesthesia by producing a 50 mM concentration at the site of action. The superimposition of 100 atmospheres of hydrostatic pressure might decrease the concentration produced by a partial pressure of 1 atmosphere of gas X to 25 mM—a concentration which would be insufficient to cause anesthesia. To produce anesthesia at 100 atmospheres total pressure, gas X would have to be increased to 2 atmospheres. However, this example exaggerates the effect of pressure on solubility: the effect is probably relatively small.

The reduction in anesthetic solubility induced by pressure indirectly antagonizes the effect of the anesthetic. It appears that there also is a direct antagonism of anesthesia by pressure. This effect may be explained by some of the previously suggested mechanisms of anesthesia. For example, if anesthetics act by expanding critical areas of the cell membrane (fig. 3, 8*c*), this expansion might be reversed by the compressive effect of increased hydrostatic pressure. The importance of expansion and compression is enhanced by evidence that the same molar concentration of an anesthetic expands a biological membrane about 10 times more than it expands an imitation site such as olive oil (41).

Finally, the results from the pressure reversal studies also argue against the importance of molar volume to the potency of an anesthetic. Hydrogen is significantly more potent than neon which, in turn, is more potent than helium. This would be predicted from their respective lipid solubilities but when molar volume times solubility is calculated, the order of predicted potency is neon, helium and (least potent) hydrogen. However, the argument is not conclusive because there are several assumptions that must be made in the calculation of molar volume.

Exceptions to the Correlation of Potency and Lipid Solubility. The lipid solubility of carbon dioxide suggests that it should produce anesthesia at 1.7 atmospheres whereas a third of an atmosphere suffices in dogs or man. This greater than predicted potency can be explained by the ability of CO_2 to lower cerebrospinal fluid pH (see Chapter 1). Oxygen at increased pressures should theoretically be anesthetic whereas, in fact, it produces convulsions. However Paton (42) has shown that suppression of the convulsive activity of oxygen uncovers its anesthetic activity at high pressures. The anesthetic partial pressure of oxygen extrapolated from these results is about 11 atmospheres which is close to that predicted from its lipid solubility. Similarly, a number of other gases are known to produce convulsions but are not known to produce anesthesia. As with oxygen, their anesthetizing partial pressures may exceed those pressures required to produce convulsions.

Another possible exception to the lipid correlation is normal decane which is not an anesthetic despite an apparently high (but unmeasured) lipid solubility. This fact suggested to Mullins (31) the possible importance of molecular size to anesthetic requirement. He postulated that there is a critical size associated with the site of action. If an agent is small, it can fit into the site but the closeness of fit is poor and the agent therefore is relatively impotent. Larger agents also fit into the site and their relatively better fit increases their potency. But if the agent is too large it cannot fit into the site and therefore is impotent. This is illustrated in figure 3, 12. Mullins suggested that normal decane fits in the "too large" category. However, this argument is complicated by the extremely low water solubility of decane. This may hinder the transport of decane to its site of action. Furthermore, it is known that in certain microorganisms, hydrocarbons such as decane can be metabolized (43). If this is the case within the nervous system it may be that however long the equilibration period, decane cannot reach an anesthetizing molar concentration. Finally, the oil/gas partition coefficient is unknown and although the lipid solubility must be high, it may be insufficient to allow the maximum partial pressure which may be achieved (i.e., the vapor pressure of n-decane) to cause anesthesia. Mullins also postulated that the molar volume of halothane (138 ml/mole) should be at the threshold of the limiting molecular size for anesthetic action. However, recent evaluations of new volatile general anesthetics suggest that the threshold, if it exists at all, would be much higher. For example, the halogenated methyl ethyl ether, $CH_3O\ CF_2\ CHBrCl$, is a good experimental anesthetic at 1.25 percent and obviously is a larger molecule than halothane ($CF_3\ CHBrCl$) (44).

Although the correlation of anesthetic potency with lipid solubility is

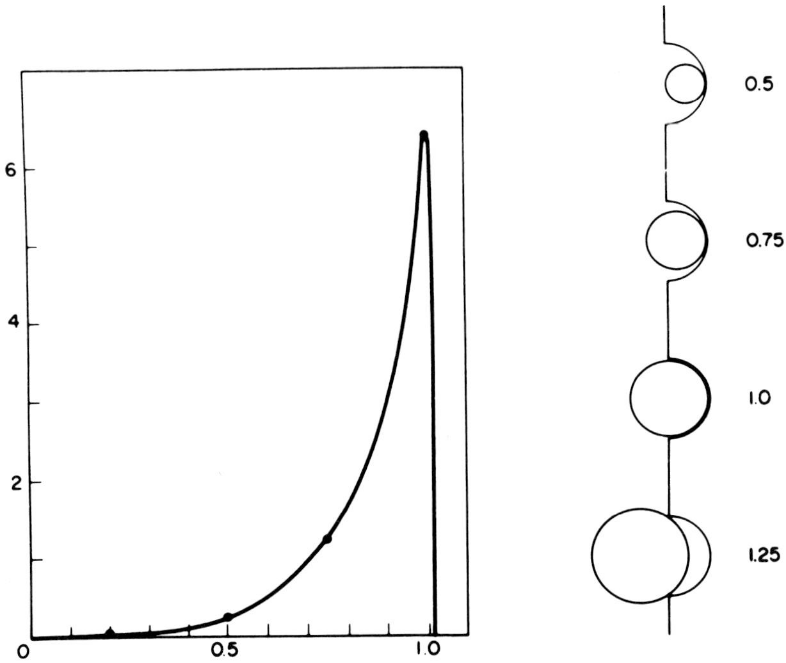

FIG. 3, 12. The closeness of fit of spherical molecules of various sizes to a hemispherical site varies with the size of the molecule. A series of molecules are considered with diameters from 0.5 to 1.25 times the diameter of the site. Assuming binding is related to the closeness of fit there is maximum binding (vertical axis in arbitrary units) for a molecule which just fits the site, and if anesthetic potency is a function of binding, then this graph also illustrates the relationship of potency to molecular size. (Reproduced with permission from Mullins, L. J.: *Anesthetics, Handbook of Neurochemistry* Edited by A. Lajtha, Vol. 6. Plenum Press, 1971.)

extremely good, it is by no means perfect. A number of factors may explain the imperfections which exist. First there is the inherent inaccuracy in the measurements of anesthetic potency. Second, some agents increase sympathetic activity whereas others are depressant, and as noted in Chapter 1, release of central catecholamines increases MAC. Nitrous oxide and fluroxene both increase sympathetic activity and both have higher MACs than would be predicted from their lipid solubility (see table 3, 1). However, cyclopropane and ether also have stimulant properties but do not deviate from the general correlation. Third, anesthetics may act at more than one molecular site. For example, the pore in the membrane may consist of 4 to 12 subunit proteins (45). If sequential or complimentary interactions between these subunits are required to produce an overall cooperative effect, then different anesthetics could act on different subunits, or groups of subunits with the same overall effect (i.e., anesthesia) (43). Minor variations in the lipid correlation would result from differences in the characteristics of the different subunits.

Model Systems. Many investigations into mechanisms of action have been conducted on "model" systems which are less complex than the human nervous system. For example, the physical changes in elastomers (elastic compounds such as silastic rubber) produced by anesthetics, may be analogous to the changes taking place at the site of action of general anesthetics (46, 47). Elastomers are not membranes or other cell parts, but other examples of model systems do approach biological reality.

The anesthetic interaction with membrane proteins which control ion fluxes is very difficult to investigate directly but other protein systems have been studied. Schoenborn (48) identified a xenon and cyclopropane binding site in myoglobin and halothane alters the structure of the beta chain of hemoglobin (49). However, it has not been possible to detect functional changes associated with these conformational alterations. Balasubramanian and Wetlaufer (50) demonstrated that six gaseous anesthetics altered the tertiary structure of beta lactoglobulin and bovine plasma albumin, and that there was a crude correlation between these effects and anesthetic potencies. Such observations suggest that anesthetics can interact with proteins *directly* and this has stimulated interest in various "protein theories" of anesthesia.

The action of anesthetics on the light-producing enzyme system in luminous bacteria has recently been studied by two groups of workers (51, 52). There is a remarkable correlation between anesthetic potencies in mammals and the inhibition of the luminescent system in bacteria. This suggests that the mechanism of general anesthesia may be more specific than has frequently been suggested and may result from the interaction of anesthetics with particuar proteins within mammalian cells.

Model systems also have been used to learn more about the effect of anesthetics on ion fluxes across membranes. Inhaled anesthetics increase the permeability of cations through artificial membrane systems such as liposomes (concentric phospholipid bilayers) (53, 54). If such increases primarily affected potassium, this might result in hyperpolarization (and inhibition) *in vivo*. On the other hand, ether and chloroform do not affect active or passive cation transport across erythrocyte membranes (55). It should be remembered that the ion fluxes across passive membranes (such as erythrocyte membranes) are at least one order of magnitude smaller than those involved in the depolarization of the neural membrane. A study of some of the new model membrane systems which mimic excitable rather than passive membranes may be particularly pertinent to understanding anesthetic mechanisms.

Biochemical Theories of Anesthesia

Verworn's (56) suggestion that narcosis results from suppression of oxygen "carriers," was the forerunner of current theories that anesthetics act by enzymatic inhibition. His "asphyxial theory" fails for there is no evidence that hypoxia or asphyxia necessarily accompany prolonged anesthesia.

Quastel and Wheatly (57) postulated that anesthesia results from depression of cerebral respiration. However, excessive anesthetic concentratins often are required to inhibit respiration in isolated tissue preparations. Furthermore, the average depression of *in vitro* resting brain oxygen consumption is small at clinically used anesthetic concentrations and the *in vivo* depression varies from agent to agent. Quastel suggested that the overall brain oxygen consumption might fail to reveal profound inhibition in vital local areas. In support of this notion a small number of cells in fish retina called "controller cells" respond within seconds to anoxia or hypercapnia or to alcohols and several volatile anesthetics (58). If "controller cells" in the central nervous system modify the activity of other cells, anesthesia might inhibit the metabolism and action of these "controller cells" without manifesting this inhibition in the total brain metabolism.

In vitro studies of brain carbohydrate metabolism suggest that anesthetics inhibit electron transport between cytochrome oxidase and a flavoprotein concerned with the oxidation of (i.e., electron transport to) reduced nicotine adenine dinucleotide (NADH) (57). Since oxidation of NADH allows phosphorylation of adenosine diphosphate (ADP) to adenosine triphosphate (ATP), it follows that anesthetics might inhibit oxidative phosphorylation. However, suppression of ATP formation may result from lowered utilization of ATP. Since ATP inhibits its own synthesis the lowered utilization would discourage further formation, and suppression of formation therefore would not necessarily prove a direct effect of the anesthetic. Finally, the *in vivo* concentration of brain ATP is unchanged during anesthesia, implying that lack of formation is not the cause of anesthesia (59).

If anesthetics act by inhibiting metabolism, then a likely site of action is the mitochondria. Major functions of mitochondria include those of energy transfer and storage. One of several models proposed for these functions is a "conformational" model (60). Tripartite repeating units form the inner membrane of the mitochondrion. Each unit undergoes a conformational change (a change in shape) on altering from a low to a high energy state. Anesthetics can prevent the conformational change and thereby prevent the mitochondria from acting as a high energy (ATP) reserve source. However, as noted previously, cerebral ATP levels do not decrease as a result of anesthesia and furthermore, anesthetics fail to influence the mitochondrial conformational change at clinically relevant concentrations.

As well as affecting many cellular biochemical systems, anesthetics can also be metabolized themselves by man. It has been suggested that this metabolic degradation might be essential for the agent's anesthetic effect. Although this may be true for some of the noninhaled agents (e.g., chloral hydrate must be metabolized to trichloroethanol to achieve anesthesia), it is unlikely to be relevant to the inhaled agents because the onset of anesthesia is far more rapid than the rise in anesthetic metabolites.

All the biochemical theories of anesthesia leave one question unresolved. Are the effects observed the primary cause of anesthesia or simply secondary effects? The old analogy is the chicken or egg—which came first? Do biochemical changes *cause* inhibition of synaptic transmission or are they themselves *caused* by the general depression of the nervous system?

Microtubule Theory

Microtubules are filaments in the cytoplasm of axons which may be important to the intraneural transport of neurotransmitters. Allison and Nunn (61) speculated that anesthetics "depolymerize microtubules and thereby impair nerve impulse transmission." One difficulty with this suggestion is that microtubules are not required for axonal or synaptic conduction of nerve action potentials. For example, the cytoplasm of an axon may be replaced by a high potassium-low sodium salt solution without impairment of impulse transmission.

The main evidence for the microtubule theory was the correlation of anesthetic potency with anesthetic concentration causing reversible dissolution of microtubules in a mold, *Actinosphaerium nucleofilum*. However, the later finding that diethyl ether did not cause microtubular dissolution severely undermined this correlative support. Another difficulty with the theory is that although pressure also causes depolymerization of microtubules it does not potentiate the action of anesthetics (see previous section on Pressure Reversal of Anesthesia).

Hydrate Theories

The brain is more water (78 percent) than lipid (12 percent) or protein (8 percent). This fact led several workers to consider an aqueous site of anesthetic action. However, the poor correlation between anesthetic potency and aqueous solubility ruled out a simple physical interaction.

In 1961, Pauling and S. L. Miller (62, 63) independently proposed that anesthesia results from the formation of gas hydrates or "icebergs" at crucial brain sites. Gas hydrates are gas molecules encaged by water molecules. The presence of the gas molecules enhances the stability of the water structure and therefore the tendency of hydrates to form. Depending on the number of water molecules per cage, there are two sizes of cavity which can be occupied and stabilized by gas molecules (fig. 3, 13). Small (structure 1) gas molecules such as nitrous oxide or xenon fit into cages which have a ratio of 5¾ water molecules per gas molecule. Larger (structure II) gas molecules such as halothane or chloroform fit into larger cages which have a ratio of 17 water molecules to each anesthetic molecule. Since all pure gas hydrates are unstable at 37°C, the hydrate theory required one further speculation. Pauling and Miller suggested that the hydrates form at membrane surfaces where the polar side chains of proteins might contribute the additional stabilization required to form the hydrates at body temperature.

How might these hydrates produce anesthesia? Pauling noted that hydrate formation might decrease the conductance of the nervous tissue and hence the energy of the "electrical oscillations." If such a decrease lowered the nerve action potential at the nerve terminal, it would reduce the number of quanta of transmitter released. While Pauling suggested that whole crystals were formed during anesthesia, Miller conceived of fragments of hydrates constantly forming and decomposing at the cell membrane. Miller suggested that those fragments might "stiffen-up" the lipid membrane or occlude pores in the membrane.

The way in which a protein folds up (i.e., its tertiary structure) depends not only on forces between the protein parts but also on forces

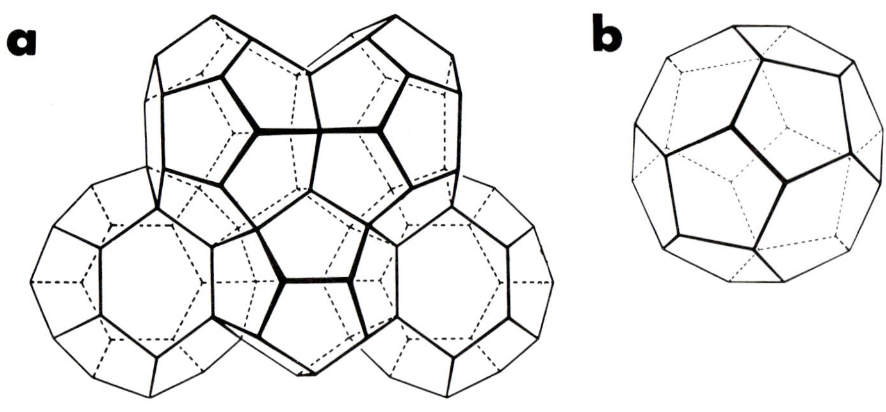

FIG. 3, 13. Part of the unit cell of the Structure I hydrate is drawn (*a*). Lines correspond to hydrogen bonds and the corners correspond to oxygen atoms. Each corner thus indicates one water molecule. An anesthetic molecule of small (Structure I) size (such as nitrous oxide) might occupy any of the cavities represented here. Larger molecules will not fit. A larger cavity may be constructed with a greater number of water molecules (*b*). This cavity can hold a larger (Structure II) gas molecule such as chloroform. (Adapted with permisson from Miller, S. L.: Effect of anesthetics on water structure. Fed. Proc. 27: 879–883, 1968.)

between the protein and the surrounding solvent (water). The balance between these two sets of forces can be upset by the conversion of free water to gas hydrates. Since the biological activity of a protein molecule is strongly dependent on its tertiary structure, the derangement of the protein-water interaction could impair protein function. Gas hydrates thus also might affect the protein structure required for enzyme activity or the release of neurotransmitters.

A change in the solvent surrounding an enzyme also might affect reaction rates. Conversion of water to ice greatly accelerates certain reactions. This may result partly from a concentration of the reactants due to freezing (since ice is mainly made from pure water, the solutes which remain behind in the unfrozen water are more concentrated) and partly from the ability of ice to function as a general catalyst. On the other hand, the ordering of water around dissolved macromolecules and at interfaces might slow the penetration of substrates to reacting groups. These effects on protein function or enzyme activity may influence the processes relevant to neurotransmitter storage and release.

The main evidence for the hydrate theories was the approximate correlation between the potency of an anesthetic and its hydrate dissociation pressure (i.e., the partial pressure of an anesthetic required to form a hydrate). Pauling restricted this correlative test to those anesthetics which could not form hydrogen bonds. He suggested that agents which did form hydrogen bonds (such as diethyl ether) might alter solvent structure independently of the formation of hydrates and that this could cause (and explain) potential deviations from the overall correlation. With this restriction, the only compound that deviated considerably from the correlation was the gas sulfur hexafluoride. Furthermore, both the temperature and pressure effects noted previously would support the hydrate theory. The potency of anesthetics and their hydrate stability concomitantly decrease with increasing temperature or with increasing hydrostatic pressure.

However, there is now considerable evidence against the hydrate theory. The correlation between the anesthetic potency and the hydrate dissociation pressure is far poorer than originally thought (fig. 3, 5, table 3, 1). This is particularly true for fluorinated compounds not commonly considered to be anesthetics, and for several clinical anesthetics. Pure hydrates of fluroxene, diethyl ether, halothane and methoxyflurane are not known. Thus, their hydrate dissociation pressures must exceed the vapor pressure of the pure anesthetic.

Less conclusive evidence against the hydrate theories are additivity studies. If the structure I and structure II hydrates occur concomitantly, the presence of each may strengthen the other and therefore produce stability at a lower anesthetic partial pressure. An analogy might be the reinforcement of concrete with iron rods. This led Pauling to predict that synergism should result when two anesthetics forming different hydrate structures are combined. But mixtures of xenon and halothane and also ethylene and halothane (see Chapter 1) are simply additive in their effects and therefore fail to confirm the Pauling prediction. Although these studies alone do not disprove the hydrate theory, they do suggest that if hydrates form, they do so as discrete independent structures rather than as a continuous ice cover.

Summary

A unique macroscopic site of anesthetic action cannot be located with certainty. A cortical, reticular, activating or spinal cord site all appear to be possible sites. The synapse is probably the cellular site of action but it is not known whether the nerve terminal (and quantal release), the subsynaptic membrane or some other site is affected primarily. The correlation between anesthetic potency and lipid solubility suggests that the molecular site of action has hydrophobic properties. This implicates lipid areas of the neuronal membrane or local hydrophobic areas within proteins or enzymes.

The most likely mechanisms of action of anesthetics involve pre- or postsynaptic membranes. The release of neurotransmitter could be affected directly either by altering the stability of the synaptic vesicle or by interrupting its exocytosis. The formation and activation of neurotransmitter receptors could be upset by anesthetics. Synaptic transmission might be blocked through obstruction of membrane pores. Transmission could be 1) directly interrupted through a reduction of subsynaptic depolarization; or 2) indirectly interrupted through a reduction in transmitter released. The latter might result from a reduced NAP at the nerve terminal.

Anesthetic molecules may block membrane pores directly by lodging in the hole, or indirectly by squeezing the pore through lateral expansion of the rest of the membrane. Alternatively, the gate mechanism of the pore (such as a lecithin bridge or deformable spiral helix) could be inactivated. Finally, the new ideas about the dynamic state of membranes suggest that pores may be formed by the aggregation of proteins which would otherwise be moving freely in the plane of the membrane. If anesthetics prevent the aggregation process, no pores would be formed at all!

Recent experimental evidence provides a framework within which any proposed theory must fit. The pressure reversal of anesthesia gives some indication of the formal changes of the molecular site of action, while exceptions to the correlation of anesthetic potency with lipid solubility suggest further factors that must be taken into account.

The possible biochemical changes associated with anesthesia may be important if it can be demonstrated that they are the primary cause of anesthesia rather than simply secondary changes following a general depression of the nervous system. The balance of evidence is now against the microtubule and hydrate theories of anesthesia.

QUESTIONS

1. Suggest three macroscopic sites of anesthetic action.
2. What evidence indicates that the synapse is a more likely site of action than the nerve axon?
3. Why does the interaction between anesthetics and lipid solubility more likely reflect the forces between anesthetics and their site of action than the interaction between anesthetics themselves (for example as measured by anesthetic vapor pressure)?
4. What are the implications of the variations of anesthetic potency with temperature and pressure?
5. Defend the "unitary hypothesis of anesthesia."
6. If the unitary hypothesis is correct, why should certain specific anesthetic agents increase sympathetic activity whereas others act as depressants?
7. Compare and contrast the pharmacological effects of convulsants and anesthetics. How might the mechanism of action of these two groups of compounds be related?
8. How might anesthetics act to block ion pores in the neural membrane? How might such blockages cause anesthesia?
9. In what ways might anesthetics reduce transmitter release?
10. MAC times oil/gas partition coefficient equals a constant for all gases except helium, neon and hydrogen. Explain the deviation of these gases from this correlation. What are the implications of "pressure reversal of anesthesia" to theories of narcosis?
11. In what ways could hydrate formation explain the diffuse effects of anesthesia?
12. Induction of anesthesia is often associated with an initial excitement of the nervous system. What different mechanisms can you postulate for this on macroscopic, microscopic and molecular levels?
13. Explain how parts of the nervous system (e.g., the respiratory center) continue to function during surgical anesthesia.
14. "It is unlikely that examination of anesthetic dose-response curves per se will shed much light on mechanism of action." Is it?.
15. "MAC is a universal characteristic of anesthesia." So what?

REFERENCES

1. Miller, K. W., Paton, W. D. M., and Smith, E. B.: The anesthetic pressures of certain fluorine-containing gases. Brit. J. Anaesth. 39: 910–918, 1967.
2. Halsey, M. J., and Kent, D. W.: *The Anesthetic Effects of Inert Gases*, pp. 105–106. Abstracts of American Society of Anesthesiologists Annual Meeting, 1972.

3. Atkinson, R. M., Davis, B., Pratt, M. A. et al.: Action of some steroids on the central nervous system of the mouse. II. Pharmacology. J. Med. Chem. 8: 426–432, 1965.
4. French, J. D., Verzeano, M., and Magoun, H. W.: A neural basis of the anesthetic state. Arch. Neurol. Psychiat. 69: 519–529, 1953.
5. Davis, H. S., Collins, W. F., Randt, C. T. et al.: Effect of anesthetic agents on evoked central nervous system responses: gaseous agents. Anesthesiology 18: 634–642, 1957.
6. Darbinjan, T. M., Golovchinsky, V. B., Plehotkina, S. I.: Effects of anesthetics on reticular and cortical activity. Anesthesiology 34: 219–229, 1971.
7. Crawford, J. M.: Anesthetic agents and the chemical sensitivity of cortical neurons. Neuropharmacology 9: 31–46, 1970.
8. Biebuyck, J. F.: Metabolic effects of halothane with particular reference to the liver. Ph.D. Thesis. Oxford, 1971.
9. Freund, F. G., Martin, W. E., and Hornbein, T. F.: The H-reflex as a measure of anesthetic potency in man. Anesthesiology 30: 642–647, 1969.
10. Galindo, A.: Effects of procaine, pentobarbital and halothane on synaptic transmission in the central nervous system. J. Pharmacol. Exp. Ther. 169: 185–195, 1969.
11. Somjen, G.: Effects of anesthetics on spinal cord of mammals. Anesthesiology 28: 135–143, 1967.
12. De Jong, R. M., Robles, R., Corbin, R. W. et al.: Effect of inhalational anesthetics on monosynaptic and polysynaptic transmission in the spinal cord. J. Pharmacol. Exp. Ther. 162: 326–330, 1968.
13. Larrabee, M. G., and Posternak, J. M.: Selective action of anesthetics on synapses and axons in mammalian sympathetic ganglia. J. Neurophysiol. 15: 91–114, 1952.
14. De Jong, R. H., and Nace, R. A.: Nerve impulse conduction and cutaneous receptor responses during general anesthesia. Anesthesiology 28: 851–855, 1967.
15. Fink, B. R.: In the Proceedings of the Conference on Neurophysiology in Relation to Anesthesiology. Anesthesiology 28: 127, 1967.
16. Clark, D. L., and Rosner, B. S.: Neurophysiological effects of general anesthetics. Anesthesiology. To be published.
17. Miller, R. D., Way, W. L., Dolan, W. M. et al.: The dependence of pancuronium and d-tubocurarine-induced neuromuscular blockades on alveolar concentrations of halothane and Forane. Anesthesiology 37: 573–581, 1972.
18. Schmidt, R. F.: Pharmacological studies on the primary afferent depolarization of the toad spinal cord. Pfluger Arch. Ges. Physiol. 227: 325–346, 1963.
19. Gissen, A. J., Karis, J. M., and Nastuk, W. L.: Effect of halothane on neuromuscular transmission. J. A. M. A. 197: 116–120, 1966.
20. Løyning, Y., Oshima, T., and Yokota, T.: Site of action of thiamylal sodium on the monosynaptic spinal reflex pathway in cats. J. Neurophysiol. 27: 408–428, 1964.
21. Crawford, J. M., and Curtis, O. R.: Pharmacological studies of feline Betz cells. J. Physiol. 186: 121–138, 1966.
22. Bloom, R. F., Costa, E., and Salmoiraghi, G. C.: Anesthesia and the responsiveness of individual neurons of the caudate nucleus of the cat to acetylcholine, norepinephrine, and dopamine administered by microelectrophoresis. J. Pharmacol. Exp. Ther. 150: 244–252, 1965.
23. Eger, E. I., II, Lundgren, C., Miller, C. L. et al.: Anesthetic potencies of sulfur hexafluoride, carbon tetrafluoride, chloroform, and Ethrane in dogs: correlation with hydrate and lipid theories of anesthetic action. Anesthesiology 30: 129–135, 1969.
24. Hasley, M. J., and Kent, O. W.: Molecular mechanisms of anesthesia. Anesthesiology 36: 313–315, 1972.
25. Adamson, R. H.: Correlation of parachor with anesthetic potency. Life Sci. 3: 1131–1134, 1964.

26. Wulf, R. J., and Featherstone, R. M.: A correlation of van der Waal's constants with anesthetic potency. Anesthesiology 18: 97–105, 1957.
27. Ferguson, J.: The use of chemical potentials as indices of toxicity. Proc. Roy. Soc. Lond. (Biol) 127: 387–404, 1939.
28. Miller, K. W., Paton, W. D. M., Smith, E. B., et al.: Physiochemical approaches to the mode of action of general anesthetics. Anesthesiology 36: 339–351, 1972.
29. Di Fazio, C. A., Brown, R. E., Call, C. G., et al.: Additive effects of anesthetics and theories of anesthesia. Anesthesiology 36: 57–63, 1972.
30. Stoelting, R. K., Longnecker, D. E., and Eger, E. I., II: Minimal alveolar concentrations on awakening from methoxyflurane, halothane, ether and fluroxene in man: MAC awake. Anesthesiology 33: 5–9, 1970.
31. Mullins, L. J.: Anaesthetics. In *Handbook of Neurochemistry*, edited by A. Lajtha, Vol. 6, pp. 395–421. 1971.
32. Clements, J. A., and Wilson, K. M.: The affinity of narcotic agents for interfacial films. Proc. Nat. Acad. Sci. U.S.A. 48: 1008–1014, 1962.
33. Allison, A. C.: Analogies between triggering mechanisms in immune and other cellular reactions. In *Cell Interactions*, edited by L. G. Silvestri, pp. 156–161. North Holland, Amsterdam, 1972.
34. Bass, L., and Moore, W. J.: Electrokinetic mechanism of miniature postsynaptic potentials. Proc. Nat. Acad. Sci. U.S.A. 55: 1214–1217, 1966.
35. Del Castillo, J., and Katz, B.: La base "quantale" de la tranmission neuromusculaire. Microphysiologie comparee des elements excitables. Coll. Int. C.N.R.S. Paris 67: 245–258, 1957.
36. Hubbard, J. I.: Mechanisms of transmitter release. Progr. Biophys. 21: 33–124, 1970.
37. Seeman, P., and Roth, S.: General anesthetics expand cell membranes at surgical concentrations. Biochim. Biophys. Acta 255: 171–177, 1972.
38. Johnson, F. H., Eyring, H., and Polissar, M. J.: *The Kinetic Basis of Molecular Biology*. Wiley, New York, 1954.
39. Halsey, M. J., Kent, D. W., and Eger, E. I., II: Pressure studies with mice up to 270 ATA. In *Proceedings of 5th Symposium on Underwater Physiology*, 1973. In press
40. Battino, R., and Clever, H. L.: The solubility of gases in liquids. Chem. Rev. 66: 395–463, 1966.
41. Seeman, P.: The membrane actions of anesthetics and tranquilizers. Pharmacol. Rev. 24: 583–655, 1972.
42. Paton, W. D. M. Experiments on the convulsant and anaesthetic effects of oxygen. Brit. J. Pharmacol. Chemother. 29: 350–366, 1967.
43. Gillette, J. R. (Ed.): Microsomes and drug oxidations. In *Symposium Proceedings*. Academic Press, New York, 1969.
44. Terrell, R. C., Speers, L., Szur, A. J. et al.: General Anesthetics I: Halogenated methyl ethyl ethers as anesthetic agents. J. Med. Chem. 14: 517–519, 1972.
45. Hill, T. C.: Comments on the theory of ion transport across the nerve membrane. To be published.
46. Larsen, E. R., Van Dyke, R.A., and Chenoweth, M. B.: Mechanisms of Narcosis. In *Drugs Affecting the Central Nervous System*, edited by A. Burger, Vol. 2 pp. 1–24. Arnold, London, 1968.
47. White, D. C., Wardley-Smith, B., and Halsey, M. J.: Elastomers as analogues of anaesthetic receptors. Brit. J. Anaesth. 44: 1020–1024, 1972.
48. Schoenborn, B. P.: Binding of anesthetics to protein: an X-ray crystallographic investigation. Fed. Proc. 27: 888–894, 1968.
49. Laasberg, L. H., and Hedley-White, J.: Optical rotatory dispersion of hemoglobin and polypeptides: effect of halothane. J. Biol. Chem. 246: 4886–4893, 1971.

50. Balasubramanian, D., and Wetlaufer, D. B.: Reversible alteration of the structure of globular proteins by anesthetic agents. Proc. Nat. Acad. Sci. U.S.A. 55: 762–765, 1966.
51. White, D. C., and Dundas, C. R.: Effect of anaesthetics on emission of light by luminous bacteria. Nature 226: 456–458, 1970.
52. Halsey, M. J., and Smith, E. B.: Effects of anaesthetics on luminous bacteria. Nature 227: 1363–1365, 1970.
53. Bangham, A. D., Standish, M. M., and Miller, N.: Cation permeability of phospholipid model membranes: effect of narcotics. Nature 208: 1295–1297, 1965.
54. Johnson, S. M., and Miller, K. W.: Antagonism of pressure and anaesthesia. Nature 228: 75–76, 1970.
55. Halsey, M. J., Smith, E. B., and Wood, T. E.: Effects of general anaesthetics on Na^+ transport in human red cells. Nature 225: 1151–1152, 1970.
56. Verworn, M.: Narcosis. Harvey Lect. 7: 52–75, 1912.
57. Quastel, J. M.: Effects of drugs on metabolism of the brain *in vitro*. Brit. Med. Bull. 21: 49–56, 1965.
58. Negishi, K., and Svaetichin, G.: Effects of alcohols and volatile anaesthetics on S-potential producing cells and on neurons. Pfluger Arch. Ges. Physiol. 292: 218–228, 1966.
59. Michenfelder, V. D., Van Dyke, R. A., and Theye, R. A.: The effects of anesthetic agents and techniques on canine cerebral ATP and lactate levels. Anesthesiology 33: 315–321, 1970.
60. Green, D. E.: The conformational basis of energy transductions in membrane systems. In *Cellular biology and toxicity of anesthetics*, edited by B. R. Fink, pp. 79–92. Williams & Wilkins, Baltimore, 1972.
61. Allison, A. C., and Nunn, J. F.: Effects of general anaesthetics on microtubules. Lancet 2: 1326–1329, 1968.
62. Pauling, L.: A molecular theory of general anesthesia. Science 134: 15–21, 1961.
63. Miller, S. L.: A theory of gaseous anesthetics. Proc. Nat. Acad. Sci. U.S.A. 47: 1515–1524, 1961.

Chapter 4

Uptake of Inhaled Anesthetics: The Alveolar to Inspired Anesthetic Difference

Previous chapters described some characteristics of anesthesia and suggested various mechanisms by which anesthetics exert their effects. We have yet to learn how anesthetics arrive at their site of action. The anesthetic concentration in the vaporizer far exceeds the concentration required to produce anesthesia. The anesthetic partial pressure progressively decreases at the several steps between machine and patient. The partial pressure is reduced by dilution with oxygen or nitrous oxide before it flows into the anesthetic system. The gas offered the patient from the anesthetic system is diluted further by the gas already present in the lungs. Another reduction in anesthetic pressure accompanies the transfer from lungs to blood and from blood to brain or other tissues. The rational control of the brain anesthetic concentration requires an appreciation of the factors governing each of these steps.

The decrease in anesthetic partial pressure from inspired to alveolar gas is the most important step between machine and brain. On one hand, the anesthetist precisely may control the inspired concentration by use of a nonrebreathing system or high inflow rates. On the other hand, the alveolar anesthetic partial pressure is the limit approached by all anesthetic partial pressures in the body. Because of its importance, the relationship of the alveolar concentration to the concentration inspired is the theme of the next several chapters.

Factors Raising the Alveolar Concentration

The Inspired Concentration and Ventilation (1–5)

Assuming a constant inspired anesthetic concentration (nonrebreathing system), what determines the rate of rise of the alveolar concentration? The inspired concentration itself is of obvious importance: the absolute alveolar rate of rise must bear some direct relation to the concentration inspired. A second factor governing the alveolar rate of rise is alveolar ventilation ($\dot{V}_A$). The greater the ventilation the more rapid the approach of the alveolar to the inspired concentration. The effect of $\dot{V}_A$ is limited by the volume of the functional residual capacity (FRC). The larger the FRC, the slower the washin of a new gas.

A normal ratio of $\dot{V}_A$/FRC produces a rapid rate of alveolar anesthetic rise. A simple example illustrates this (fig. 4, 1). Imagine a lung with an FRC of 2 liters and $\dot{V}_A$ of 4 liters/minute. How fast will the alveolar concentration of a newly respired gas (for example 100 percent nitrous oxide) rise in the absence of anesthetic absorption by lung or blood? In the first minute, 4 liters of new gas flow through the lungs. If all 4 liters enter in one breath, then the alveolar concentration rises to 67 percent of the inspired concentration (i.e., 4 liters of new gas diluted in a total of 4 liters plus 2 liters FRC). Dividing the 4 liter breath into smaller breaths increases the rate of change. If the 4 liters are split into 2 equal breaths, then the first breath raises the alveolar concentration to 50 percent of that inspired (2 liters of new gas diluted in a total of 2 liters plus the 2 liter FRC), and the second breath increases the alveolar concentration to 75 percent (2 liters of 50 percent plus 2 liters of 100 percent). Subdivision of the $\dot{V}_A$ to 8 breaths of 500 ml tidal volume further increases the rate of rise of alveolar concentration so that at 1 minute the alveolar concentration is 83 percent of inspired. Greater subdivision of breaths causes little additional increase in the washin rate. Maximum efficiency occurs with infinitely small breaths (continuous flow) and produces an 86 percent rise at 1 minute.

Three lessons follow from figure 4, 1. First, the alveolar washin of a new gas is rapid, normally being over 80 percent complete in 1 minute if no gas if lost from lung to blood. Second, for a given $\dot{V}_A$ the maximum rate of washin is approached with normal tidal volumes; large tidal volumes decrease the rate but the decrease is small. Third, figure 4, 1 illustrates the time constant (2). *The time constant is the time required for the flow through a container to equal the capacity of the container. It is also the time required for a 63 percent washin or washout of a new gas from the lungs.** The time constant in our example is ½ minute, since in ½ minute the flow (4 liters/minute $\dot{V}_A$) through the container (the 2 liter FRC) equalled the container capacity. In ½ minute, a 63 percent rise in alveolar concentration was obtained (500 ml breaths or continuous flow). Doubling the time caused a 63 percent rise in the remaining difference between 63 and 100 percent. Similarly, each succeeding time constant

---

* The time constant is calculated from $1 - 1/e^{KT}$ where e is the base of the natural logarithms. K is a constant equalling F/V where F is the flow through the container, and V is the capacity of the container. T is time, and for 1 time constant T is a value such that KT equals 1 (that is T equals V/F).

would have reduced the remaining difference by 63 percent. Thus, at 1 minute the change in alveolar concentration was 86 percent complete [63 + (63/100) (100–63)]. At 1½ minutes the change would have reached 95 percent [86 + (63/100) (100−86)] and at 2 minutes 98 percent [95 + (63/100) (100–95)]—that is, virtually complete washin. The time constant is useful both because it is easy to calculate and because it describes the maximum rate of change in many systems important to uptake of anesthetic gases. To calculate the time constant you need only know flow and capacity: capacity divided by flow gives the time constant. Limitations to its use lie in the assumptions on which it is based: these are a constant inflow of constant gas concentration and complete mixing within a container of constant capacity.

Uptake of Anesthetic at the Lungs

Relative Effects of Uptake and Ventilation (1–5)

Alveolar concentrations of anesthetics fail to rise as rapidly as predicted by a time constant derived from normal $\dot{V}_A$ and FRC values. The gain in alveolar concentration promoted by ventilation is opposed by a minor anesthetic loss to lung tissue and a major loss to blood passing

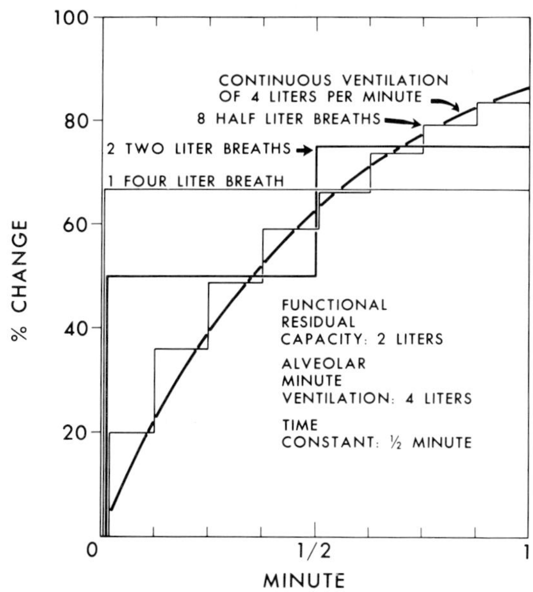

FIG. 4, 1. The rate of rise in the alveolar concentration of an insoluble gas expressed as a percent of the inspired concentration depends on the relationship between the alveolar ventilation and the functional residual capacity. The larger the ratio of these two, the faster the rate of rise. As illustrated here, the size of the tidal volume is of relatively little importance. Two 2 liter breaths produce almost as much of an increase in the alveolar concentration after 1 minute as 8 half liter breaths. Both are nearly as effective as an infinite number of small breaths totaling 4 liters. In all cases, the rate of rise is very rapid.

through the lung. Ventilation introduces anesthetic into the lungs while uptake removes it. The relationship between input and removal determines the alveolar concentration. Uptake of one-half the entering anesthetic reduces the alveolar concentration to one-half of that inspired and uptake of two-thirds the entering agent reduces the concentration to one-third of that inspired.

Factors Determining Uptake by Blood

Three factors determine anesthetic uptake: 1) solubility (blood/gas partition coefficient); 2) cardiac output; and 3) the alveolar to mixed venous anesthetic partial pressure difference. An increase in any of these factors will increase anesthetic uptake.

Solubility

Figure 4, 2 illustrates the derivation of the blood/gas partition coefficient (6). An 80 percent alveolar concentration of a mythical agent achieves a 40 percent concentration in arterial blood when the 2 phases (alveolar gas and blood) are in equilibrium. Equilibrium means the same anesthetic partial pressure exists in both phases. Notice that equality of partial pressures (remember that pressure is defined as the tendency of a gas to leave a phase) in the 2 phases does not mean equality of concentrations or content in the 2 phases. In figure 4, 2 the gas concentration is double that in blood. Thus, our mythical agent has a blood/gas solubility or partition coefficient of 40/80 or 0.5. Solubility of an anesthetic describes the relative capacity per unit volume of two solvents such as blood and gas for that anesthetic. In our example, the blood has half the capacity per unit volume to hold anesthetic compared

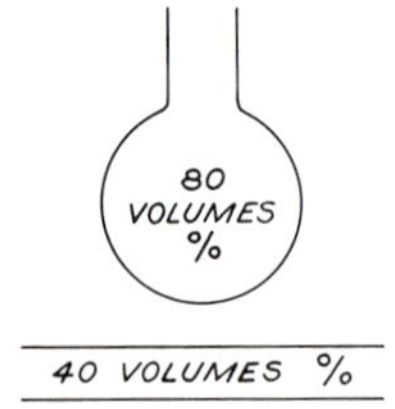

$$\frac{\text{BLOOD}}{\text{GAS}}\ \text{PARTITION COEFFICIENT} = \frac{40}{80} = 0.5$$

FIG. 4, 2. If at equilibrium an arterial concentration of 40 volumes percent results from an alveolar anesthetic concentration of 80 volumes percent then the blood/gas partition coefficient is 0.5. Note that although the concentrations in the gas and blood phases are different, the partial pressures are identical. (Reproduced with permission from Eger, E. I., II: Inhalation anaesthesia: Pharmacokinetics. In *General Anaesthesia*, edited by T. Cecil Gray and J. F. Nunn, Ed. 3, Ch. 30, London, Butterworths, London, 1971.)

to the gas phase. To indicate this relative capacity requires that we name the two solvents or phases *and* the phase ratio. By convention we reference the capacity of blood to gas rather than the reverse. But it would be just as correct (though uncommon) to say that figure 4, 2 illustrates a gas/blood partition coefficient of 80/40 or 2. The meaning is unchanged: a gas/blood partition coefficient of 2 indicates that blood has half the capacity per unit volume of the gas phase (or that gas has twice the capacity per unit volume of blood).

The use of partition coefficient is not limited to gas and blood but extends to any 2 phases. Blood/gas, tissue/blood and oil/gas partition coefficients are given in table 4, 1. Note that both phases and the phase ratio are stated. As with the blood/gas partition coefficient the tissue/blood and oil/gas partition coefficients describe the relative capacity per unit volume of each phase for the anesthetic.

Figure 4, 3 further illustrates the development of the distribution of an anesthetic with a blood/gas partition of 0.5. The lung gas (lower "box") is filled with 3 volumes percent of an anesthetic (*A*). This equilibrates with an equal volume of blood (upper "box") which represents the cardiac output. The final ratio of the concentration in blood to that in gas must equal 0.5 (*B*). Figure 4, 3, *C* and *D*, demonstrates the effect of a greater solubility on alveolar anesthetic concentration. Again, imagine filling the lung with 3 percent of a second mythical anesthetic (*C*). Unlike the previous anesthetic, this mythical agent has a blood/gas partition coefficient of 2 so that after equilibration, the blood concentration must be twice that in the alveoli (*D*). Note that the greater blood/gas partition coefficient of 2 produces half the alveolar concentration found with a

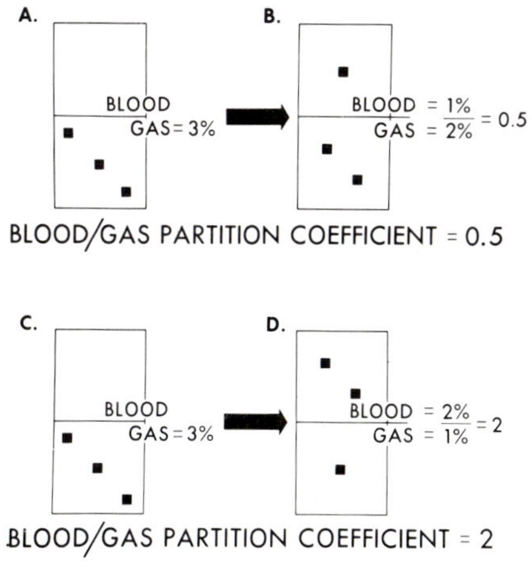

FIG. 4, 3. Three volumes percent of anesthetic are introduced into a lung (*lower* "gas" *boxes*, *A* and *C*). The anesthetic then equilibrates (*B* and *D*) between the lung gas and an equal volume of blood (*upper boxes*) as indicated by the indicated blood/gas partition coefficient.

TABLE 4, 1

*Partition coefficients at 37°C (7–12)**

Anesthetic	Blood/Gas	Tissue/Blood							Oil/Gas
		Brain (Grey)	Brain (White)	Liver	Kidney	Muscle	Fat	Lung	
Cyclopropane	0.4 to 0.6† (8)	0.76‡ (8)	1.5‡ (8)	1.16‡ (8)	0.62‡ (8)	1.16‡ (8)	12.9§		11.8
Nitrous oxide	0.47	1.06 (average grey and white)		0.80 (9)		1.15 (9)	2.3§	1.0 (10)	1.4
Fluroxene	1.37	1.43	1.43	1.37	1.05 (8)	2.3	23.0§		47.7
Isoflurane	1.41 (11)	2.6 (average grey and white) (12)		2.5 (12)		4.0 (12)	45.0§		98 (11)
Enflurane	1.78 (12)	1.45 (average grey and white) (12)		2.1 (12)		1.7 (12)	36.2§		98 (13)
Halothane	2.3	2.3	3.5	2.6	1.6	3.5	60		224
Divinyl ether	2.8	1.80 (8)	1.62 (8)	1.15 (8)	0.76 (8)	1.11 (8)	13.8§		58
Chloroform	8.4	1.38 (8)	2.39 (8)	1.98 (8)	1.22 (8)	1.89 (8)	30.8§		394
Diethyl ether	12.1	1.03 (8)	1.12 (8)	1.01 (8)	1.06 (8)	0.98 (8)	3.7§		65
Methoxyflurane	12.0	1.70	2.34	1.90 (8)	0.93 (8)	1.34	48.8§		970

* Numbers in parentheses indicate reference for the value. If no reference is cited, the value is taken from the compilation made by Eger and Larson (7).

† The variable nature of the solubility of cyclopropane in blood will be discussed in Chapter 8.

‡ Assuming a blood/gas partition coefficient of 0.565 (from Lowe and Hagler (8)).

§ Estimated from the assumption that fat consists of 65 percent fat (oil) and 35 percent whole blood.

coefficient of 0.5. If all other things are equal, the greater the blood/gas partition coefficient, the greater the uptake of anesthetic and the lower the alveolar concentration. Table 4, 1 lists the anesthetics in order of increasing blood/gas partition coefficients. Those at the top of the list achieve their effects rapidly compared to those at the bottom. A higher coefficient results in a slower induction. This impediment to rapid induction may be partly or completely overcome by raising the inspired concentration to levels well in excess of MAC. However, because of their very large blood/gas partition coefficients, ether or methoxyflurane induce anesthesia slowly despite elevation of the inspired concentration. The limitation on rate of induction imposed by halothane's moderate blood/gas partition coefficient can be overcome with an inspired concentration of 3 to 5 times MAC. Some anaesthetists actually use 10 to 15 times MAC for induction with halothane (14), but we shall see that this has a potential for disaster. Since cyclopropane is so poorly soluble in blood, a rapid cyclopropane induction is achieved with an inspired concentration only modestly higher than that used for maintenance of anesthesia.

Many different terms describe the same or nearly the same equilibrium distribution of anesthetic between gas and liquid phases. Partition coefficient is the most fitting for use with inhaled anesthetics. The less commonly used Ostwald solubility coefficient (λ) equals the volume of gas absorbed per unit volume of solvent at the temperature of the measurement when the partial pressure of the dissolved gas equals 760 torr. Thus, the Ostwald solubility coefficient always presumes that one phase is pure gas thus giving a fractional concentration of 1 or 100 percent. The gas phase is always the denominator of the ratio. The Ostwald solubility coefficient numerically equals the partition coefficient: an Ostwald blood solubility coefficient of 0.5 is the same as a blood/gas partition coefficient of 0.5. The Bunsen solubility coefficient (α) is an Ostwald coefficient corrected to standard temperature (273°A) and therefore is obtained by multiplying the Ostwald coefficient by 273A/the absolute temperature at which solubility was determined. Were the above partition coefficient of 0.5 obtained at body temperature the Bunsen solubility coefficient would be 0.44 (equals 0.5 times 273A/310A). In the jargon of medical writing, "blood solubility" has come to mean a blood/gas partition coefficient and "tissue solubility" a tissue/blood partition coefficient. Such "slang" frequently will be used in the remainder of the book.

Cardiac Output

Since blood carries anesthetic away from the lungs, the greater the cardiac output, the greater the uptake (1–5). Imagine in figure 4, 3*A* that the box representing the blood passing through the lung per unit time increased 4 fold without any change in the volume of the gas phase (that is, cardiac output quadrupled with no change in alveolar ventilation). With a blood/gas partition coefficient of 0.5, the 3 volumes of gas must distribute so that 1 volume remains in the gas phase while the remaining 2 dissolve in the 4 volumes of blood.* Compare this with the distribution resulting from equal cardiac output and alveolar ventilation (fig. 4, 3*B*). Quadrupling the cardiac output halved the alveolar concentration.

Alveolar to Venous Anesthetic Difference

The difference between the alveolar anesthetic partial pressure and the partial pressure in the returning venous blood is the third determinant of uptake (2–5). During induction the tissues remove nearly all the anesthetic brought to them. This lowers the venous anesthetic partial pressure far below the partial pressure delivered from the alveoli in arterial blood. The result is a large alveolar to venous anesthetic partial pressure difference which causes a maximum anesthetic uptake. As time passes, the increasing tissue anesthetic concentrations reduce the rate of uptake and more anesthetic appears in venous blood. The resulting rise in the venous anesthetic partial pressure narrows the alveolar to venous difference and thereby reduces uptake.

The factors determining uptake from the lung (U_L) may be resummarized as

$$U_L = \lambda_B \dot{Q} \, (P_A - P_v)/BP \tag{1}$$

where λ_B is the blood/gas partition coefficient, $\dot{Q}$ is the cardiac output, $P_A - P_v$ is the alveolar to venous anesthetic partial pressure difference and BP is the barometric pressure.† An increase in any of these factors increases uptake. However, if any factors equal zero, then uptake is zero.

---

* At first glance, this appears to conflict with a blood/gas partition coefficient of 0.5. Twice as many anesthetic molecules reside in the blood phase. However, the partition coefficient is not defined as the relative volumes of anesthetic in two phases but as their relative concentrations. Thus, 2 molecules per 4 volumes of blood are in equilibrium with 1 molecule per 1 volume of gas as required by a blood/gas partition coefficient of 0.5.

† The proof for equation 1 is as follows. From the Fick equation

$$U_L = (C_a - C_v) \, \dot{Q} \tag{2}$$

where C_a is the anesthetic concentration in arterial blood and C_v the concentration in venous blood. By definition

$$\lambda_B = C_a/C_A \tag{3}$$

where C_A is the alveolar gas concentration in equilibrium with C_a. Then

$$C_a = \lambda_B C_A = \lambda_B P_A/BP \tag{4}$$

where BP is the barometric pressure. Similarly

$$C_v = \lambda_B P_v/BP \tag{5}$$

substituting 4 and 5 into 2 gives equation 1.

Tissue Uptake of Anesthetic

Tissue uptake determines the uptake at the lung. The two are equal: uptake from the alveoli is the sum of uptakes by the individual tissues. If anesthetic were not removed by the tissues (as in an arteriovenous shunt or after saturation of the tissues), then the blood would return to the lungs with as much anesthetic as it carried away. The alveolar to venous difference would be zero, there would be no uptake, and the alveolar concentration would quickly approach the concentration inspired.

Uptake by a tissue (U_t) is governed by factors analogous to those that determined uptake at the lungs: tissue solubility, tissue blood flow ($\dot{Q}_t$) and the arterial (P_a) to tissue (P_t) anesthetic partial pressure difference. Thus

$$U_t = \lambda_B \dot{Q}_t \, (P_a - P_t)/BP^* \tag{6}$$

and, as at the lungs, an increase in any of these factors will increase tissue uptake and a decrease will reduce uptake. Notice that each factor may limit uptake: if any factor approaches zero, then uptake must approach zero regardless of the magnitude of the remaining factors. Thus, as tissues become saturated (meaning the tissue anesthetic partial pressure approaches that in arterial blood) uptake must approach zero. Let us look at the factors which determine how rapidly the tissue anesthetic partial pressure rises.

Tissue Capacity and Blood Flow

The capacity of a tissue to hold anesthetic depends both on the size of the tissue and on the affinity of the tissue for the anesthetic. Thus, the capacity of a tissue equals the product of tissue solubility (tissue/blood partition coefficient) and tissue volume. The greater the solubility or tissue volume, the greater the capacity of that tissue for anesthetic.

The tissue capacity relative to blood flow determines the rate at which the tissue anesthetic partial pressure rises. In a tissue which has a large capacity and a small blood flow the rate of rise is slow, permitting the

---

* From the Fick equation,

$$U_t = (C_a - C_v)\,\dot{Q}_t \tag{7}$$

where C_a is the arterial anesthetic concentration, and C_v is the venous concentration. Since the alveolar (P_A) and arterial (P_a) anesthetic partial pressures are in equilibrium, from equation 4,

$$C_a = \lambda_B P_a/BP \tag{8}$$

Similarly, venous (P_v) and tissue (P_t) anesthetic partial pressures are assumed to be in equilibrium and

$$C_v = \lambda_B P_t/BP \tag{9}$$

Substituting 8 and 9 into 7 gives equation 6.

tissue to continue to extract anesthetic for a long time. Conversely, the rate of rise usually is rapid in a highly perfused tissue and uptake by such a tissue soon ceases. With the exception of fat, tissue/blood partition coefficients vary far less than blood/gas partition coefficients (table 4, 1). The lowest is slightly less than 1 while the highest (muscle/blood or brain white matter/blood for halothane) is only 3.5 to 4—roughly a 4 fold range as compared to the 29 fold range for blood/gas partition coefficients. This means that the rate at which a tissue anesthetic partial pressure approaches a given arterial anesthetic partial pressure is fairly uniform for all anesthetics.

Tissue Time Constants

From the relationship of tissue capacity to blood flow we can derive a time constant describing the rate of rise of the tissue anesthetic partial pressure. Recall that a time constant is the time required for the flow into a container to equal the capacity of the container. Consider 100 ml of a tissue which receives a blood flow of 100 ml/minute, and has a tissue/blood partition coefficient of 1. Such a tissue might be the grey matter of brain and the anesthetic might be nitrous oxide or ether. The time constant is 1 minute. That is, in 1 minute, the flow through the container (100 ml/minute) equals the capacity of the container (1 times 100 ml). In 1 minute, then, the anesthetic partial pressure in grey matter reaches 63 percent of that in arterial blood. In 2 minutes, it rises to 86 percent and in 3 minutes, 95 percent. Thus, any difference between arterial and tissue anesthetic partial pressures quickly disappears, and in a very short time the tissue ceases extracting anesthetic from blood. Consider the same tissue but increase the tissue/blood partition coefficient to 2.3 as would be the case for halothane (see table 4, 1). Although neither blood flow nor tissue volume has changed, the increase in tissue solubility increases the tissue capacity 2.3 fold. Instead of 1 minute, the time constant is 2.3 minutes. That is, it takes 2.3 minutes to achieve a 63 percent change in the tissue concentration. Despite the 2.3 fold delay in the rise to equilibrium, the rate of rise of anesthetic partial pressure still is rapid. Much longer delays can be expected in tissues with low perfusions per capacity. For example, resting muscle has a blood flow of 3 ml/minute for each 100 ml of tissue. Such a flow gives a time constant of 33 minutes if nitrous oxide (tissue/blood partition coefficient about 1) is the anesthetic. That is, it takes 33 minutes for 100 ml of blood to pass through the 100 ml capacity tissue. Halothane, with a muscle/blood partition coefficient of 3.5, has a muscle time constant 3.5 times greater (116 minutes) than nitrous oxide. Equilibrium of anesthetic between muscle and arterial blood is approached more slowly than in the brain. Conversely, removal of anesthetic by muscle continues far longer. The time constant for fat exceeds that of all other tissues. Although the blood flow per unit volume of fat is comparable to resting muscle, the fat solubility of anesthetics is far greater. For halothane, the fat/blood partition coefficient is 60, giving a time constant of 2 days. Uptake of halothane by fat continues unabated long after brain and muscle stop removing halothane from the arterial blood. This eventual primacy of fat uptake applies to all anesthetics.

Estimation of the Relative Contribution of Each Tissue to Central Venous Anesthetic Tension

The relative contribution of each tissue to the average anesthetic partial pressure in venous blood is determined by the anesthetic partial pressure in that tissue times the fraction of the cardiac output perfusing that tissue. This means that a low tissue anesthetic saturation or a low blood flow may limit the contribution of a tissue to the venous anesthetic tension. The importance of saturation and flow as determinants of the fixed venous partial pressure is illustrated in table 4, 2. A mythical body has a cardiac output divided between 2 tissues. Tissue X receives 10 percent of the cardiac output and tissue Y receives 90 percent. In example A, the anesthetic partial pressures in tissues X and Y are 1 and 10 torr, respectively, while in example B they are reversed, 10 and 1. In B, despite the fact that tissue X has a high anesthetic partial pressure, the low perfusion limits its contribution. Tissue Y, with its low venous anesthetic partial pressure predominates because of its more generous perfusion. As illustrated here, the mixed venous partial pressure is greatest when the higher numbers multiply each other (example A). If either number (fractional flow or partial pressure) is small, then the product has little influence on the mixed venous partial pressure. This is demonstrated by comparison of example C with A. The large increase in tissue partial pressure assigned to X in example C causes little rise in the mixed venous partial pressure because of the small fractional flow given to X.

TABLE 4, 2

Effect of tissue blood flow and tissue anesthetic partial pressure on mixed venous anesthetic partial pressure

(1) Example	(2) Tissue	(3) Fraction of Cardiac Output	(4) Tissue (venous) Partial Pressure (torr)	(5) Torr Contribution to Mixed Venous Partial Pressure ((3) × (4))	(6) Mixed Venous Partial Pressure (torr) (sum of (5))
A	X	0.1	1	0.1	9.1
	Y	0.9	10	9.0	
B	X	0.1	10	1.0	1.9
	Y	0.9	1	0.9	
C	X	0.1	10	1.0	10.0
	Y	0.9	10	9.0	

Tissue Groups Arranged by Solubility and Perfusion Characteristics

The diverse tissue volumes, blood flows and solubilities make it impractical to examine each individual tissue contribution to the mixed venous anesthetic pressures. Nor is it necessary to do so to account for uptake from the lungs. Instead, we can assign each body tissue to groups defined by blood flow per unit tissue volume and by solubility characteristics. Division of the body into three to four such groups permits a prediction of total body uptake which accords well with measured values (table 4, 3) (3, 4). Increasing the number of groupings does not improve agreement with measured values (3).

The vessel rich group (VRG), the muscle group (MG) and the vessel poor group (VPG) have similar tissue/blood partition coefficients but very different blood flows per unit volume of tissue. The VRG includes the highly perfused tissues such as brain, heart, kidney, splanchnic bed (including liver) and endocrine glands. Although these tissues make up only 9 percent of the body, they receive 75 percent of the cardiac output. The high flow per unit volume produces a small time constant and these tissues soon equilibrate with the arterial anesthetic partial pressure. They cease removing appreciable volumes of anesthetic 5 to 15 minutes after induction. Muscle and skin form the MG. These tissues fill half the body mass, but require less than a fifth of the cardiac output at rest. The MG time constants for various anesthetics are large, indicating a slow approach to equilibration and a slow decrease in the rate of anesthetic removal. The VPG, including bony, ligamentous and cartilaginous tissues, has little effect on uptake although it makes up almost a quarter of the body mass. Despite a continuing uptake as indicated by the sizeable time constants, its perfusion is so low that the small volumes of

TABLE 4, 3

Tissue group characteristics

	VRG (Vessel-Rich)	MG (Muscle)	FG (Fat)	VPG (Vessel-Poor)
Body mass (percent)	9	50	19	22
Volume (liters) in a 70 kg man	6	33	14.5	12.5
Perfusion as percent of cardiac output	75	18.1	5.4	1.5
Perfusion (liter/minute with a 6 liter/minute cardiac output)	4.5	1.09	0.32	0.08
Time constant (minutes) for nitrous oxide*	1.3	30	100	160
Time constant (minutes) for halothane†	3.3	106	2720	390

* Presumes a VRG, MG or VPG/blood partition coefficient of 1 and a FG/blood partition coefficient of 2.2.

† Presumes a VRG or VPG/blood coefficient of 2.5, a MG/blood of 3.5, and a FG/blood of 60.

anesthetic it removes cannot appreciably modify total body uptake. The fraction of cardiac output the VPG receives times its venous anesthetic partial pressure is too small to influence the mixed venous anesthetic partial pressure. For this reason we will ignore its effect on anesthetic uptake. The high solubility of the fat group (FG) distinguishes it from the VRG, MG and VPG. Although the perfusion per unit volume of fat is similar to muscle, the time constants for the FG are far greater because of the far greater capacity for anesthetic.

Changes in Tissue Uptake with Duration of Anesthesia

Uptake from the lungs reflects and equals the sum of uptake by the 4 tissue groups. Figure 4, 4 displays the uptake by individual tissue groups and their sum (total uptake) for nitrous oxide and halothane. Uptake by the VRG predominates in the initial minutes of anesthesia because of the high blood flow to the VRG. By speeding tissue equilibration, the high blood flow causes effective uptake to cease in 5 to 15 minutes—leaving the MG and FG as the sole determiners of uptake. In 1 to 3 hours, extraction by the MG wanes, and after 3 hours, uptake by fat predominates. As suggested above, VPG uptake is omitted because it is negligible.

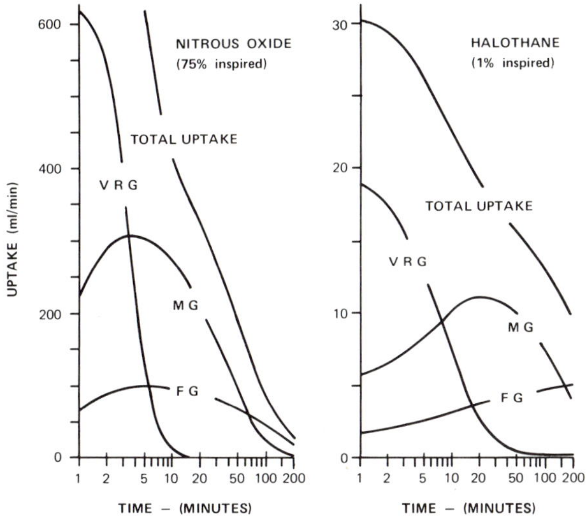

FIG. 4, 4. Total uptake is the sum of uptake by individual body tissues. The uppermost curve for each anesthetic is the sum of the three curves beneath it (with a slight time lag). The curves for nitrous oxide and halothane are identical in shape to those for all anesthetics. Uptake progressively decreases with duration of anesthesia and with saturation of the tissue depots. The order of saturation is always VRG first then MG, and FG last. As noted in the illustration, the inspired concentration is constant at 75 percent nitrous oxide or 1 percent halothane.

Effect of Tissue Uptake on Alveolar Rate of Rise

A knowledge of the time course of uptake by the tissues allows us to describe the rate of rise of the alveolar anesthetic concentration. The relationship between the alveolar (F_A) and inspired concentrations (F_I) is given by:

$$F_A/F_I = 1 - \dot{U}_L/F_I\dot{V}_A \quad (10)$$

where $\dot{U}_L$ is uptake at the lungs and $\dot{V}_A$ is alveolar ventilation.* Since F_I is constant, the larger the ratio of $\dot{U}_L/\dot{V}_A$ the smaller F_A/F_I—that is, the lower the alveolar anesthetic concentration. Since $\dot{U}_L$ is a function of solubility, cardiac output and the alveolar to venous partial pressure difference (see equation 1), a decrease in any of these factors raises the alveolar concentration. Similarly, an increase in $\dot{V}_A$ also raises the alveolar concentration.

Figure 4, 5 describes the approach of the alveolar to the inspired concentration for 4 anesthetics: ether, halothane, cyclopropane and nitrous oxide. Dissimilarities in uptake caused by differences in solubility determine the position of each curve: as demonstrated by equation 10 the greater the solubility (uptake), the lower the alveolar concentration. Though the ether, halothane and cyclopropane curves vary in position, they have a common shape. The alveolar concentration initially rises rapidly regardless of solubility. Even the start of the ether curve shows this quick upswing. The reason is that at the start of anesthesia, the alveolar concentration is zero and low after the first few breaths. The alveolar to mixed venous anesthetic partial pressure difference at this time is too small to permit a significant uptake of anesthesia (see equation 1). Without uptake, the effect of ventilation to produce a rapid increase in alveolar concentrations is unopposed.

However, within 1 to 2 minutes the alveolar concentration rises and thereby develops a significant anesthetic partial pressure difference between alveolar gas and venous blood. Uptake increases in proportion to this difference. When the removal of anesthetic from the alveoli by uptake equals the input of anesthetic by ventilation, a rough balance is achieved and the rapid initial rise in alveolar concentration slows drastically. This results in the first bend or "knee" in the curves (see first arrow, fig. 4, 5). If uptake continued unchanged from these initial levels,

---

* The uptake of anesthetic equals the volume of anesthetic delivered to the lungs by alveolar ventilation minus the volume lost from the lung by ventilation (the whole equals the sum of its parts). Thus

$$\dot{U}_L = F_I\dot{V}_A - F_A\dot{V}_A \quad (11)$$

Rearranging gives equation 10. This relationship ignores one important aspect of the development of F_A/F_I which is the washin of the alveolar gas space. That is, it describes F_A/F_I in the absence of any need for washin.

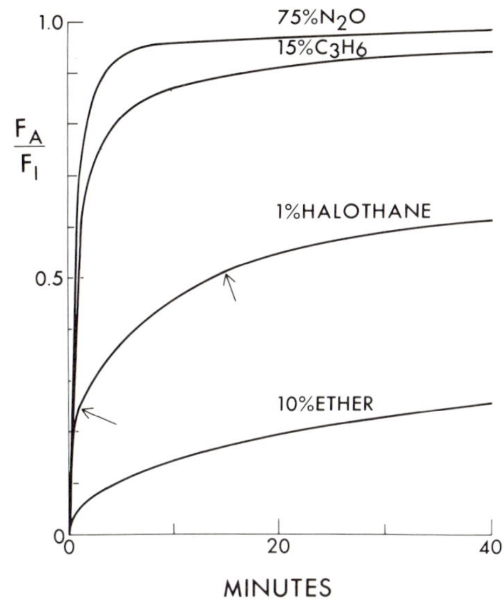

FIG. 4, 5. The approach of the alveolar (F_A) concentration to the concentration inspired (F_I) varies inversely with solubility. It is slow with a very soluble agent such as ether but quickly nears 100 percent (1.0) with nitrous oxide or cyclopropane. Despite differences in their heights, the curves for ether, halothane and cyclopropane follow the same three part pattern: a rapid upswing (to the first arrow in the case of halothane), a slower continuing upsweep (to the second arrow), and a continuing slower rise thereafter. The first part of the sequence results from unopposed or partially opposed ventilatory input of anesthetic, the second part results from equilibration with VRG, and the third part results from the continuing approach to equilibration of MG and FG. The volume percent (%) before each agent indicates the inspired concentration and is the F_A value reached when F_A/F_I reaches 1. The inspired concentration for any one anesthetic is constant at all times.

then the alveolar curves would rise no further as indicated in figure 4, 6. This is what would occur if all tissues were of infinite capacity. P_v then would always be zero. In figure 4, 6 the height to which each curve would rise is readily calculated from the blood/gas partition coefficient (λ_B), the ventilation ($\dot{V}_A$) and the cardiac output (Q) (2):

$$F_A/F_I = \dot{V}_A/(\lambda_B\dot{Q} + \dot{V}_A) \tag{12}$$

where F_A/F_I is the ratio of alveolar to inspired concentration.*

---

* By definition:

$$\lambda_B = F_B/F_A \tag{13}$$

where F_B is the blood concentration and F_A the gas concentration after equilibration. Let F_I be the concentration in the entering gas before equilibration. The volume of gas transferred to blood by equilibration (X) plus the amount remaining in the gas phase ($\dot{V}_AF_A$) must equal the original amount introduced by ventilation ($\dot{V}_AF_I$) (the whole equals the sum of its parts) or

$$X + \dot{V}_AF_A = \dot{V}_AF_I \text{ or } X = \dot{V}_AF_I - \dot{V}_AF_A \tag{14}$$

Note that the larger the blood/gas partition coefficient (λ_B), the lower the height to which the alveolar concentration rises.

But the curves do rise further. The initial uptake is not sustained because of the progressive and rapid approach to saturation by the VRG. As this tissue group approaches equilibration with the arterial anesthetic partial pressure, 75 percent of the blood returning to the lungs contains the same partial pressure as when it left (fig. 4, 7). This reduction in the difference between alveolar and mixed venous blood partial pressure thereby reduces uptake (fig. 4, 4). The reduction in uptake permits ventilation to drive the alveolar concentration higher. Within 5 to 15 minutes, equilibration of the VRG with the arterial anesthetic partial pressure is nearly complete and the rapid reduction in uptake slows. A

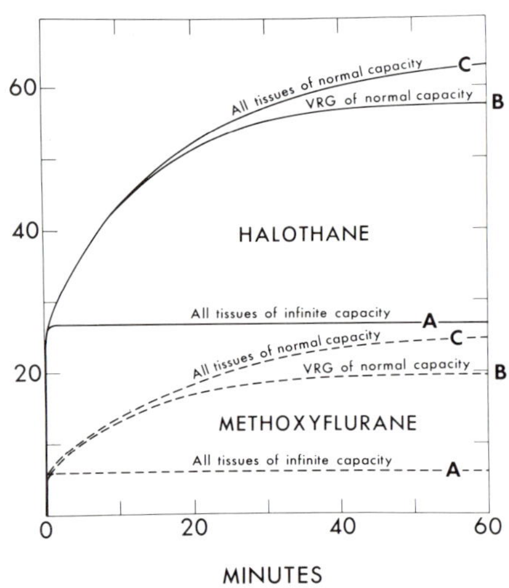

FIG. 4, 6. The alveolar rate of rise toward the inspired concentration is illustrated for three circumstances: *A*) If all tissues (except blood) have an infinite capacity, then the blood returning to the lungs contains no anesthetic. The alveolar level attained is described by equation 12 and is the lowest curve for each anesthetic. *B*) If all tissues except VRG have an infinite capacity but VRG capacity is normal, then the alveolar concentration rises to a far higher level than in *A* before a plateau is reached. Note the similarity of these curves to the curves immediately above them where, *C*) all tissues are assumed to have a normal capacity. The blood flow to the VRG exerts the major influence on the mixed venous anesthetic partial pressure and hence on the alveolar anesthetic concentration.

By definition,

$$F_B = X/\dot{Q} \tag{15}$$

This presumes no recirculation of anesthetic—an assumption which follows from our original assumption that uptake is unchanged from the initial levels.
Substituting 14 into 15 and 15 into 13:

$$\lambda_B = (\dot{V}_A F_I - \dot{V}_A F_A)/\dot{Q} F_A \tag{16}$$

Rearranging gives equation 12.

second bend or "knee" is seen (second arrow, fig. 4, 5). Uptake after this is by the MG and FG. Were uptake to these groups to continue unabated, there would be no further rise in the curves. Note however, that equilibration of muscle and fat has little influence on the alveolar anesthetic partial pressure during the first hour of anesthesia (fig. 4, 6). The VRG saturation is of overwhelming importance during this time.

Summary

Ventilation causes a rapid rise in the alveolar anesthetic partial pressure. Such a rise does not reach the inspired partial pressure because of the action of anesthetic uptake which removes gas from the lungs. Uptake from the lungs is directly related to 3 factors: blood solubility, cardiac output and the alveolar to systemic venous anesthetic partial pressure difference. Uptake by any tissue similarly is governed by solubility, blood flow to the tissue and the arterial to tissue partial pressure difference. Uptake from the lungs and uptake by the body tissues are directly related since uptake from the lungs is simply the sum of uptake by the tissues. The arterial to tissue difference and thus tissue

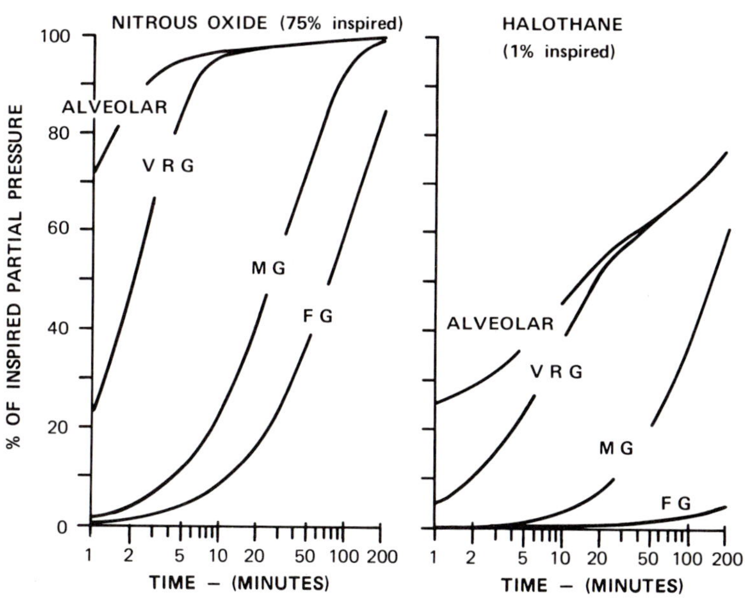

FIG. 4, 7. Those tissue groups having a higher perfusion and lower solubility equilibrate sooner with the alveolar (i.e., arterial) anesthetic partial pressure. Thus, the VRG partial pressure rises more rapidly than that in the MG and the MG partial pressure rises more rapidly than that in the FG. Tissue uptake may be obtained from these graphs as the alveolar to tissue partial pressure difference times the tissue perfusion. Peak uptake (see fig. 4, 4) results from the peak difference between alveolar and tissue values and is therefore a function both of the alveolar and of the tissue rate of rise. Note the logarithmic time scale.

uptake decreases with time, eventually reaching zero for all tissues. The rate of decrease in uptake is directly related to tissue blood flow and inversely related to the capacity of the tissue for anesthetic. The capacity in turn equals the product of tissue solubility and volume. The relative rates of decrease in uptake for different tissues may be estimated from their time constants which are a function of tissue solubility, volume and blood flow.

Tissue uptake affects uptake at the lung by controlling the rate of rise of the mixed venous anesthetic partial pressure. The mixed venous anesthetic partial pressure equals the sum of the contributions of venous partial pressures from each of the body tissues. Each tissue's contribution equals the tissue anesthetic partial pressure times the fraction of the total cardiac output delivered to that tissue. When either factor (tissue anesthetic partial pressure or fraction of the total cardiac output) is small, then the tissue's contribution to the rise in mixed venous partial pressure is small.

We have spent much time exploring ways of viewing the factors influencing the alveolar anesthetic concentration because they are the foundation for all that follows.

QUESTIONS

1. Where do anesthetic partial pressure differences appear between vaporizer or tank and the brain? Why is the difference between inspired and alveolar anesthetic partial pressures of pivotal importance?
2. What makes the alveolar concentration rise?
3. In figure 4, 1, if ventilation were taken in 400 ml breaths, what percent change in alveolar concentration would occur in a ½ minute?
4. Define the time constant. What do you need to know to calculate it? What is it an index of? What units is it expressed in? Given an FRC of 4 liters and a V_A of 4 liters/minute, what is the time constant? If a patient with these variables breaths an insoluble gas, how long will it take for the alveolar concentration to reach 95 percent of the concentration inspired?
5. Why does the rate of rise of alveolar anesthetic concentration normally fail to be simply a function of FRC and V_A?
6. What are the factors which determine uptake at the lungs? At the tissue?
7. What does a blood/gas partition coefficient describe? What does a tissue/blood partition coefficient describe?
8. Define the term "pressure" as it applies to an anesthetic. How does pressure relate to equilibration between 2 phases? If the pressure of an anesthetic in 2 phases is identical, must the anesthetic concentrations in those phases also be identical?
9. Imagine that you filled the FRC with 15 volumes percent of a hypothetical agent having a blood/gas partition coefficient of 0.5. This gas phase is now

brought into contact with an equal volume of blood, (as in fig. 4, 3). When equilibrium is achieved what will be the concentrations in the gas and blood phase? What will the concentrations be if the blood/gas partition coefficient is 1? 2? 4? 9? 14?

10. Why does ether act more slowly than cyclopropane?
11. What factors limit the rate of rise of the venous anesthetic partial pressure?
12. What 2 factors determine the capacity of a tissue to hold anesthetic?
13. A tissue has a blood flow at rest of 20 ml/100 ml/minute. What is the time constant for this tissue for an anesthetic with a tissue/blood partition coefficient of 1.43? of 3.5? of 2.34? What is the tissue, and what are the anesthetics?
14. On what basis were the 4 tissue groups (VRG, MG, FG, VPG) selected?
15. Why does the peak uptake by the VRG exceed that by the MG (see fig. 4, 4)?
16. When a constant concentration of anesthetic is inspired, at what points during the course of anesthesia is uptake smallest?
17. Of what significance are the 2 arrows on the halothane curve in figure 4, 5?
18. Using equation 12 what is the F_A/F_I ratio for nitrous oxide? Isoflurane? Halothane? Methoxyflurane? (assume a cardiac output of 5 liters/minute and an alveolar ventilation of 4 liters/minute) What do these figures indicate?
19. Equilibration of the VRG means that 75 percent of the blood leaves and returns to the lungs with the same anesthetic partial pressure. That is, only 25 percent of the cardiac output takes up anesthetic at the lung. Recalculate the F_A/F_I ratios determined for question 18, but assume a cardiac output of 1.25 liters/minute. How do these answers and the answers obtained to question 18 relate to figure 4, 6?
20. Explain the differences between the curves for nitrous oxide versus halothane in figure 4, 7.

REFERENCES

1. Kety, S. S.: Theory and application of exchange of inert gas at the lungs and tissues. Pharmacol. Rev. 3: 1–41, 1951.
2. Severinghaus, J. W.: Role of lung factors. In *Uptake and Distribution of Anesthetic Agents*, edited by E. M. Papper and R. J. Kitz, Ch. 6. McGraw-Hill, New York, 1963.
3. Mapleson, W. W.: An electric analogue for uptake and exchange of inert gases and other agents. J. Appl. Physiol. 18: 197–204, 1963.
4. Eger, E. I., II: A mathematic model of uptake and distribution. In *Uptake and Distribution of Anesthetic Agents*, edited by E. M. Papper and R. J. Kitz, Ch. 7. McGraw-Hill, New York, 1963.
5. Eger, E. I., II: Applications of a mathematical model of gas uptake. In *Uptake and Distribution of Anesthetic Agents*, edited by E. M. Papper and R. J. Kitz, Ch. 8. McGraw-Hill, New York, 1963.
6. Eger, E. I., II: Inhalation anaesthesia: pharmacokinetics. In *General Anaesthesia*, Ed. 3, edited by T. Cecil Gray and J. F. Nunn, Ch. 30. Butterworths, London, 1971.
7. Eger, E. I., II, and Larson, C. P., Jr.: Anaesthetic solubility in blood and tissues: values and significance. Brit. J. Anaesth. 36: 140–149, 1964.
8. Lowe, H. J., and Hagler, K.: Determination of volatile organic anaesthetics in blood,

gases, tissues and lipids: partition coefficients. In *Gas Chromatography in Biology and Medicine, a Ciba Foundation Symposium*, edited by R. Porter. pp. 86–112. J. and A. Churchill, Ltd., London, 1969.

9. Assali, N. S., and Ross, M.: Nitrous oxide solubility in fetal and uterine tissues in human pregnancy. Proc. Soc. Exp. Biol. 100: 497–498, 1959.
10. Cander, L. Solubility of inert gases in human lung tissue. J. Appl. Physiol. 14: 538–540, 1959.
11. Cromwell, T. H., Eger, E. I., II, Stevens, W. C., and Dolan, W. M.: Forane uptake excretion and blood solubility in man. Anesthesiology 35: 365–373, 1971.
12. Lowe, H. J.: Personal communication.
13. Stevens, W. C.: Unpublished data.
14. Johnstone, M., and Nisbet, H. I. A.: Ventricular arrhythmia during halothane anaesthesia. Brit. J. Anaesth 33: 9–16, 1961.

Chapter 5

Mysterious Models: Uptake by Intuition

The curves of uptake in the previous chapter, and many in the chapters ahead, were obtained from models which simulated anesthetic uptake. Several theories of uptake were developed with such models and their predictions usually have preceded *in vivo* substantiation of new ideas (1). Models of uptake may be exceedingly complex or surprisingly simple. They include elegant equations digestible only by digital computers or active analog circuits. Simpler models may be constructed from resistors, capacitors and a flashlight battery, or even from pipes, reservoirs and water. The latter, a hydraulic model, is usually ignored because it is cumbersome, difficult to build, inflexible and messy. However, as Mapleson (2) has suggested, the hydraulic model presents the ideas of uptake and distribution in a manner which may be more readily understood. For this reason, it will serve as our example of how computers simulate uptake and distribution. In so doing, it also may increase our appreciation of the factors which govern uptake and distribution.

Analogy of the Model to Human Parts and Functions

The hydraulic model consists of a set of reservoirs connected by pipes (fig. 5, 1). Each reservoir represents a part of the body or anesthetic equipment. The capacity of each reservoir represents the capacity of that part of the body (or equipment) to hold anesthetic. The capacity of a reservoir is proportional to and is indicated by its cross-sectional area (not by its height). The capacity of a gas containing reservoir (i.e., the lungs) is determined by its volume, whereas the capacity of a tissue is determined by its volume times the tissue/gas partition coefficient. These relationships will be detailed later. The fluid in the reservoirs represents the anesthetic agent itself and the fluid height in any vessel represents the anesthetic partial pressure. Thus, the height of the fluid level in the inspired reservoir represents the inspired anesthetic partial pressure. Constancy of the inspired partial pressure is conferred by

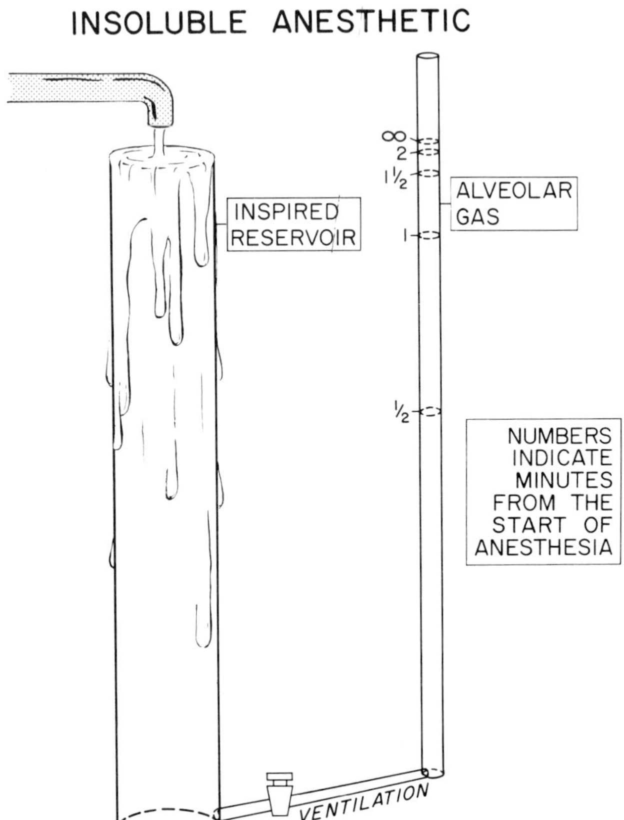

FIG. 5, 1. A constant fluid level is maintained in the inspired reservoir and represents a constant inspired anesthetic partial pressure. When the tap in the ventilation pipe is opened, fluid (representing anesthetic) flows from the inspired reservoir into the alveolar gas reservoir. The rate of rise of fluid in the alveolar gas reservoir represents the rate of rise of the alveolar anesthetic partial pressure. The larger the cross-section of the ventilation pipe (i.e., the larger the ventilation) and the smaller the cross-section of the alveolar gas reservoir (i.e., the smaller the lung capacity (FRC)) the faster does the alveolar concentration rise. In this example alveolar ventilation is 4 liters/minute and the FRC is 2.7 1, giving the rapid rise indicated.

constancy of the fluid level in the reservoir. The partial pressure is maintained by continually flowing an excess of anesthetic (indicated by the fluid issuing from the faucet) into the reservoir. Overflow of the surplus anesthetic prevents the inspired partial pressure from rising above the rim of the reservoir.

The pipes connecting the reservoirs represent the systems which carry anesthetic within the body. Both the respiratory and circulatory systems are represented. We shall assume that their capacity to convey anesthetic from one reservoir to another (i.e., their conductance) is directly proportional to their cross-sectional area. That is, doubling the cross-section doubles the conductance and hence doubles the flow. The fastidious rightly may complain that this ignores some physical laws; that is, that laminar flow is a function of the fourth power of the diameter of the pipe. We have, however, sacrificed accuracy for the sake of clarity and ease in illustration.

Induction begins when the tap in the pipe connecting the inspired and lung reservoirs is opened. This pipe simulates alveolar ventilation ($\dot{V}_A$) and the larger the pipe, the larger the ventilation. The capacity of a given alveolar ventilation to carry anesthetic does not differ from one anesthetic to another and the conductance (and therefore the diameter) of the ventilatory pipe is the same for all anesthetics. Similarly, since the capacity of the alveolar gas space (FRC) to hold anesthetic is identical for all anesthetics, the diameter of the alveolar gas reservoir is the same for all.

The Alveolar to Inspired Relationship in the Absence of Uptake

When we open the tap in figure 5, 1, consider how rapidly the fluid level (i.e., the anesthetic partial pressure) in the alveolar gas reservoir rises. Since a relatively large diameter ventilation pipe connects the inspired and alveolar gas reservoirs and since the alveolar gas reservoir is small, the fluid level in the alveoli rapidly approaches that in the inspired reservoir. Within 2 minutes there is essentially no difference. This describes the alveolar rate of rise of gases of very limited blood solubility and illustrates the rise achieved with normal ventilation when uptake is zero. Gases such as nitrogen or helium or even (though not quite as well) the anesthetics ethylene or xenon would show this rapid approach of alveolar to inspired partial pressure. The rate of change is that of the simple lung washin previously illustrated in figure 4, 1.

The Effect of Uptake by Blood

However, the lung does not live in isolation. Uptake by the blood perfusing the alveoli prevents the rapid rise in alveolar anesthetic partial pressure. To describe the uptake by blood with the hydraulic model requires addition of a "blood" pipe exiting from the lungs (fig. 5, 2). Note that the fluid issuing from the open end of the "blood" pipe is not blood but is the anesthetic carried away by that pipe. The cross-sectional area of the pipe represents the capacity of pulmonary blood flow to carry away anesthetic just as the cross-sectional area of the ventilation pipe represents the capacity of ventilation to deliver anesthetic. This capacity of pulmonary blood flow is a function of the volume of blood passing through the lungs per unit time (cardiac output) and the capacity of each

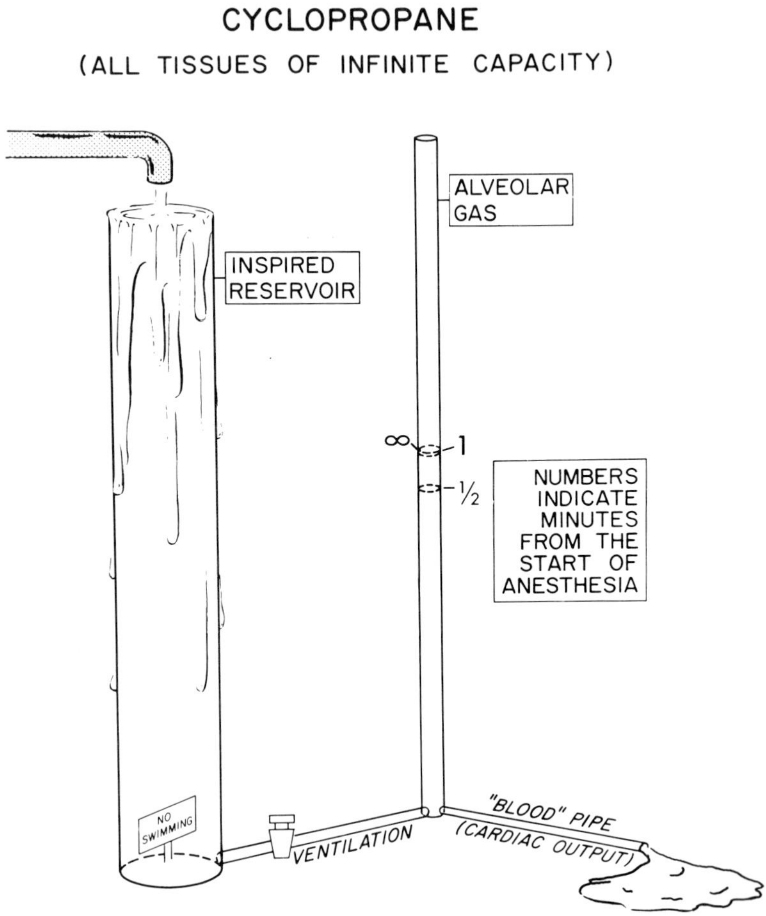

FIG. 5, 2. Figure 5, 1 illustrates the alveolar rate of rise of an anesthetic, without escape from the lung, by uptake into blood. To illustrate uptake requires addition of a "blood" pipe which carries anesthetic away from the lungs. The capacity of the blood to remove the anesthetic is determined by blood solubility and by cardiac output. The product of these two factors determines the size of the "blood" pipe relative to the ventilation pipe. Notice that the addition of the "blood" pipe does not prevent a rapid initial rise in the alveolar anesthetic partial pressure but does limit the height of rise.

liter of blood to hold anesthetic (blood solubility). Now what must be the size of the "blood" pipe draining the lungs for an anesthetic such as cyclopropane? If we assume as blood solubility of 0.47, then each liter of cardiac output carries only 0.47 times as much cyclopropane as a liter of alveolar ventilation. If ventilation and cardiac output in liters per minute were equal then the cross-section of the "blood" pipe would have to be 0.47 times or about half as large as the cross-section of the ventilation pipe. Notice that differences in solubility between anesthetics will require a different "blood" pipe size to represent the different conductance for each anesthetic. The fact that liters per minute of cardiac output exceeds ventilation makes the "blood" pipe a bit larger: if the cardiac output were 50 percent greater (1.5 times) than ventilation, then the "blood" pipe diameter would be 1.5 times 0.47, or 0.7 times as large as the ventilation pipe.

The drain through the "blood" pipe does not prevent a rapid initial rise in alveolar anesthetic partial pressure, although it limits the height to which the fluid level eventually may rise. To lose anesthetic requires an alveolar fluid level (partial pressure) which is high enough to drive anesthetic out through the "blood" pipe. The zero or low alveolar pressure during the first few moments of anesthesia means that little anesthetic is lost at this time and the effect of the ventilatory input of fluid to raise the alveolar level is essentially unopposed.

The alveolar level reached after the first 1 to 2 minutes of anesthesia is determined by the relative conductances of the ventilation and cardiac output pipes. Equality of inflow and outflow conductances would allow the alveolar level to rise half way toward the level in the inspired reservoir. This results when half the anesthetic brought into the alveoli by ventilation is removed by uptake. In the example illustrated by figure 5, 2, the conductance of the admitting ventilation pipe is greater than that of the exiting "blood" pipe and the alveolar level at equilibrium is therefore more than half of the inspired partial pressure. If, as in our example, the conductance of the outflow pipe is half the conductance of the inflow pipe then the alveolar partial pressure approaches two-thirds of the inspired pressure.

Although the blood leaves the lungs in a common conduit it soon divides into the sections that perfuse different tissues. Thus, the single "blood" pipe must split into 3 smaller pipes which convey anesthetic to 3 tissue groups: the VRG, MG and FG. We will ignore the VPG since its perfusion is so low. The cross-section of each pipe again reflects flow and blood solubility (fig. 5, 3). For any one anesthetic the pipe to the VRG is 4 times greater in cross-section (twice the diameter) than the pipe to the MG since blood flow to the VRG is 4 times that to the MG. Similarly, the MG pipe has 3 times the conductance of the FG pipe. Greater variations in conductance are produced by differences between the blood solubility of anesthetics. The solubility of methoxyflurane in blood is 25 to 30 times the solubility of cyclopropane and accordingly would require a 25 to 30 fold greater conductance in this model.

Splitting the cardiac output into 3 parts does not alter the alveolar level reached (fig. 5, 3). Notice that this is the level attained when all tissues have an infinite capacity to hold anesthetic. In figures 5, 2 and 5,

3, infinite capacity is simulated by having open pipe ends. This permits all the fluid (anesthetic) entering the pipes to escape without building up back pressure.

The Effect of Tissue Uptake

But the pipes draining the lung are not open-ended. They lead to reservoirs, which are of finite capacity (figs. 5, 4; 5, 5 and 5, 6). The flow of fluid (anesthetic) into these reservoirs raises their fluid level, creates a back pressure, and thereby decreases the pressure difference between

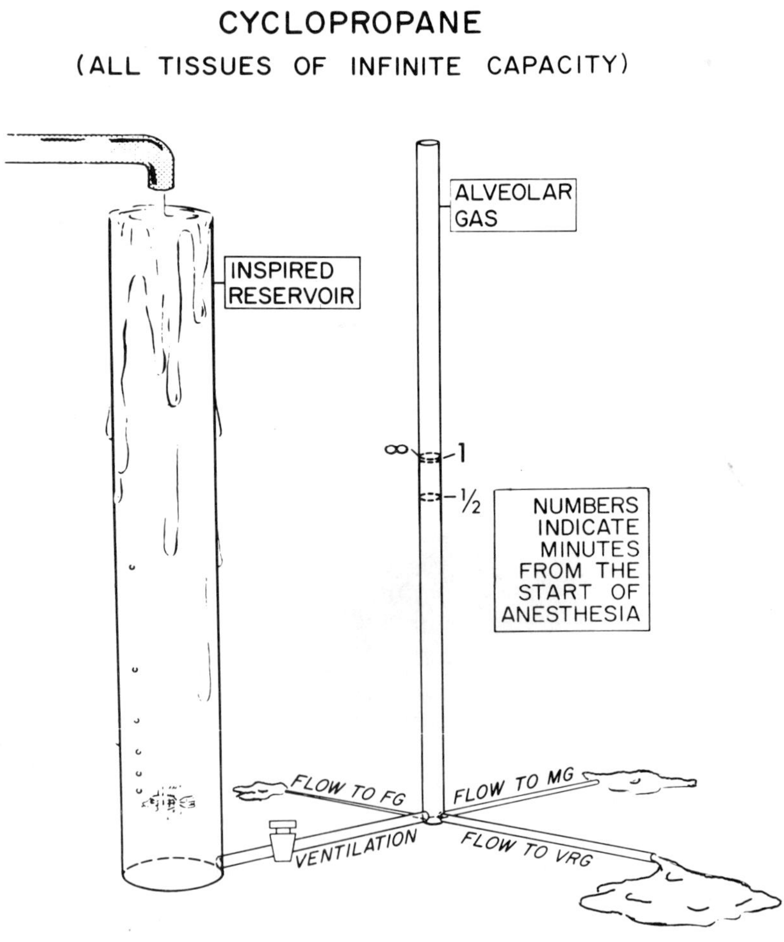

FIG. 5, 3. The "blood" pipe in figure 5, 2 has been divided into 3 pipes, simulating the division of blood flow to the 3 major recipients of the cardiac output: the vessel rich group, the muscle group and the fat group. This division does not alter the alveolar rate of rise or the level reached.

alveoli and tissue. The decreased pressure difference reduces the rate of fluid loss (uptake) from the alveoli which in turn permits the ventilatory input to raise further the alveolar fluid level.

The rate at which a tissue reservoir fills up is directly related to the pipe size leading to it (perfusion and blood solubility) and inversely related to the capacity (cross-sectional area) of the reservoir: that is, the bigger the pipe, the faster the reservoir is filled; and the bigger the reservoir, the slower it fills. The connection of alveolar and tissue reservoirs suggests that their capacity to hold anesthetic must be given in the same units. Thus, the capacity of a tissue reservoir is determined by its absolute volume times the tissue/gas partition coefficient (the tissue/gas coefficient equals the tissue/blood coefficient times the blood/gas coefficient, table 4, 1). It is the tissue/gas partition coefficient which converts the tissue capacity unit to that possessed by the alveolar gas. Thus, although the absolute volume of the VRG is slightly more than twice the volume of the FRC, the small VRG/gas partition coefficient (about 0.5) for cyclopropane makes the capacity of the alveolar and VRG reservoirs approximately equal for that gas (fig. 5, 4). In contrast, the methoxyflurane VRG/gas partition coefficient of 17.4 makes the VRG reservoir 40 to 50 times as large as the alveolar reservoir (fig. 5, 6). The enormous differences in solubility between anesthetics therefore produce proportionately enormous differences in the capacity of the same tissue group. Similarly, great differences may exist between tissue groups for the same anesthetic. Notice the huge capacity of the halothane and methoxyflurane fat reservoirs—so big that they extend beyond the edge of the illustrations (figs. 5, 5 and 5, 6). Compare these capacities with those of the MG. The far greater FG capacities are entirely due to the greater fat solubility.

As noted above, the tissue fluid level rises at a rate which is directly proportional to the pipe size emptying into it and inversely related to the reservoir capacity. Thus, the relatively large inflow pipe and small capacity of the VRG reservoir permit the fluid level in the VRG reservoir rapidly to approach the fluid level in the alveolar gas reservoir: when the levels are equal (i.e., the anesthetic partial pressures are equal) the VRG ceases to accept fluid. Conversely, the small pipe conveying anesthetic to fat, and the large cross-sectional area of the fat reservoir results in a slow filling of that reservoir—and a prolonged drain on the alveolar fluid. The importance of this prolonged drain is related to how small the flow pipe to fat really is. Remember that although the absolute blood flow to fat is only 5 percent of the cardiac output, the capacity of that 5 percent to carry anesthetic is modified by solubility. For example, methoxyflurane blood solubility is so great that the pipe conveying anesthetic to fat equals in cross-section the ventilation pipe (fig. 5, 6). Similarly, the

CYCLOPROPANE

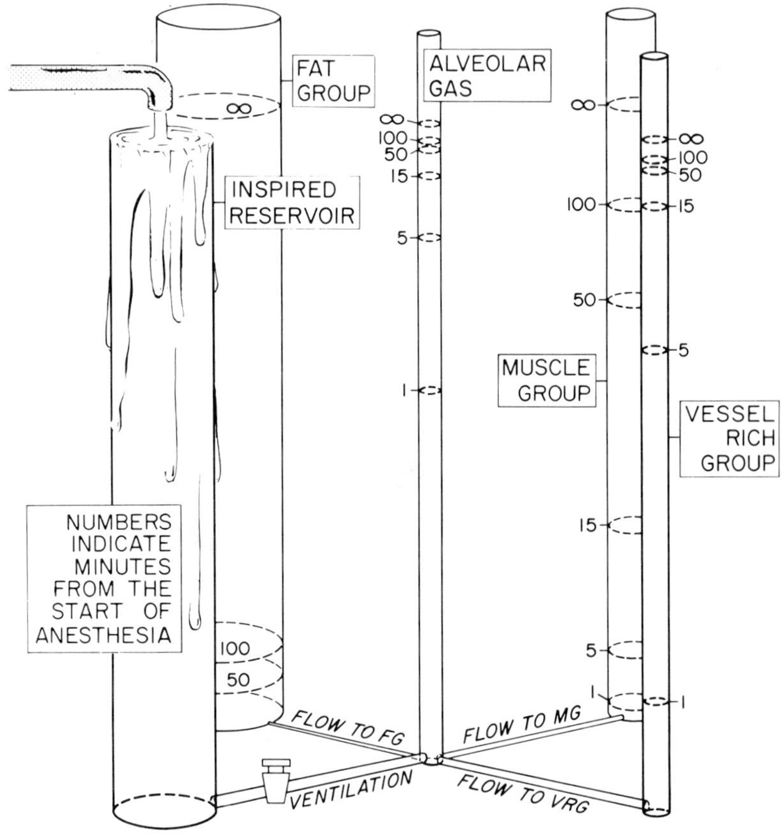

FIGS. 5, 4; 5, 5 and 5, 6. The addition of tissue reservoirs permits the development of an anesthetic back pressure from the tissues. This back pressure simulates the return of blood to the lungs containing anesthetic—that is, it simulates P_v. The capacity of each tissue reservoir expressed as its cross-sectional area is determined by the product of its absolute volume and its tissue/gas partition coefficient. The rate at which the fluid rises in each reservoir simulates the tissue anesthetic rate of rise. The rate is fastest with the VRG since the flow to the VRG is greatest (biggest flow pipe) and the tissue capacity smallest. The rate of rise is next most rapid with the MG and least rapid with the FG, this progression being due to a decrease in the flow pipe size and increase in the tissue reservoir capacity. The figures differ by virtue of differences in blood and tissue solubility. An increase in blood solubility causes a proportional increase in the cross-section of the flow pipes. An increase in the tissue/gas partition coefficient causes a proportional increase in tissue capacity. These increases cause a greater drain from the alveolar reservoir and therefore slow the alveolar rate of rise. The increases progress from cyclopropane (5, 4) to halothane (5, 5) to methoxyflurane (5, 6) and therefore their respective alveolar rates of rise are progressively ventilation pipe is only 5 times larger than the halothane pipe to fat. Such sizeable drains have an appreciable effect on the alveolar anesthetic partial pressures. After 100 minutes of methoxyflurane anesthesia the only fluid level not aligned or nearly aligned with the alveolar level is that in the fat—and the drain to fat alone is sufficient to keep the alveolar level less than half the inspired level for over 100 minutes from the start of induction (fig. 5, 6).

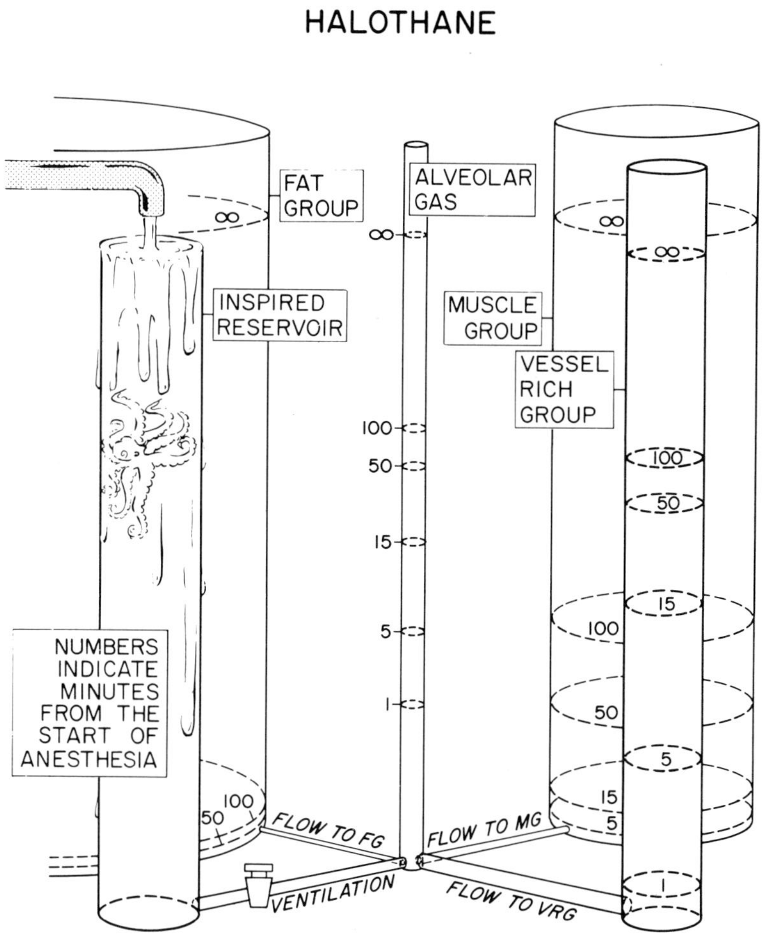

Fig. 5, 5

slower. Notice that the rapid alveolar anesthetic rise to a fixed level seen in figures 5, 1 through 5, 3 is replaced in figures 5, 4 through 5, 6 by a rapid initial rise (first minute) followed by a progressively slower, continuing rate of rise which is determined by the decreasing loss of fluid (anesthetic) to the tissue reservoirs.

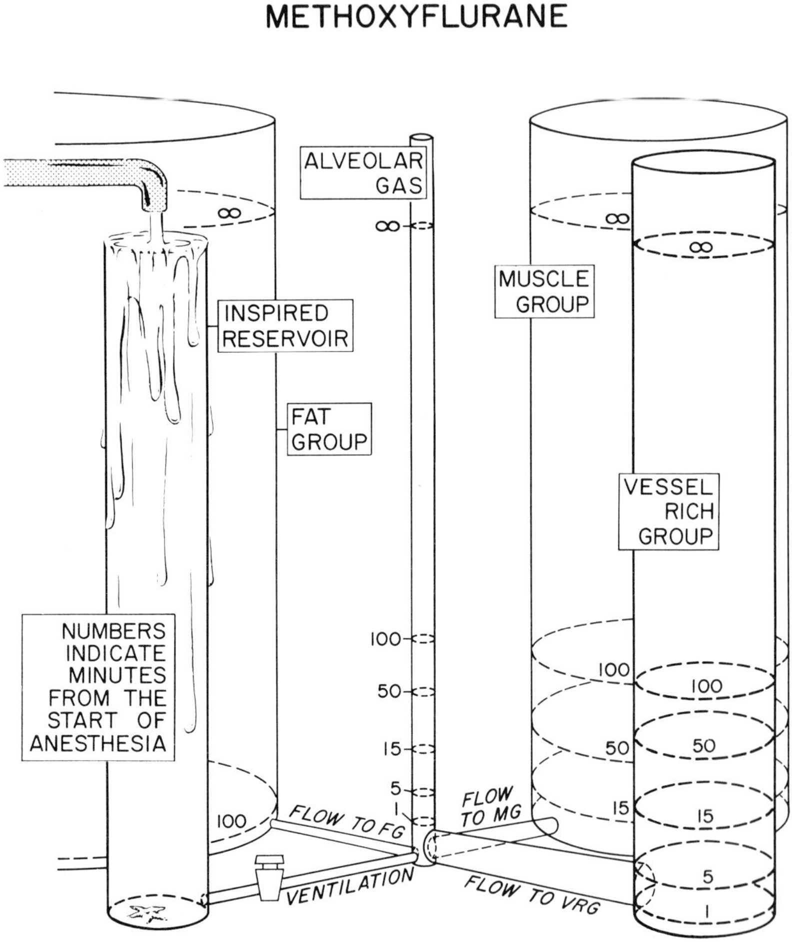

Fig. 5, 6

The Interaction of Ventilation, Blood Uptake and Tissue Uptake

Anesthesia begins with a rapid initial rise in fluid level in the alveolar gas reservoir with all anesthetics (figs. 5, 4; 5, 5 and 5, 6). Remember that uptake requires the development of an anesthetic pressure in the alveolar gas reservoir. Without this pressure there can be no drain of fluid to the tissue reservoirs. Since there is initially no alveolar fluid level and hence no uptake, the anesthetic input via the ventilation pipe is unopposed and results in a rapid fluid rise in the alveolar reservoir. The progressive development of an alveolar anesthetic pressure causes a progressive increase in the loss to the tissue reservoirs. Within ½ to 2 minutes a balance is struck between the fluid flowing in via the ventilation pipe and the fluid exiting via the pipes to the tissue groups. The alveolar level that results is low for methoxyflurane where the exiting pipes are large, and high for cyclopropane where the exiting pipes are small. The alveolar level for halothane lies between these two extremes. During the first few minutes of anesthesia the empty tissue reservoirs act as nearly infinite reservoirs. Thus, the cyclopropane alveolar level at 1 minute in figure 5, 4 is only slightly greater than that at the same time in figures 5, 2 or 5, 3 where the tissue reservoirs are indeed infinite in capacity.

As the tissue reservoirs fill, the drain from the alveolar reservoir lessens and allows the alveolar level to be forced upward by the ventilation input. Initially the drain to the VRG reservoir is larger than that to both of the other reservoirs since the flow pipe to it is largest. The VRG reservoir fills first as expected from the large blood flow pipe and small capacity. The elimination of the large drain initially directed to the VRG permits a considerable increase in the alveolar level. The cessation of uptake by the VRG leaves only the drain to muscle and fat. In the case of cyclopropane (fig. 5, 4), this rate of loss is limited by the smallness of the pipes leading to these tissues. Furthermore, the smallness of the cyclopropane fat and muscle reservoirs permits an appreciable back pressure to develop from these reservoirs in the first ½ to 1 hour of anesthesia. In contrast, the halothane (fig. 5, 5) and methoxyflurane (fig. 5, 6) muscle and fat groups continue to drain large volumes of anesthetic through their blood flow conduits which equal or exceed the ventilatory conduit. The capacious MG and especially FG reservoirs for halothane and methoxyflurane preclude their rapid filling and thereby permit only a prolonged slow rise in alveolar anesthetic pressure.

Students of anesthetic uptake often ask; "If most of the entering methoxyflurane or any highly soluble agent is taken up and reaches the brain, why isn't anesthesia rapidly achieved?" The answer may be readily grasped from this hydraulic model. First, uptake of a large amount of agent prevents the development of a partial pressure sufficient to achieve anesthesia. The brain partial pressure cannot exceed the alveolar partial pressure and this is very apparent in a hydraulic model. High uptake keeps the alveolar partial pressure low. Second, although most of the methoxyflurane reaching the lungs is taken up, the tissue capacity (including the brain) is too large to be rapidly filled by the limited ventilatory input, even if *all* the agent inspired were taken up.

The Effect of Changes in Ventilation, Cardiac Output or the Inspired Partial Pressure

The hydraulic model may be used to illustrate the effect of changes in alveolar ventilation or cardiac output on the alveolar anesthetic rate of rise. A doubling of ventilation doubles the cross-section of the ventilation pipe. The increased conductance of anesthetic permitted by the larger cross-section causes a more rapid rise which is most obvious early in anesthesia (compare figs. 5, 6 and 5, 7). A reduction in cardiac output may be simulated by reducing the cross-section of the pipes leading to tissues. In figure 5, 8 the flow pipes (and hence cardiac output) are one-third normal. The smaller pipes decrease the drain from the alveoli and allow a more rapid rise in the alveolar pressure. Compare figures 5, 6 and 5, 8: notice that the alveolar fluid level rises more rapidly in 5, 8 while the fluid levels in the tissue reservoirs rise more slowly—an

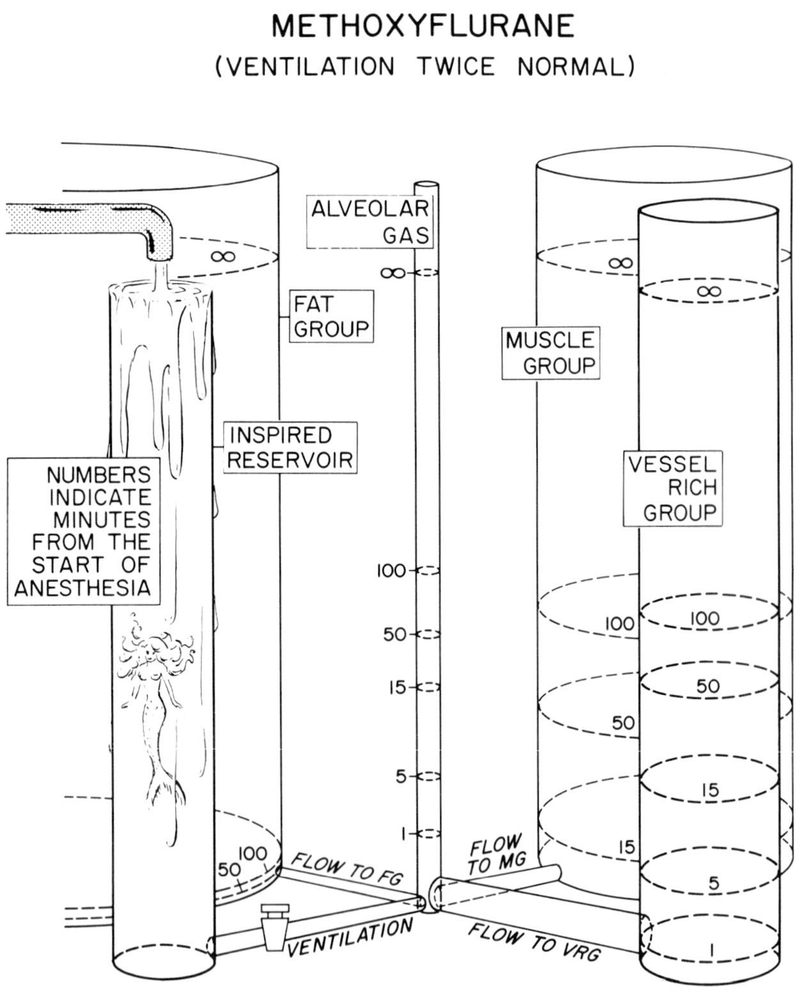

FIG. 5, 7. This figure differs from the preceeding one by the doubled cross-section of the ventilation pipe (alveolar ventilation twice normal). The result is a more rapid rise in the alveolar level which is particularly apparent during the first 15 minutes of anesthesia.

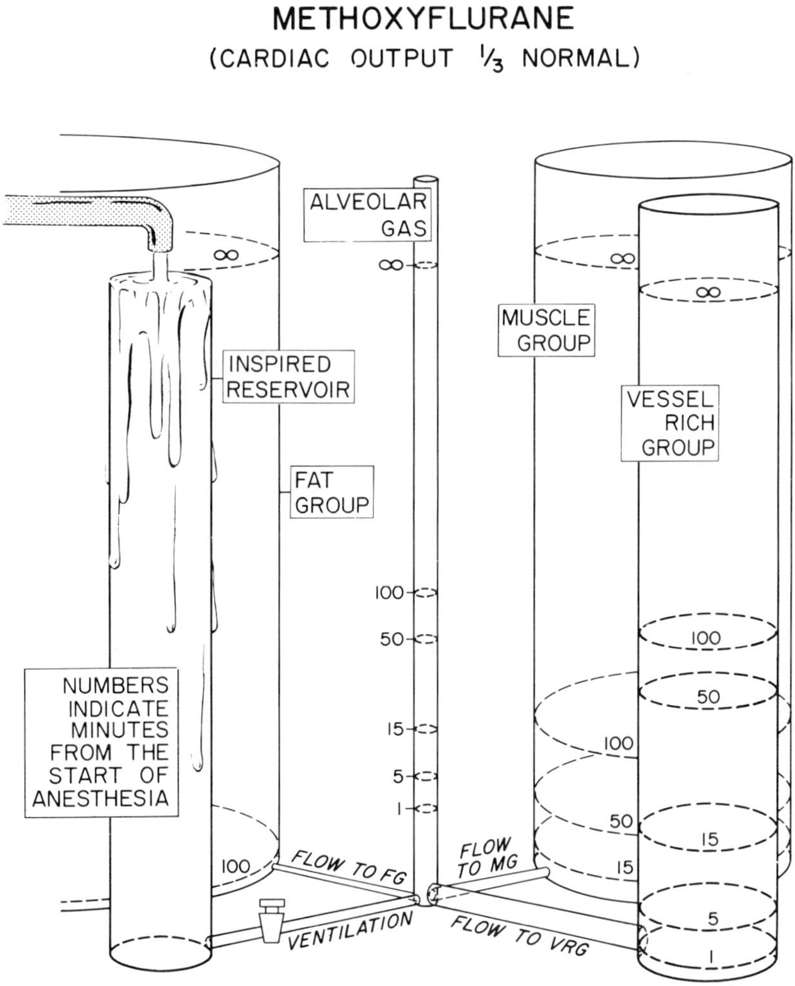

FIG. 5, 8. This figure differs from figure 5, 6 in that the flow pipes to the tissues are reduced by two-thirds reflecting a reduction of cardiac output to one-third of normal. The result is a less rapid drain from the alveolar reservoir to tissues thus producing a more rapid rise in fluid level in the alveoli and a slower rise in the tissues.

observation which is particularly apparent early in the course of anesthesia. Finally, the hydraulic model may be used to show how the anesthetist overcomes the limitation to alveolar rate of rise imposed by high solubility. To decrease the time required to attain anesthesia with methoxyflurane the anesthetist raises the fluid level in the inspired reservoir. Although the alveolar rate of rise toward the inspired anesthetic pressure may remain unchanged (that is, the alveolar/inspired ratio is unaltered), the absolute alveolar partial pressure is increased.

Equality of Hydraulic and Resistance-Capacitor Analogs

The hydraulic model has an identical counterpart in a conductance-capacitor circuit powered by a flashlight battery (fig. 5, 9). The inspired anesthetic partial pressure is simulated by the electrical voltage (electrical pressure) of the battery and is equivalent to the fluid pressure given by the inspired reservoir. The conductance (reciprocal of resistance and measured in micromhos) is analogous to the cross-section of pipe. Actual anesthetic flow is simulated by electrical current. One liter/minute gas flow is usually obtained with 1 micromho conductance. The reservoir capacity is described by a capacitor whose dimensions are usually in microfarads, 1 microfarad equalling 1 liter of capacity. The filling of a tissue is simulated by the voltage rise in the capacitor. The voltage rise across the capacitor parallels the rise in fluid pressure seen above for the hydraulic model.

Summary and Cautions

The story told by the hydraulic model is identical to the one related in the previous chapter. Initially, the alveolar anesthetic partial pressure

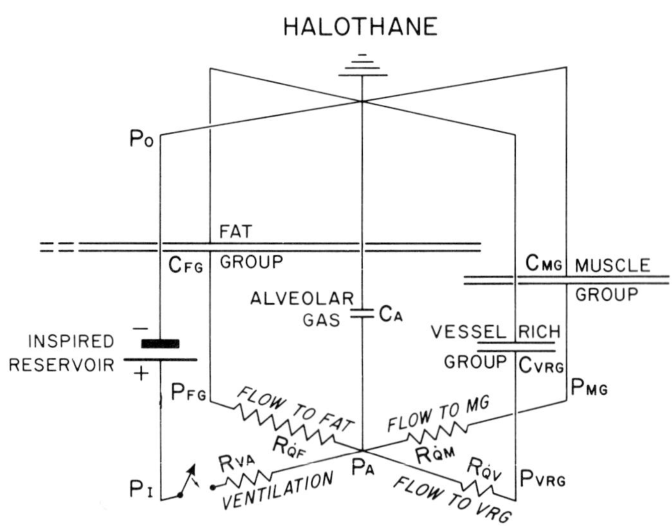

FIG. 5, 9. This electrical analog is functionally identical to the hydraulic models of the 5 previous figures. The battery produces a constant electrical pressure (voltage P_I) representing the inspired anesthetic partial pressure. The ventilatory conductance ($1/R_{\dot{V}A}$) represents the ventilation flow pipe and the flow conductances to the tissues ($1/R_{\dot{Q}V}$, $1/R_{\dot{Q}M}$ and $1/R_{\dot{Q}F}$) represent the "blood" flow pipes to the VRG, MG and FG. The electrical pressures (voltages) P_A, P_{VRG}, P_{MG} and P_{FG} are analogous to the fluid level pressures (anesthetic partial pressures), respectively, in the alveoli, VRG, MG and FG reservoirs. The respective capacities of these reservoirs are represented by the capacitors C_A, C_{VRG}, C_{MG} and C_{FG}.

rises rapidly since the effect of ventilatory input is unopposed by uptake until a lung to mixed venous or lung to tissue partial pressure difference appears—a difference which cannot appear until the alveolar pressure rises. Within 1 to 2 minutes the alveolar pressure is sufficient to produce an uptake which balances the net ventilatory input (that is, the inspired input less the expired output). The alveolar pressure required to produce this balance nearly reaches the inspired pressure for a poorly soluble agent but is only a small fraction of the inspired pressure for a highly soluble agent. Because of the large conduit connecting the VRG to the lung the VRG receives most (about 75 percent) of the early uptake. However, the limited capacity of the VRG causes its rapid filling and hence the development of a back pressure which rapidly approaches the pressure in the lung. This eliminates uptake by the VRG which in turn permits a further rise in the alveolar pressure. During and after equilibration between lung and the VRG, a further slow rise in alveolar anesthetic pressure is occasioned by the development of a significant back pressure (i.e., a fall in uptake) in the muscle and fat groups.

The validity of analog simulation is supported by the work of Mapleson (3) and Eger (4), who demonstrated that simple electrical or digital analogs accurately describe the *in vivo* alveolar rate of rise for anesthetics of diverse solubilities. The simple electrical analog has provided the basis for many of the theories of anesthetic uptake described in the coming chapters. It unfortunately has limitations. It cannot predict the concentration or second gas effects (Chapter 6). It ignores limitations on equilibration that may be imposed by diffusion (Chapter 15). It cannot readily simulate the effect of changes during the course of a given anesthetic such as alterations in solubility (Chapter 9) or in physiological variables such as respiration or circulation (Chapters 7 and 8). For these simulations, electrical analogs with "active circuits" or digital computers are required. Such complex models, however, are still basically the simple pipes and puddles we have just waded through.

Acknowledgment

Many of the ideas for this chapter were suggested by Dr. W. W. Mapleson. His advice, inspiration and encouragement have been gratefully received.

QUESTIONS

1. What do these parts of the hydraulic model simulate: a) reservoir; b) pipe; c) fluid level in a reservoir; d) fluid volume in a reservoir?
2. How are these factors represented in the hydraulic model: a) inspired anesthetic partial pressure; b) ventilation; c) perfusion; d) blood solubility; e) tissue solubility?

3. What determines how rapidly the alveolar reservoir fills? What determines how rapidly a tissue reservoir fills?
4. What would happen to the fluid level in the alveoli if the ventilation tap in figure 5, 5 were turned off at 5 minutes? How would this differ from what would happen if it were turned off at 100 minutes? What does turning off the ventilatory tap simulate?
5. Calculate the dimensions of a hydraulic model for fluroxene from the following information: the ventilatory pipe has a cross-section of 4 cm^2 and represents a $\dot{V}_A$ of 4 liters/minute. The alveolar gas reservoir has a cross-section of 2 cm^2 and represents an FRC of 2 liters. What are the cross-section areas of the pipes to the VRG, MG and FG assuming absolute flows of 4.5, 1.1 and 0.3 liters/minute, respectively, and a blood solubility of 1.4? What are the cross-section areas of the VRG, MG and FG reservoirs assuming absolute volumes of 6, 33 and 14.5 liters, respectively, and tissue/gas partition coefficients of 1.9, 3.1 and 29.2, respectively?
6. If all the tissues in the above question were of infinite capacity, how high would the alveolar fluid level rise relative to the level in the inspired reservoir?
7. How would you change the model in problem 5 to a model where ventilation was doubled? What changes would be required to simulate shock in which blood flow to all body tissues was reduced by half? How would these changes in ventilation or circulation affect the fluid level rise in the alveoli? In the tissues?
8. What values of a resistance-capacitor circuit would describe the pipes and reservoirs determined in problem 5?
9. Which parts of the hydraulic model for a given anesthetic would have to be variable if the model were to describe accurately all that might occur in clinical practice?
10. How could you account for metabolism of the anesthetic using a hydraulic model (assume metabolism is proportional to anesthetic partial pressure in the liver)? An electrical model?
11. How could you calculate the mixed venous anesthetic tension in the hydraulic model?

REFERENCES

1. Eger, E. I., II, and Halsey, M. J.: Dimensions of anesthetic uptake. Anesthesiology 33: 381–382, 1970.
2. Mapleson, W. W.: The uptake and distribution of inhaled anesthetics—the broad picture. In *Progress in Anaesthesiology*. Proceedings of the Fourth World Congress of Anesthesiologists. Excerpta Medica International Congress Series 200, Amsterdam, 1968.
3. Mapleson, W. W.: Quantitative prediction of anesthetic concentrations. In *Uptake and Distribution of Anesthetic Agents*, edited by E. M. Papper and R. J. Kitz, pp. 104–119. McGraw-Hill, New York, 1963.
4. Eger, E. I., II: A mathematic model of uptake and distribution, Chapter 7 In *Uptake and Distribution of Anesthetic Agents*, edited by E. M. Papper and R. J. Kitz, Ch. 7, pp. 72–87. McGraw-Hill, New York, 1963.

Chapter 6

Uptake of Inhaled Anesthetics: The Concentration and Second Gas Effects

The Concentration Effect

Our previous discussion suggests an error in figure 4, 5. Despite the near identity of the cyclopropane and nitrous oxide blood/gas partition coefficients (0.46 versus 0.47) used to calculate these curves, the nitrous oxide curve rises more rapidly. No difference should appear if the alveolar concentration resulted solely from a balance between ventilatory input and loss through uptake since the similar solubilities should cause relatively equivalent uptakes.* However, the inspired concentration modifies the relationship between ventilatory input and uptake. In figure 4, 5 the alveolar nitrous oxide approaches its inspired concentration of 75 percent faster than the alveolar cyclopropane approaches a 15 percent inspired concentration because the inspired nitrous oxide concentration is higher. *The "concentration effect" rules that the higher the inspired concentration, the more rapid the relative rise in alveolar concentration* (1, 2).

Two elements cause the concentration effect. The first is a *concentrating effect* which is illustrated as follows. Imagine a lung filled with 1 percent nitrous oxide (fig. 6, 1*A*). If half is taken up then the remaining concentration (fig. 6, 1*B*) is halved (0.5 parts in 99.5 parts). Now imagine the same lung filled with 80 percent nitrous oxide (fig. 6, 1*C*). Suppose that half the nitrous oxide is taken up (fig. 6, 1*D*). The total volume decreases by the amount taken up and this reduction in total volume

* Relatively equivalent uptake means that the 5 fold difference in inspired partial pressures (75 percent nitrous oxide versus 15 percent cyclopropane) would produce a 5 fold greater nitrous oxide uptake. Thus, the same fraction of inspired nitrous oxide or cyclopropane should be removed by uptake.

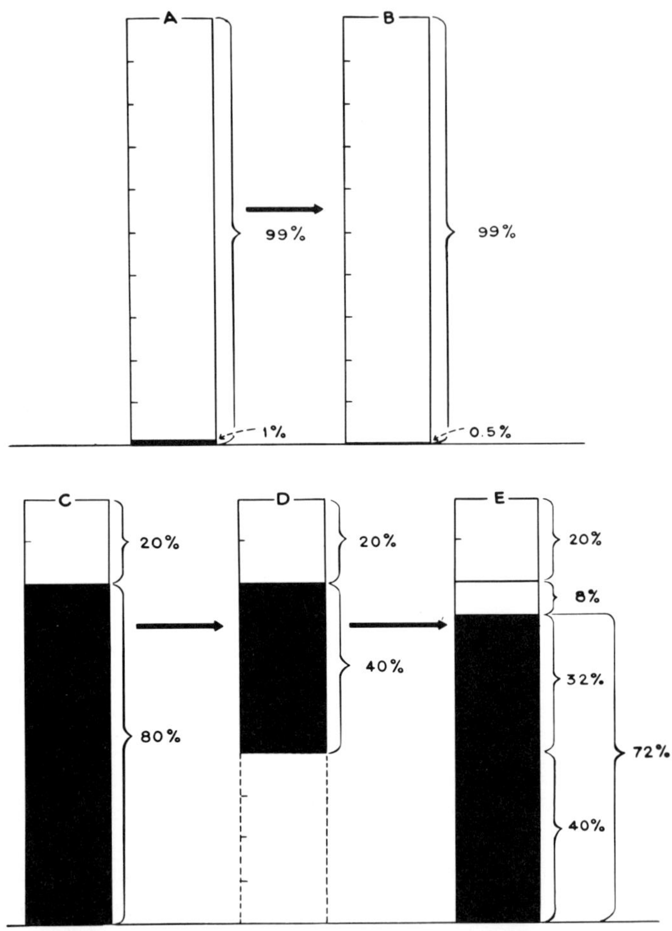

FIG. 6, 1. Each rectangle (*A* to *E*) illustrates the lung gas concentrations. The *filled areas* represent anesthetic and the *open areas*, oxygen. At a low concentration, uptake of half the anesthetic halves the alveolar anesthetic concentration (*A* to *B*). At a high concentration, uptake of half the anesthetic reduces the concentration by a far smaller amount (*C* to *D*) and even this amount is further decreased by the drawing in of sufficient gas to replace that taken up (*D* to *E*). Thus, uptake of half the anesthetic reduces an 80 percent starting concentration by a tenth instead of a half. (Reproduced with permission from Eger, E. I., II: Effect of inspired anesthetic concentration on the rate of rise of alveolar concentration. Anesthesiology 24: 153–157, 1963.)

concentrates the remaining gas. Instead of halving the alveolar concentration, the uptake of half the nitrous oxide causes a fall in concentration from 80 to 67 percent (40 parts in a total of 60). The same point may be made at a still greater extreme.

Imagine a lung filled with 100 percent of any anesthetic. No matter how much anesthetic is taken up, what remains is still 100 percent since nothing dilutes the residual anesthetic.*

The second element of the concentration effect is *an increase in input or inspired ventilation*. When appreciable volumes of anesthetic are taken up as in figure 6, 1*C* and *D*, the lungs do not collapse. Instead the negative pressure created by anesthetic uptake causes the inspiration of additional gas which replaces that lost by uptake (fig. 6, 1*E*). Since the inspired gas contains 80 percent anesthetic, this additional inspiration further raises the alveolar nitrous oxide concentration: the 67 percent nitrous oxide in figure 6, 1*D* increases to 72 percent (40 plus 32) in figure 6, 1*E*. The result of both the concentrating effect and the increase in inspired ventilation is that uptake of half the nitrous oxide causes the alveolar concentration to decrease only by a tenth.

The concentration effect modifies the influence of uptake on the rate of rise of alveolar concentration toward the concentration inspired. At low inspired concentrations the alveolar concentration results from a balance between uptake and ventilatory input: if uptake removes half of the anesthetic introduced by ventilation then the alveolar concentration is half that inspired. The influence of uptake diminishes as the inspired concentration increases. At 100 percent inspired concentration, uptake ceases to influence the alveolar concentration, and the relationship of ventilation to the functional residual capacity alone determines the rate of alveolar rise. At 100 percent inspired concentration the rate of rise for both highly soluble or totally insoluble anesthetics follows the "washin" curve illustrated by figure 4, 1.

The above reasoning suggests that the "spread" between the rate of rise at low and at high inspired concentrations must relate to solubility (fig. 6, 2). At 100 percent inspired concentration the rate of rise is the same for all agents. At lower inspired concentrations the rate of rise results from a balance between ventilatory input of anesthetic and removal by uptake, and uptake varies as a function of solubility. As we saw in Chapter 4 lower curves are produced by greater solubility. In clinical practice the concentration effect is significant for anesthetics taken up in large volumes. This would exclude halothane, enflurane, isoflurane or methoxyflurane because the low concentrations required for anesthesia limit their uptake. Ethylene also would be excluded because its low solubility limits its uptake even at high concentrations. Anesthetics which might show a significant "spread" in clinical practice are nitrous oxide, ether, cyclopropane and fluroxene.

---

* This ignores water vapor and carbon dioxide. They do not significantly influence the concentration effect.

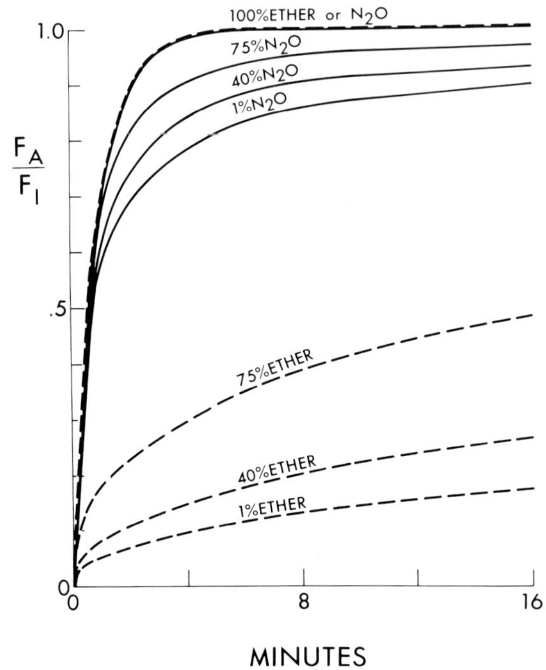

FIG. 6, 2. Increasing the inspired concentration (indicated by the percent figures) from 1 to 40 to 75 to 100 percent, increases the rate of rise of the alveolar concentration of both ether and nitrous oxide. At 100 percent inspired concentration, the rate of rise is identical for both agents and equals the washin rate of the lungs.

The Second Gas Effect

Epstein *et al.* (3) suggested that *uptake of large volumes of a first or primary gas (usually nitrous oxide) accelerates the alveolar rate of rise of a second gas given concomitantly. This is known as the second gas effect.* Since the uptake of the first gas increases the inspiratory volume (see above), Epstein reasoned that this increase in ventilation should increase the alveolar concentration of all concomitantly inspired gases regardless of their inspired concentration. To test this he administered 0.5 percent halothane to dogs, first with 70 percent nitrous oxide and next with 10 percent nitrous oxide. As expected from the concentration effect, the alveolar nitrous oxide rose more rapidly toward the inspired concentration when 70 percent was administered than when 10 percent was administered (fig. 6, 3). In addition, the alveolar halothane concentration rose more rapidly when administered with 70 percent nitrous oxide, proving that the higher inspired nitrous oxide concentration accelerated the alveolar rate of rise of a second gas given concomitantly.

However, an increase in inspired ventilation alone cannot explain the second gas effect (4). Stoelting suggested that uptake of the primary gas reduced the total gas volume and thereby concentrated any gas given concomitantly. He demonstrated that this concentrating effect influenced the concentration of a second gas *without any increase in inspired ventilation*. To do this he caused the tissues of a dog to equilibrate with a second gas (ethylene, cyclopropane or halothane) so that the inspired and alveolar concentrations were identical. Then, keeping constant the inspired concentration of the second gas, he changed the primary gas from oxygen to 70 percent nitrous oxide. The alveolar concentration of the second gas promptly rose *above* the inspired concentration (fig. 6, 4). An increase in inspired ventilation cannot explain this rise since the inspired concentration was less than that attained in the alveoli.

Figure 6, 5 illustrates Stoelting's reasoning. Eighty percent nitrous oxide plus 1 percent of a second gas are introduced into a "lung." Uptake of half the nitrous oxide (*A*) reduces the volume and concentrates the second gas to 1.7 percent (1 part second gas in 60 total parts) without any replacement of the lost gas. Restoration of the lung volume by drawing in

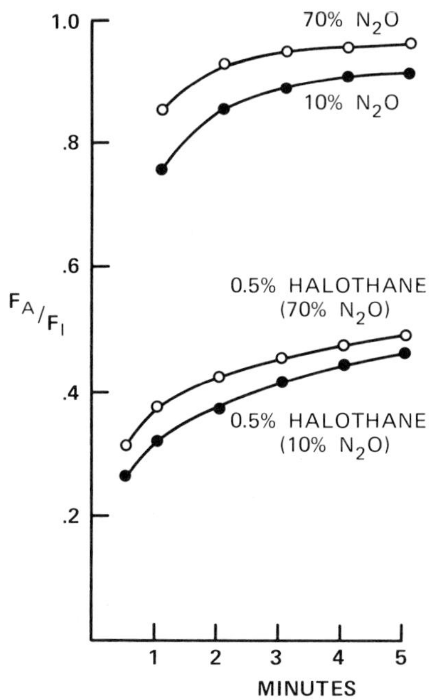

FIG. 6, 3. Half percent halothane was administered to dogs under 2 conditions: 1) with 70 percent nitrous oxide; and 2) with 10 percent nitrous oxide. The alveolar rate of rise of both nitrous oxide and of halothane were more rapid with the higher nitrous oxide concentration. (Adapted with permission from Epstein, R. M., Rackow, H., Salanitre, E., and Wolf, G. L.: Influence of the concentration effect on the uptake of anesthetic mixtures: the second gas effect. Anesthesiology 25: 364–371, 1964.)

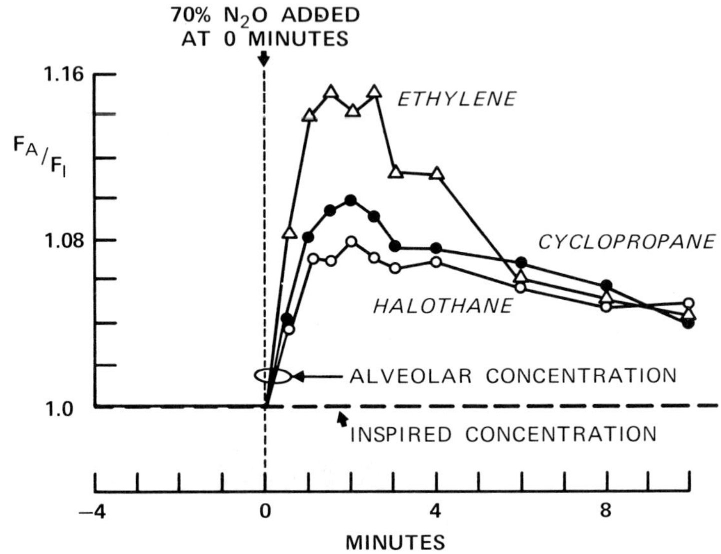

FIG. 6, 4. The body tissues of a dog were equilibrated with low concentrations of ethylene, cyclopropane and halothane so that the alveolar and inspired concentrations were identical. At "zero" minutes 70 percent nitrous oxide was added to these gases without altering their inspired concentrations. The subsequent alveolar concentrations rose above the inspired concentrations. (Reproduced with permission from Stoelting, R. K., and Eger, E. I., II: An additional explanation for the second gas effect: A concentrating effect. Anesthesiology 30: 273–277, 1969.)

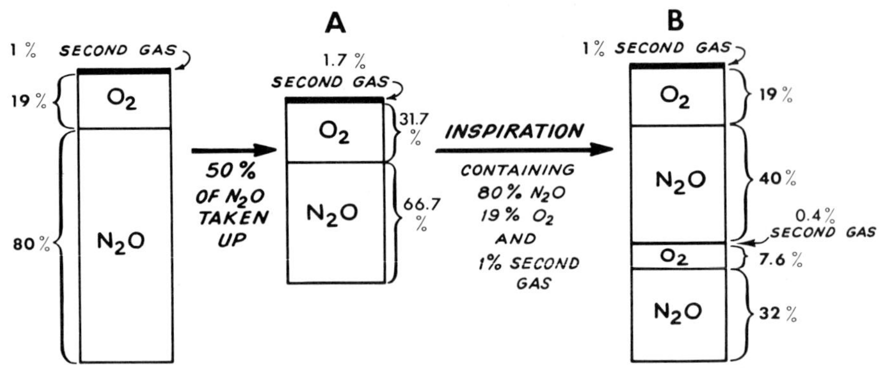

FIG. 6, 5. A lung is filled with 80 percent nitrous oxide and 1 percent of a second gas. Uptake of 50% of the nitrous oxide increases the concentration of the second gas to 1.7 percent (*A*). Restoration of the lung gas volume by addition of more of the original 80% to 1% mixture changes the second gas concentration to 1.4%. (Reproduced with permission from Stoelting, R. K., and Eger, E. I., II: An additional explanation for the second gas effect: A concentrating effect. Anesthesiology 30: 273–277, 1969.)

additional gas (an increase in inspired ventilation) not only fails to increase further the concentration of the second gas but actually produces a decrease to 1.4 percent (*B*)! However, this does not disprove the contribution of an increase in inspired ventilation since the example ignores the concomitant uptake of the second gas. When the alveolar second gas concentration is less than inspired (as it would be if the fraction of second gas taken up exceeded the fractional uptake of the first gas) then both an increase in ventilation and concentrating of the residual gas act to raise the alveolar second gas concentration.

The fractional uptake of the second gas determines the relative importance of increased ventilation versus concentrating effect. Increased ventilation plays the greater role in raising the second gas concentration when the fraction of second gas removed by uptake is large (i.e., with more soluble second gases). The concentrating effect plays the greater role when the uptake is small (i.e., with less soluble agents). The reason for the differential impact of solubility is best seen at the extremes. If almost all the second gas is taken up (high solubility), then concentrating the residual second gas cannot add appreciably to its arterial concentration. For example, if 95 percent of the second gas is taken up by blood, then a maximum of 5 percent more can be added to blood by concentration of the residual gas. Since concentration is proportional to partial pressure (Henry's Law) arterial anesthetic partial pressure cannot rise by more than 5 percent in the above example—and then only if *all* the remaining anesthetic were taken up. However, if the inspired ventilation increased by 40 percent (as in fig. 6, 5*B*) then 40 percent more of the second gas becomes available for uptake. Since most of this gas will be taken up, the increase in inspired ventilation may increase the arterial (and alveolar) anesthetic partial pressure by roughly 40 percent—a figure far in excess of the effect achieved by concentration of the residual gas. On the other hand, if the second gas is poorly soluble, the alveolar and inspired concentrations will be close. Then, as shown by Stoelting's experiment (see fig. 6, 5*C*) an increase in inspired ventilation will be less likely to increase the alveolar concentration than the concentrating effect.

Clinical Implications of the Concentration and Second Gas Effects

The concentration and second gas effects both hasten induction. Although simultaneous introduction of nitrous oxide and a second gas will hasten induction it may be more effective to introduce the nitrous oxide a few minutes after beginning administration of the second gas (terminology confuses the issue for now we are giving the second gas first!). A delayed introduction of the nitrous oxide may accelerate induction through the period when excitement is most likely to occur. Excitement is produced by concentrations of 0.5 to 1 MAC. If used from the start, the rapidly obtained effect of 50 to 80 percent nitrous oxide (0.5 to 0.8 MAC) may cause entry into but not passage through this "zone of excitement." If, however, the rapidly obtained effect of nitrous oxide is superimposed on a level of halothane which is just below the "zone of excitement," the combination may quickly carry the patient through excitement to anesthesia.

The second gas need not be anesthetic. The reduction in lung gas volume that results from the absorption of nitrous oxide also concentrates companion gases of physiological importance. Heller and Watson (5) have shown that arterial oxygen partial pressure rises on changing from breathing air to breathing 21 percent oxygen and 79 percent nitrous oxide.

We have presumed that an increase in inspired ventilation prevented the decrease in lung volume that otherwise would attend absorption of large volumes of nitrous oxide. However, collapse of the lung volume also may be prevented by exhaling less gas. This should reduce elimination of CO_2. Consonant with this argument Kitahata *et al.* (6) found that alveolar CO_2 rises on induction of anesthesia with nitrous oxide.

Summary

Uptake of large volumes of anesthetic, usually nitrous oxide, concentrates the remaining gases regardless of whether they are nitrous oxide (concentration effect) or a second gas concomitantly administered (second gas effect). Uptake of large volumes also increases inspired ventilation. The concentrating action and increase in inspired ventilation both tend to increase the concentration of nitrous oxide and any second gas. Since uptake of large volumes of nitrous oxide is limited to the first 5 to 10 minutes of induction, these effects are of moment only during this time.

QUESTIONS

1. Define and explain the basis for the concentration effect. How does it modify the effects of ventilation and uptake on the alveolar anesthetic pressure?
2. Define and explain the basis for the second gas effect.
3. In the illustration 6, 1 why is 72 percent nitrous oxide really not the final concentration attained? After considering the effect of water vapor, carbon dioxide and oxygen, what other factors remain?
4. We are inducing anesthesia with 60 percent nitrous oxide, 25 percent ether and 15 percent oxygen. Assuming no laryngospasm, why is hypoxia unlikely in the first few minutes of induction? How may the nitrous oxide affect the

alveolar rate of rise of ether? How may the ether affect the alveolar rate of rise of nitrous oxide? In this case, which is the first and which is the second gas?

5. a) A lung is filled with 90 percent of gas X. If half of gas X is taken up, what concentration remains? b) If the lung were filled with 50 percent gas X and half were removed what would be the remaining concentration? c) What if the initial concentration were 1 percent? What would be the resultant alveolar concentrations in the above examples relative to the initial concentrations? (Divide the final by the initial concentration which filled the lungs.)
6. The example in question 5 suggested that the alveolar volume decreased by the volume of gas taken up. If the taken up gas were replaced by the gas used originally to fill the lungs, what would be the final absolute and relative concentrations?
7. Would the concentration effect be more or be less apparent if the patient's total ventilation were increased? What about the second gas effect?
8. Why would ethylene be a poor gas to use as the "first" gas if you wished to produce a large "second gas effect?" Why would methoxyflurane also be a poor choice?
9. In Stoelting's experiment (fig. 6, 5) why does the halothane rise less than cyclopropane after introduction of 70% nitrous oxide?
10. a) Presume that 1 percent of a second gas, Y, was present prior to the uptake suggested in question 5. a) Presuming none of Y were taken up, what would be the Y concentration after the replacement suggested in question 5? b) Assume that the volume of blood traversing the lung equals the total initial volume of gas in the lung. Assume that Y has a blood/gas partition coefficient of 0.5. What would be the final concentration of Y if no X were taken up? If half of X were taken up but not replaced by further inspiration? If half of X were taken up and was replaced by further inspiration? c) Presume the same conditions as in b, except that Y has a blood/gas partition coefficient of 9.

REFERENCES

1. Eger, E. I.: Application of a mathematical model of gas uptake. Chapter 8 In *Uptake and Distribution of Anesthetic Agents*, edited by Papper, E. M. and Kitz, R. J., Ch. 8, pp. 88–103, McGraw-Hill, New York, 1963.
2. Eger, E. I., II: Effect of inspired anesthetic concentration on the rate of rise of alveolar concentration. Anesthesiology 24: 153–157, 1963.
3. Epstein, R. M., Rackow, H., Salanitre, E., and Wolf, G. L.: Influence of the concentration effect on the uptake of anesthetic mixtures: the second gas effect. Anesthesiology 25: 364–371, 1964.
4. Stoelting, R. K. and Eger, E. I., II: An additional explanation for the second gas effect. Anesthesiology 30: 273–277, 1969.
5. Heller, M. L., and Watson, T. R., Jr.: The role of preliminary oxygenation prior to induction with high nitrous oxide mixtures. Anesthesiology 23: 219–230, 1962.
6. Kitahata, L. M., Taub, A., and Conte, A. J.: The effect of nitrous oxide on alveolar carbon dioxide tension: a second gas effect. Anesthesiology 35: 607–611, 1971.

Chapter 7

Ventilation, Circulation and Uptake

Our preceding analyses assumed the existence of a standard man with an average ventilation, average cardiac output and average distribution of blood flow. It is no surprise that this assumption deviates from reality. Drugs, disease, aging, anxiety, sleep or anesthesia itself may change both respiration and circulation and thereby, anesthetic uptake. Depressant medication, normal sleep or anesthesia may reduce breathing and cardiac output, whereas fever or hyperthyroidism cause both to increase. How do these and similar examples affect the alveolar anesthetic rate of rise?

Effect of Change in Ventilation without Change in Circulation

An increase in alveolar ventilation causes a more rapid rise in the alveolar concentration (1–6) of ether, halothane or nitrous oxide (fig. 7, 1). However, although the qualitative change is the same for all 3 anesthetics there are quantitative differences. The more soluble the anesthetic the greater the effect of a ventilatory change. Thus, alveolar nitrous oxide is least affected by alterations in ventilation, halothane more affected, and ether, most affected. For example, 20 minutes after the start of anesthesia the alveolar halothane concentration is 35 percent of inspired when alveolar ventilation is 2 liters/minute, and 72 percent when ventilation is 8 liters/minute—a 2 fold difference in the dose delivered to the tissues. At the same time the alveolar ether concentrations are 11 and 33 percent—a 3 fold difference. Notice that the difference for nitrous oxide is inconsequential. Thus, low solubility confers greater predictability in the presence of ventilatory variations. An increase in ventilation cannot appreciably change the dose of cyclopropane or nitrous oxide; but may considerably increase the dose of methoxyflurane, ether, and to a lesser extent, halothane.

The influence of solubility becomes evident at the extremes. The alveolar concentration of a gas which is totally insoluble will normally

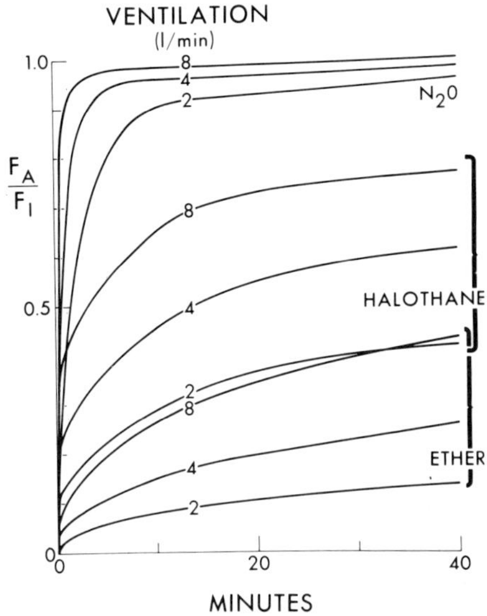

FIG. 7, 1. The alveolar rate of rise toward the inspired concentration (F_A/F_I) is accelerated by an increase in alveolar ventilation from 2 to 4 and from 4 to 8 liters/minute (constant cardiac output). The ratio of lowest to highest anesthetic dose produced by these differences in ventilation is greatest with the most soluble anesthetic, ether; less with the anesthetic of intermediate solubility, halothane; and least with the least soluble anesthetic, nitrous oxide.

approach 98 percent of the inspired concentration within 2 minutes, (fig. 4, 1). Even if ventilation is halved, the 86 percent mark is reached in 2 minutes and the 98 percent mark in 4 minutes. Thus, changes in ventilation cannot appreciably affect the alveolar concentration of a poorly soluble agent except for the first 1 to 3 minutes of washin: an increase in ventilation can but trivially raise an alveolar concentration which already nearly equals that inspired.

In contrast to poorly soluble agents, a change in ventilation causes a nearly equal change in the alveolar concentration of a highly soluble agent: doubling ventilation approximately doubles the concentration, halving ventilation nearly halves the concentration. The alveolar concentration of an extremely soluble anesthetic is far below inspired because most of the anesthetic is taken up. If an anesthetic were infinitely soluble it would all be taken up. A doubling of alveolar ventilation doubles the input of anesthetic into the lung. Because most of the anesthetic is taken up, this increase in ventilation must nearly double the arterial anesthetic concentration and partial pressure (twice the volume of anesthetic in the same volume of blood: this presumes of course, that cardiac output remains constant). Halving ventilation does the opposite and through the same line of reasoning can be shown to approximately halve the arterial and alveolar concentrations.

The same thoughts apply to less extreme examples. We can illustrate the significance of solubility in an intermediate range with the "box" examples in figure 7, 2. Imagine that we fill a lung with 10 volumes percent of a gas having a blood/gas partition coefficient of 0.5 (*A*). If the gas in the lungs is equilibrated with an equal volume of blood then 3⅓ volumes pass into the blood, leaving 6⅔ in the alveoli (*B*) (3⅓ divided by 6⅔ equals 0.5—the blood/gas partition coefficient). Now imagine that we double the ventilation, that is, we double the volume of gas relative to blood. Instead of one gas volume we have two gas volumes each containing 10 volumes percent (*C*). After equilibration with the blood, 8 volumes percent remain in each of the gas phases and 4 in the blood (*D*). Doubling ventilation increased the alveolar concentration from 6⅔ to 8, or 20 percent (8 divided by 6⅔ equals 1.20).

Now fill the same lung with 10 volumes percent of an agent having a blood/gas partition coefficient of 2 (fig. 7, 2 *E*). After equilibration with an equal volume of blood, 6⅔ volumes percent move into the blood leaving 3⅓ volumes percent in the lungs (*F*). But if ventilation doubles (*G*) then the final volumes percent in blood and lungs are 10 and 5 (*H*). Doubling ventilation increased the alveolar concentration from 3⅓ to 5, or 50 percent. Compare this to the 20 percent increase achieved with the anesthetic having the lower blood/gas partition coefficient of 0.5 (fig. 7, 2 *A* to *D*). Again the importance of solubility to the effect of changes in ventilation is evident.

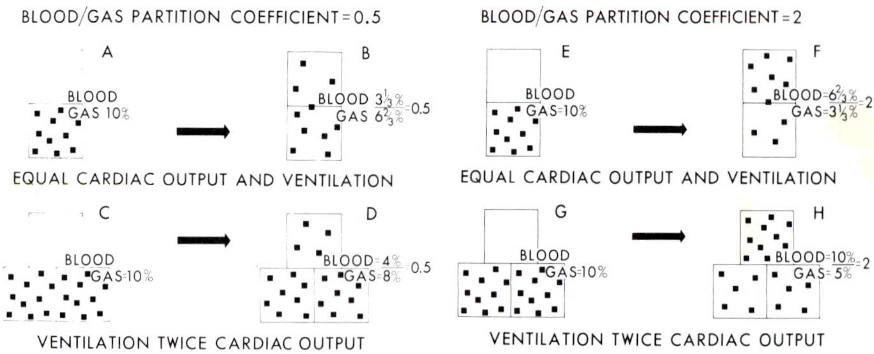

FIG. 7, 2. These "box" diagrams illustrate the importance of solubility to the effect of an increase in ventilation on alveolar rate of rise. The *lower boxes* in each diagram indicate the lung gas space and the *upper boxes*, the blood passing through the lungs. Note that a relatively larger increase in either the alveolar or the arterial concentration is produced by an increased ventilation with a more soluble anesthetic.

Hyperventilation and Cerebral Blood Flow

From the above discussion it would seem that hyperventilation must accelerate the rate at which induction is achieved, but this is not necessarily so (7). Hyperventilation lowers arterial CO_2 which in turn reduces cerebral blood flow. Doubling ventilation may halve both arterial CO_2 *and* cerebral flow. The reduction in cerebral perfusion delays the rise of brain anesthetic partial pressure towards the partial pressure in arterial blood. This opposes the tendency of the more rapid rise in alveolar anesthetic concentration to hasten induction. The balance between these effects differs between anesthetics of different solubilities. The effect of the modest increase in alveolar concentration of a poorly soluble agent such as cyclopropane or nitrous oxide produced by hyperventilation is more than offset by the reduction of cerebral blood flow. The result is a delay in induction (fig. 7, 3). On the other hand, the considerable rise in alveolar anesthetic concentration induced by hyperventilation with a very soluble agent cannot be offset by the reduced cerebral blood flow. Thus, induction with methoxyflurane is accelerated by hyperventilation. The intermediate solubility of halothane permits an

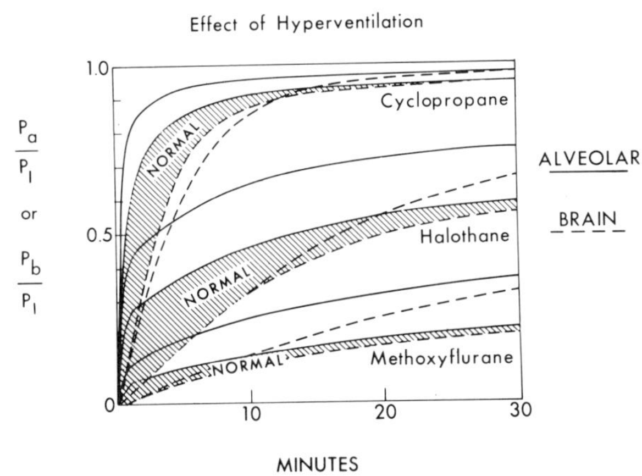

FIG. 7, 3. These graphs demonstrate the approach of the cerebral anesthetic partial pressure (*dashed lines*) to the alveolar anesthetic partial pressure (*continuous lines*) under two circumstances: 1) normal arterial CO_2 (alveolar and cerebral partial pressure connected by diagonal lines); and 2) hypocapnea induced by hyperventilation. Note that hyperventilation accelerates the alveolar anesthetic rate of rise but that the reduction of cerebral blood flow that attends hypocapnea exerts an opposing effect on the cerebral anesthetic partial pressure rate of rise. In the case of halothane, this conflict creates an almost perfect balance so that for the first 10 minutes of anesthesia the cerebral rate of rise is almost exactly the same as that obtained normally. In the case of cyclopropane, the rate of rise with hyperventilation is actually slower than normal, whereas in the case of methoxyflurane, it is faster. (Adapted with permission from Munson, E. S., and Bowers, D. L.: The effects of hyperventilation on the rate of cerebral anesthetic equilibration. Anesthesiology 28: 377–381, 1967.)

almost perfect balancing of the increased alveolar anesthetic rate or rise and reduced brain perfusion: the cerebral halothane rate of rise does not differ from normal for the first 10 minutes of induction despite a doubling of ventilation (fig. 7, 3). Note that this balance does not persist for any agent (even the least soluble) beyond the first 5 to 15 minutes of anésthesia: eventually hyperventilation does produce a higher cerebral anesthetic partial pressure. Note also that hypocapnea does not equally reduce blood flow to all tissues. Coronary perfusion is affected little. The heart therefore may perceive the more rapid rise in alveolar anesthetic before the brain when hyperventilation is present.

Preanesthetic medications may induce hypoventilation. As with hyperventilation this induces two counterbalancing effects on induction. Hypoventilation slows the rate of alveolar anesthetic rise and thereby slows induction. But the increased cerebral blood flow that accompanies hypercapnia acts to accelerate the equilibration between arterial and brain anesthetic partial pressures. This shortening of the cerebral time constant acts to hasten induction.

Anesthetic Depression of Ventilation Alters Its Own Uptake

We have considered the effects of different constant levels of ventilation on the rate of alveolar anesthetic rise but in so doing we have ignored the fact that ventilation may alter continuously as a function of anesthetic dose. All anesthetics are respiratory depressants: at some dose all produce apnea. For example, halothane and isoflurane both cause a dose-related depression of alveolar ventilation (8, 9) which progresses to apnea at an alveolar concentration of between 2 and 2.5 percent (fig. 7, 4) (10). These data were collected from young, healthy human volunteers who received no medication other than the anesthetic agent (8, 9). The alveolar levels (except for the apnea level*) were sustained for at least 15 minutes to assure equilibration with brain anesthetic partial pressures. Under these conditions cardiac output remained constant (halothane) or increased slightly (isoflurane).

Figure 7, 4 suggests that ventilation is not constant during the course of anesthesia, but progressively decreases as the alveolar and brain concentrations rise. The ventilatory depression given by higher brain anesthetic levels lowers the ingress of anesthetic and thereby hinders further rise in alveolar concentration. This limits both the rate at which deeper levels of anesthesia can be developed and the ultimate level achieved.

---

* Apnea levels were obtained as the extrapolated zero intercept of the graph of slope of ventilatory CO_2 response curves versus anesthetic dose. That is, apnea was assumed to occur at an anesthetic partial pressure which abolished any ventilatory response to an imposed increase in CO_2.

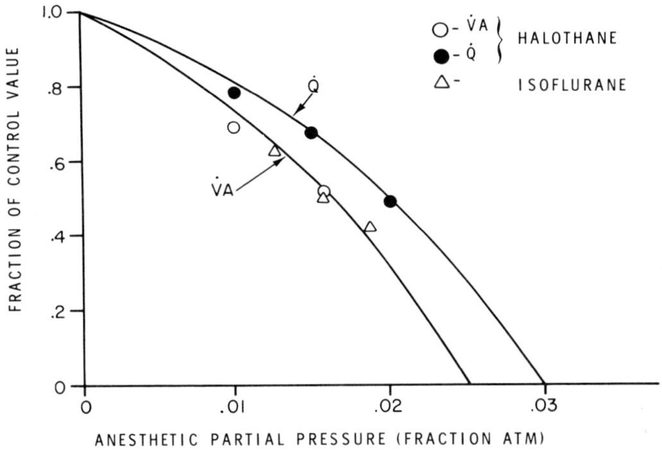

FIG. 7, 4. The results of two experiments are superimposed here. The graph labelled "V_A" indicates the changes in ventilation obtained with halothane (*open circles*) and isoflurane (*open triangles*) in young healthy males. All values are represented as a fraction of the control (awake) value. The second graph, labeled "Q" indicates the reduction in cardiac output in young healthy males induced by halothane during ventilation controlled to maintain $PaCO_2$ between 35 and 40 torr. Both the ventilatory and circulatory curves are extrapolated to zero fraction of the control value. The zero intercept for ventilation was obtained from the zero intercept of the slope of the ventilatory response to CO_2 (see footnote). The zero horizontal intercept for Q is speculative. We would guess that it must lie above the intercept for the ventilation but below a straight line extrapolation of the observed cardiac output points. However, these limits leave considerable room for error and acceptance of this intercept therefore must be tentative. (Reproduced with permission from Munson, E. S., *et al.*: Effects of anesthetic-depressed ventilation and cardiac output on anesthetic uptake. Anesthesiology 38: 251–259, 1973.)

The effect of progressive ventilatory depression induced by anesthesia may be viewed in two ways: 1) as an effect on the anesthetic dose attained in the alveoli; and 2) as an effect on the relative rate of rise of alveolar anesthetic. The anesthetic dose achieved in the alveoli increases with increasing inspired concentrations but the effect is not a proportionate one. Except for transient changes (see below), the anesthetic partial pressure causing apnea imposes an upper limit on the rise in alveolar concentration. The alveolar or brain anesthetic partial pressure cannot exceed this limit since lack of ventilatory exchange prevents addition of anesthetic to the alveoli* (10) (fig. 7, 5). Note in figure 7, 5 that the vertical coordinate is percent alveolar halothane concentration and not the alveolar fraction of inspired concentration. Thus, breathing 20 percent halothane for 10 to 30 minutes produces an alveolar concentration only slightly greater than that produced by breathing 15 or even 8 percent.

---

* Except for that gas drawn into the lungs by the uptake of anesthetic. The small ventilatory input that results from oxygen uptake is not included.

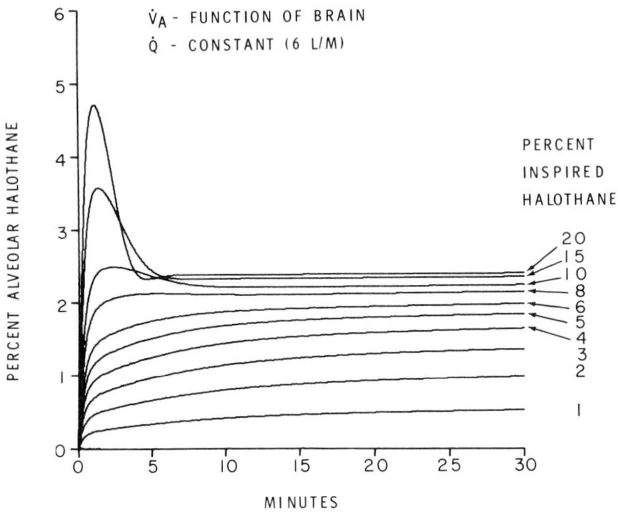

FIG. 7, 5. Alveolar ventilation decreases roughly in proportion to the brain halothane partial pressure (constant cardiac output). Thus, increases in the inspired halothane concentration do not produce proportional increases in alveolar concentration. Elevation of the inspired concentration above 8 percent does not produce an appreciable increase in the alveolar concentration. The apnea produced by an alveolar concentration of 2.5 percent halothane sets an upper limit to the attainable alveolar concentration—except for the first few minutes of anesthesia where an overshoot is possible. (Reproduced with permission from Munson, E. S., *et al.*: Effects of anesthetic-depressed ventilation and cardiac output on anesthetic uptake. Anesthesiology 38: 251–259, 1973.)

Greater differences between the effects of different inspired concentrations appear during the first 5 minutes of anesthesia. The delay in the transfer of the alveolar anesthetic to the brain postpones the development of the ventilatory depression. Thus, inspired concentrations exceeding 8 percent result in an overshoot which is halted as the brain anesthetic partial pressure approaches that in the alveoli. During the ensuing apnea, the continuing uptake of anesthetic from the alveoli causes the alveolar concentration to decrease. Eventually the brain anesthetic partial pressure falls below that partial pressure causing apnea and ventilation resumes—albeit at a low level. The resumption of ventilation halts the fall in alveolar anesthetic concentration which then stabilizes at a level slightly less than that producing apnea.

These effects on the absolute anesthetic rate of rise also appear in the relative approach of the alveolar concentration to the concentration inspired (10). In this case the position of the curves is reversed: the higher the inspired concentration, the lower the position of the curve (fig. 7, 6) (note in this figure the return of the vertical coordinate to the ratio of alveolar to inspired concentrations). Since the alveolar concentration is limited by respiratory depression, raising the inspired concentration must lower the relative rate of rise (except for the first few minutes of anesthesia where the brain perception of a depressant alveolar partial pressure is delayed).

Ventilatory depression with ether and fluroxene does not follow the pattern produced by halothane and isoflurane. Instead of reducing ventilation in proportion to dose, ether and fluroxene permit normal ventilation over a wide range of alveolar concentrations (8, 11). Depression becomes manifest only at deeper levels where normal ventilation may change to apnea following small increases in anesthetic partial pressure. This exaggerates the overshoot seen in figures 7, 5 and 7, 6 with the higher inspired concentrations of halothane. The result for ether may be oscillations in the alveolar ether concentration (fig. 7, 7) which, as for halothane, are a consequence of the lag in brain anesthetic partial pressure (10). The alveolar ether concentration reaches and passes the apnea level before this level is attained in the brain. Ventilation persists unabated and continues to drive the alveolar concentration upward until the brain anesthetic partial pressure also reaches the level producing apnea. Even after apnea occurs, the brain partial pressure continues to

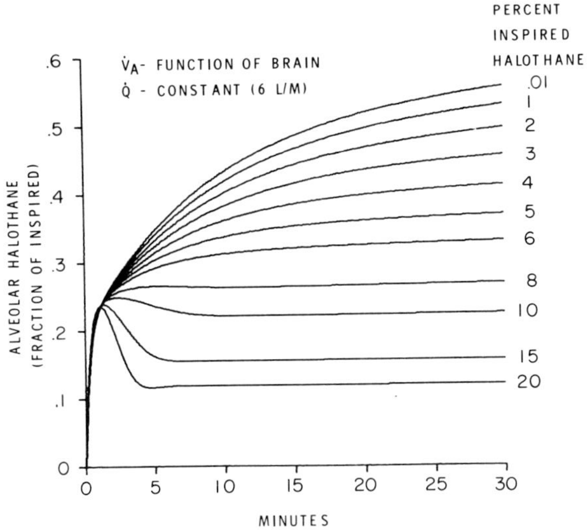

FIG. 7, 6. As a result of the greater depression of ventilation achieved at higher halothane concentrations, the rate of rise of the alveolar concentration toward the inspired concentration is progressively decreased by increasing the inspired concentration. As in figure 7, 5 alveolar ventilation decreases roughly in proportion to the brain halothane partial pressure (cardiac output constant). Both figures 7, 5 and 7, 6 show an initial overshoot at inspired concentrations above 10 percent which results from the delay in the transfer of anesthetic partial pressure from the alveoli to the brain. (Reproduced with permission from Munson, E. S., *et al:* Effects of anesthetic-depressed ventilation and cardiac output on anesthetic uptake. Anesthesiology 38: 251–259, 1973.)

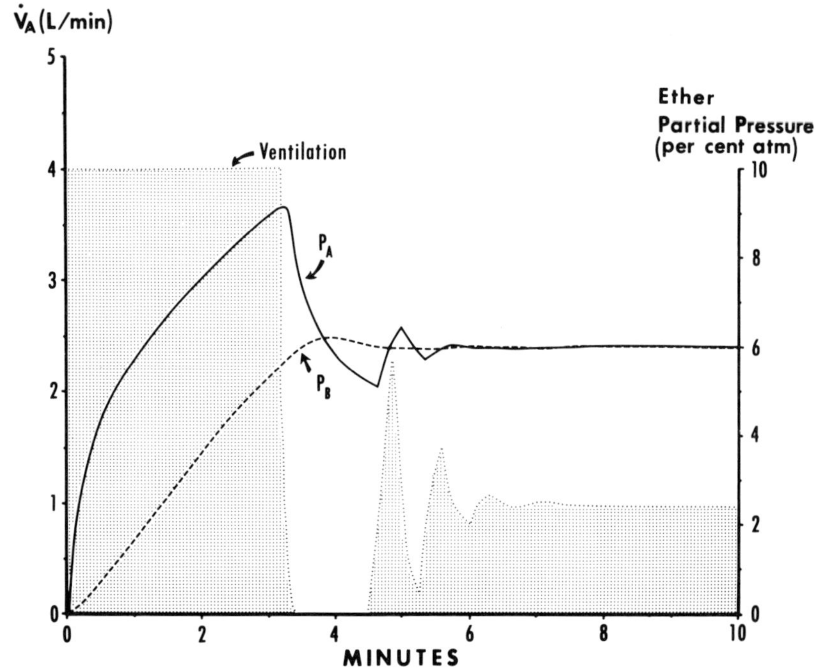

FIG. 7, 7. The inspiration of 50 percent ether causes the alveolar partial pressure (P_A) to rise rapidly. The brain anesthetic partial pressure (P_B) follows at a rate dictated by the rise in alveolar partial pressure and by the time constant for brain. Scale for P_A and P_B is the right hand vertical coordinate. Alveolar ventilation (*stippled area*) remains unaffected by the rising brain anesthetic partial pressure until that partial pressure reaches 5.9 percent of an atmosphere. Above 5.9 percent ventilation decreases and reaches zero at 6 percent. The apnea which follows (at about 3.3 minutes) persists until the redistribution of ether reduces the alveolar and hence, the brain anesthetic partial pressure to a level below 6 percent of an atmosphere. These oscillations repeat in a progressively damped fashion as indicated. (Reproduced with permission from Munson, E. S., *et al.:* Effects of anesthetic-depressed ventilation and cardiac output on anesthetic uptake. Anesthesiology 38: 251–259, 1973.)

rise (and sustain apnea) as long as the alveolar partial pressure is higher than that in the brain. However, apnea halts ventilatory input of anesthetic. Uptake and distribution to tissues such as muscle and fat then reduce the alveolar ether concentration thus permitting a reduction in the brain ether partial pressure. When the brain partial pressure falls below the point of apnea, ventilation resumes and once again raises the alveolar ether concentration. This oscillation of the alveolar ether concentration becomes progressively more damped.

Effect of Changes in Cardiac Output without Change in Ventilation

In contrast to the effect of ventilatory changes, an increase in cardiac output lowers the alveolar concentration (fig. 7, 8) (1–4, 6). An increase in output from 2 to 6 to 18 liters/minute successively lowers the alveolar rate of rise of nitrous oxide, halothane or ether. As with changes in ventilation, the magnitude of the effect is related to solubility: the dose of the most soluble anesthetic is most affected, the dose of the least soluble, nitrous oxide, is least affected.

Again, this is visualized most easily at the extremes of solubility. There can be no uptake of an insoluble agent regardless of the cardiac output, and therefore changes in cardiac output cannot affect the alveolar concentration. If an agent is highly soluble then normally most of the anesthetic molecules that reach the lungs are absorbed by the blood. Doubling the cardiac output (without changing ventilation) cannot appreciably increase the extraction of agent from the lung since most of the molecules would have been absorbed anyway. Therefore, approximately the same number of molecules must reside in twice the volume of blood—that is, the concentration (and the partial pressure) is

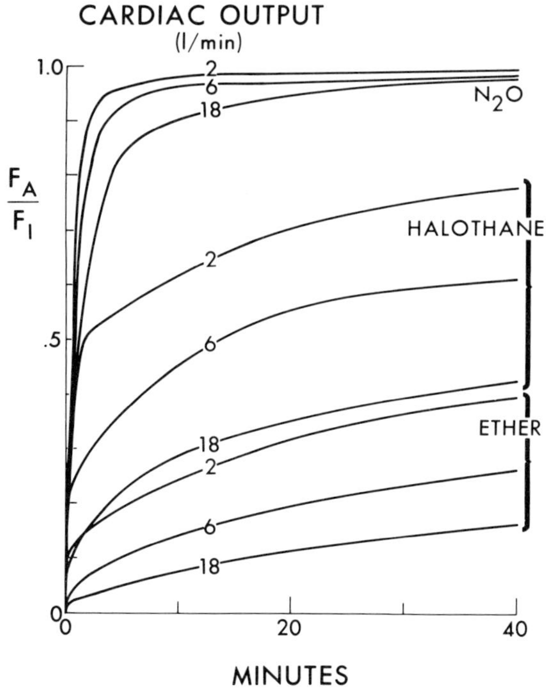

FIG. 7, 8. If ventilation is held constant, then increases in cardiac output of from 2 to 6 to 18 liters/minute will increase uptake and consequently retard the rate of rise of the alveolar concentration (F_A) toward the concentration inspired (F_I). The decrease in anesthetic dose produced by an increase in cardiac output is greatest with the more soluble anesthetic. These graphs presume that changes in cardiac output proportionately affect all tissues: that is, if cardiac output is tripled, then flows to VRG, MG, FG and VPG are all tripled.

halved. Since lungs and blood are in equilibrium, the alveolar concentration also must be halved. By a similar reasoning, halving the cardiac output doubles the alveolar concentration.

The effect of solubility in the finite range can be demonstrated with "box" examples (fig. 7, 9). As for figure 7, 2, initially assume equality of ventilation and blood flow and assume that the lung is filled with 10 volumes percent of anesthetic with a blood/gas partition coefficient of 0.5 (*A*). After equilibration of the anesthetic between blood and gas, the concentrations in each phase will be 3⅓ and 6⅔ volumes percent, respectively (*B*). If the cardiac output is doubled (*C*) then after equilibration (*D*), the blood concentration is 2.5 and the alveolar concentration 5 volumes percent. Thus, doubling the cardiac output lowers the alveolar concentration to 75 percent of the value obtained when output is normal (5 divided by 6⅔ equals 0.75).

Now examine the same relationship when the blood/gas partition coefficient equals 2. When output and ventilation are equal (*E*) the equilibration ratio (*F*) is 6⅔ volumes percent in blood to 3⅓ volumes percent in gas. When cardiac output is doubled (*G*) the blood and gas concentrations following equilibration (*H*) are 4 and 2 volumes percent, respectively. Doubling cardiac output reduced the alveolar concentration to 60 percent of the value obtained with a normal output. Note that this reduction is greater than the reduction to 75 percent achieved with the lower partition coefficient of 0.5. The higher the solubility the greater the effect of a change in cardiac output on the alveolar concentration.

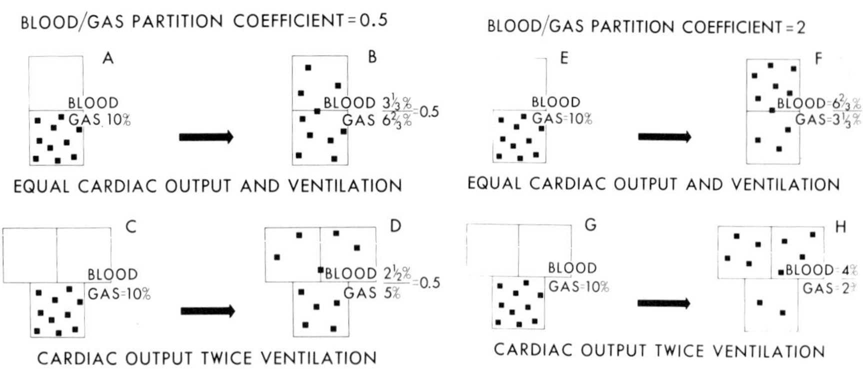

FIG. 7, 9. This illustration is similar to figure 7, 2 except that in this case these diagrams illustrate the importance of solubility to the effect of cardiac output increase on alveolar rate of rise. As in figure 7, 2 the lung gas space is simulated by the *lower box* and cardiac output (blood) by the *upper box*. The effect of an increase in cardiac output is proportionately greater with the more soluble anesthetic: a doubling of cardiac output reduces the alveolar concentration by 40 percent when the blood/gas partition coefficient is 2, but only by 25 percent when the blood/gas partition coefficient is 0.5.

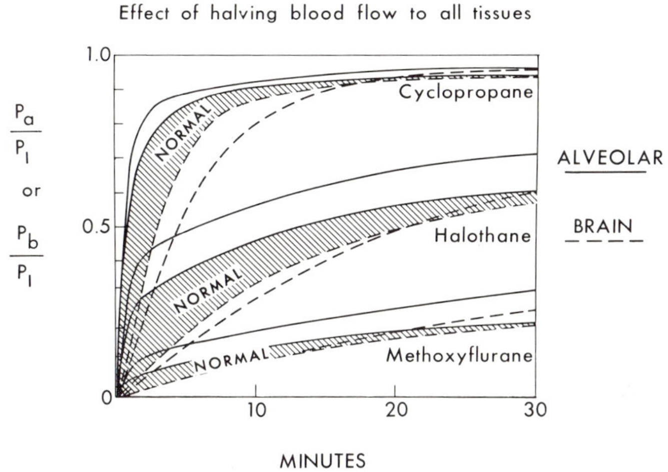

FIG. 7, 10. A halving of cardiac output reduces uptake and hence accelerates the rise in alveolar anesthetic partial pressure (P_A) toward the partial pressure inspired (P_I) for all anesthetics (continuous graphs). If (as in these graphs) the reduction in total blood flow is equally shared by all tissues, then the reduction in cerebral blood flow must delay the approach of the brain anesthetic partial pressure (P_B) to the inspired partial pressure (*dashed lines*). The lines for alveolar and brain partial pressures under normal conditions are connected by the diagonal lines. Note the similarity of the effect to that seen in figure 7, 3. (Adapted with permission from Munson, E. S., Eger, E. I., II, and Bowers, D. L.: The effect of changes in cardiac output and distribution on the rate of cerebral anesthetic equilibration. Anesthesiology 29: 535–537, 1968.)

Effect of Reduced Cerebral Blood Flow in Association with a Reduced Cardiac Output

The lesser uptake which accompanies a lower cardiac output permits a more rapid rise in alveolar anesthetic partial pressure. However, if the lower output is shared proportionately by all tissues including the brain, then the reduced cerebral blood flow slows the transfer of the higher alveolar partial pressure to the brain (fig. 7, 10) (12). The effect is similar to that whch resulted from the reduction in cerebral blood flow secondary to hyperventilation. Despite the acceleration of the alveolar rate of rise, induction with the less soluble agents is slowed by the larger brain time constant. With the more soluble agents, the acceleration of the alveolar rate of rise is sufficient to balance the effect of the reduced cerebral blood flow: the initial rise in brain anesthetic partial pressure is normal and within 10 to 20 minutes exceeds normal (see the methoxyflurane graphs, fig. 7, 10). Eventually of course, the higher alveolar anesthetic partial pressure resulting from a reduced cardiac output is transmitted to the brain regardless of differences in solubility.

The brain blood flow may not share proportionately in reductions of total blood flow. Cerebral perfusion during shock tends to be maintained at the expense of flow to other tissues (13). Anesthetics may augment this effect since they tend to cause cerebral vasodilation (14). If cerebral blood flow is sustained when total flow is reduced then the alveolar anesthetic partial pressure is transmitted as rapidly as normally to the brain (fig. 7, 11). In this case, the augmented rate of alveolar rise results in an accelerated rate of induction for all anesthetics—and the greatest acceleration continues to be found with the most soluble agent.

Implications to the Patient in Shock

The above relationships between cardiac output, ventilation and solubility suggest that the dose of anesthetic achieved in the alveoli becomes less predictable as solubility increases. Extreme alveolar anesthetic changes may occur when output and ventilation change in opposite directions. For example, ventilation increases and output falls in hemorrhagic shock. Thus, shock may permit the alveolar concentration of a highly soluble agent to reach unexpected levels, levels which may fatally depress an already compromised circulation. Safer anesthetic choices in such a patient might be less soluble agents such as nitrous oxide or cyclopropane.

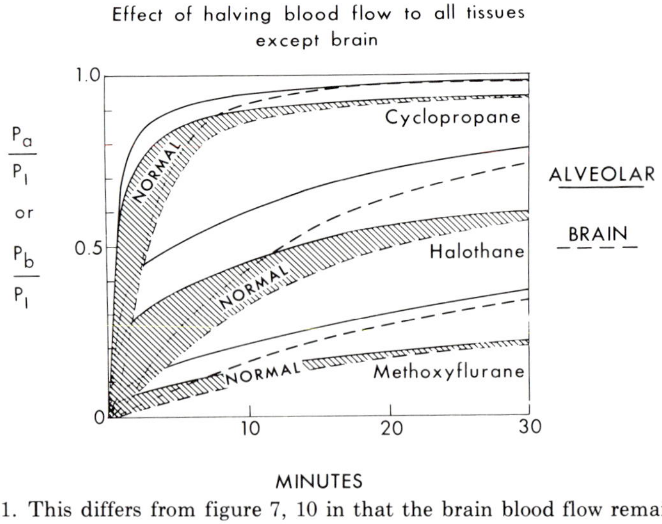

FIG. 7, 11. This differs from figure 7, 10 in that the brain blood flow remains normal when the cardiac output is halved. This permits the more rapid ascent of the alveolar anesthetic partial pressure resulting from the reduced cardiac output to be reflected in the rate of rise of the brain anesthetic partial pressure. (Adapted with permission from the article by Munson *et al.*: The effects of changes in cardiac output and distribution on the rate of cerebral anesthetic equilibration. Anesthesiology 29: 533–537, 1968.)

Anesthetic Depression of Cardiac Output Alters its own Uptake

In considering the effect of different constant levels of cardiac output, we have neglected the progressive changes in cardiac output that may be produced by increasing anesthetic doses. If alveolar ventilation is held constant (as indicated by a constant arterial PCO_2) then during halothane anesthesia the cardiac output is inversely related to the alveolar (actually vessel rich group) halothane concentration (15) (fig. 7, 4). The progressive fall in uptake that must accompany this fall in cardiac output should accelerate both the absolute and relative rate of rise of the alveolar concentration. Thus, an increase in the inspired halothane concentration results in a disproportionate increase in the absolute alveolar halothane partial pressure (fig. 7, 12) (10). For example, 30 minutes after induction, the curve for 2 percent inspired halothane is more than twice as high as the 1 percent curve. Similarly, the 4 percent curve is more than double the 2 percent curve.

Figure 7, 13 illustrates the effect of the dose-related decrease in cardiac output (and uptake) on the rate of halothane rise toward different inspired concentrations. The cardiac output decrease between the 0.01 and 1 percent curves is small and induces a slightly more rapid rate of

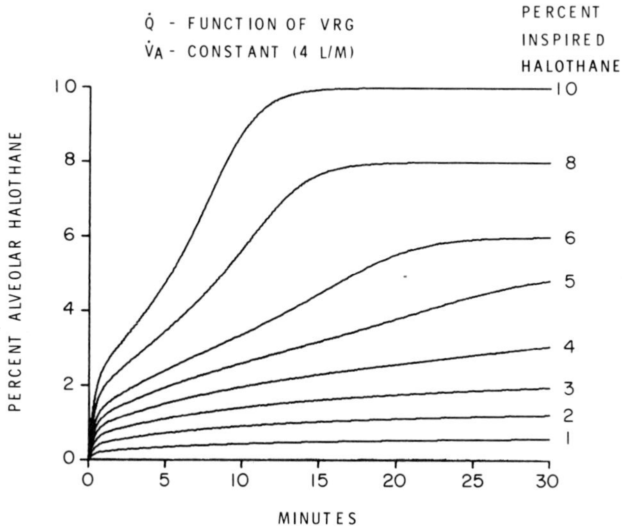

FIG. 7, 12. As indicated in figure 7, 4 cardiac output falls as the alveolar halothane concentration is raised (constant alveolar ventilation). Therefore, doubling the inspired concentration produces a more than doubling of the actual alveolar halothane concentration since the higher alveolar concentration that results will not produce a proportional increase in uptake. Note that the vertical axis indicates the absolute percent halothane achieved in the alveoli. (Reproduced with permission from Munson, E. S. *et al.*: Effects of anesthetic-depressed ventilation and cardiac output on anesthetic uptake: A computer nonlinear simulation. Anesthesiology 38: 251–259, 1973).

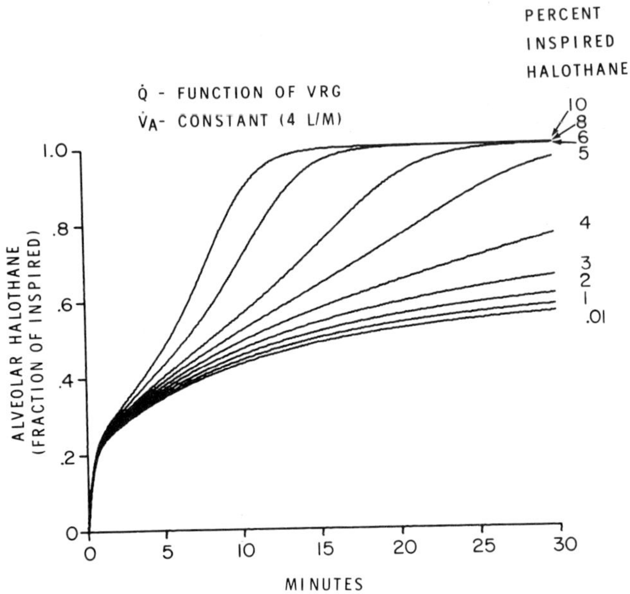

FIG. 7, 13. This figure demonstrates the relative rates of rise of alveolar halothane at different inspired halothane concentrations. Note now we have reverted to relative (F_A/F_I) rather than absolute rate of rise. As indicated for the previous figure, the rate of rise is greater for higher inspired concentrations because of the dose-related depression of cardiac output and uptake produced by halothane. Equality of alveolar and inspired concentrations (6 percent or greater inspired halothane) indicates that cardiac arrest has occurred. (Reproduced with permission from Munson, E. S. *et al.*: Effects of anesthetic-depressed ventilation and cardiac output on anesthetic uptake: A computer nonlinear simulation. Anesthesiology 38: 251–259, 1973.)

alveolar rise. The difference between the curves accords with the prediction by Ashman *et al.* (16). Further increases in inspired concentration cause a still greater decrease in cardiac output and hence a still greater acceleration of the rate at which the alveolar concentration of halothane rises. In both figures 7, 12 and 7, 13 the normal deceleration of the alveolar rate of rise is lost at the higher inspired concentrations. For example, breathing 10 percent halothane, the rate of rise of the alveolar concentrations decreases between 1 and 2 minutes, but after 2 to 3 minutes this deceleration is reversed and the rate of rise now increases. Within 10 minutes the alveolar halothane has nearly reached the inspired concentration of 10 percent. This acceleration of the alveolar rate of rise results from cardiovascular collapse and the cessation of halothane uptake. Beyond this point the alveolar rate of rise is determined solely by the ventilatory washin of halothane.

Effect of Concomitant Ventilatory and Circulatory Changes in the Same Direction

Many conditions alter ventilation and circulation in the same direction. A change in metabolic rate due to changes in body temperature or abnormalities of thyroid hormone release is probably the most common cause for such a deviation from normal. At first glance it would appear that the alveolar rate of rise should not be affected by a concomitant and equal change in ventilation and circulation: each would seem to cancel the effect of the other. This ignores the effect of changes in cardiac output on the rate of anesthetic equilibration with the tissues. An increase in blood flow accelerates the rate of equilibration. That is, the time constant for each tissue group decreases. With equilibration, the anesthetic partial pressure in the mixed venous blood is increased. The higher venous anesthetic partial pressure reduces the alveolar to venous blood partial pressure difference. This lowers uptake and thereby permits a higher alveolar concentration.

The above description suggests that a proportional increase in respiration and cardiac output eventually must cause a more rapid approach of the alveolar to the inspired concentration. However, the *initial* course of the alveolar concentration is determined by the distribution of the increase in blood flow. At least three general possibilities exist. First, if all tissues share proportionately in the increased blood flow, then the alveolar concentration is greater than normal at all times—but the difference achieved with reasonable cardiorespiratory increases is not great. Second, if the VRG or any part of the VRG is the primary recipient of the increases in blood flow then the alveolar concentration again is always above normal. In contrast to the small effect of proportionate increases in blood flow, the differences here may be considerable. Third, if the increase is directed to the MG or FG then the initial rise in alveolar concentration may be slower than normal. In this last case, the reduction from normal is small and as with the first two cases, eventually the alveolar concentration exceeds normal. Let us examine each of these possibilities.

Effect of Proportional Flow Increases to All Tissues

Assume that each tissue receives a proportional increase in blood flow. That is, if flow to the VRG is doubled then flows to the MG, FG and VPG also are doubled. In this example, ventilation likewise would be doubled. As noted above, the increase in tissue blood flow reduces the tissue time constants and causes a chain of events that accelerates the alveolar rate of anesthetic rise: the shorter time constants indicate more rapid tissue equilibration: the more rapid tissue equilibration results in a more rapid rise in tissue and hence mixed venous anesthetic partial pressure; the higher venous anesthetic partial pressure reduces the alveolar to venous partial pressure difference; this reduced difference decreases anesthetic uptake; and the reduction in uptake permits the higher alveolar anesthetic partial pressure.

Proportional increases in blood flow and ventilation accelerate the alveolar rate of rise of all anesthetics (fig. 7, 14) (17). The magnitude of this effect is related to solubility, being trivial with the poorly soluble nitrous oxide and largest with the highly soluble methoxyflurane. However, fever or hyperthyroidism rarely causes even a doubling of cardiac output and ventilation. Thus, the increase in alveolar anesthetic dose that might attend these changes—even with the highly soluble methoxyflurane—would be small. Furthermore, any increases would be matched by an increase in MAC (see Effects of Temperature and Hyperthyroidism on MAC in Chapter 1).

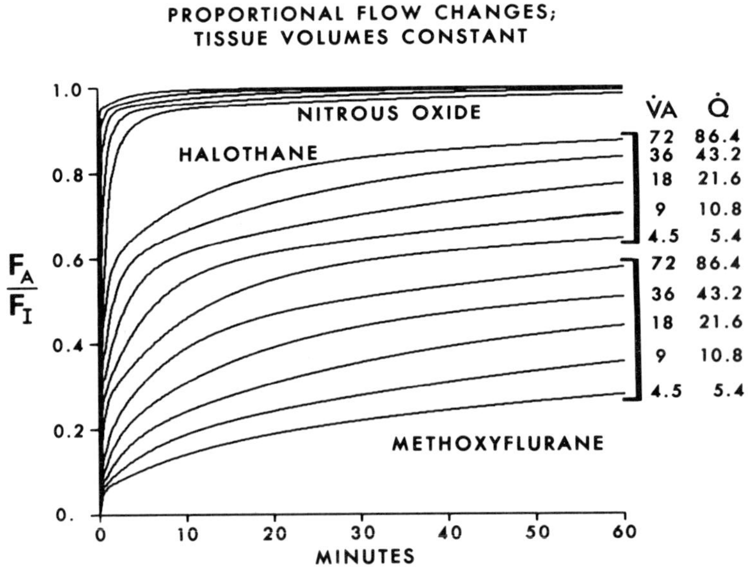

FIG. 7, 14. The vertical axis indicates the ratio of alveolar (F_A) to inspired (F_I) concentrations. These curves demonstrate that concomitant doubling of ventilation and cardiac output accelerates the rate of rise of alveolar concentration of all anesthetics. The doubling indicated for this figure is geometric (i.e., each ventilation and circulation for succeeding curves is double that of the preceding curve) and thus the 5 curves for each anesthetic cover a 16 fold variation in circulation and ventilation. As opposed to the subsequent 2 figures, the increases in cardiac output used for the simulations for this figure were distributed proportionately to all tissues. That is, a doubling of cardiac output meant a doubling of blood flow to all tissues. (Adapted with permission from Eger, E. I., II *et al.*: Effect of age on the rate of increase of alveolar anesthetic concentration. Anesthesiology 35: 365–372, 1971).

Effect of Increases in Flow Directed to the VRG

An increase in perfusion to an already well perfused tissue will raise the alveolar concentration more than the proportional increases noted above. The reason for this is apparent at the extreme exemplified by a left to right shunt. A left to right shunt increases cardiac output but since the shunted blood cannot lose anesthetic to tissue, it returns to the lung with the same anesthetic partial pressure as it took from the lung. Thus, shunted blood cannot contribute to the uptake of anesthetic. This also follows from the observation that uptake from the lungs must equal the sum of tissue uptakes. If the increase in cardiac output associated with a left to right shunt were accompanied by a proportional increase in ventilation, then the alveolar rate of anesthetic rise would be accelerated as a function of the ventilatory increases—exactly as indicated in figure 7, 1.

The above analogy is flawed by the fact that a shunt produces a negligible increase in metabolism and therefore causes a negligible increase in ventilation. One natural condition which does influence perfusion *and* ventilation in the manner described is youth. Although all tissues in the young receive a greater perfusion per kilogram than adult tissues, the principle recipients are the tissues already benefiting from a high flow, the VRG. This further hastens the already rapid equilibration of the VRG with the arterial anesthetic partial pressure. Once equilibration occurs, the increased flow to the VRG acts like the shunt described in the previous paragraph. However, in contrast to that shunt, the increased flow to VRG exists to supply a metabolic need and hence this flow is associated with a proportional ventilatory increase.*

The above reasoning suggests that the alveolar rate of anesthetic rise should be considerably greater in children (especially neonates) than in adults. Salanitre and Rackow (18) have demonstrated that this indeed is the case. The effects of differences in perfusion per kilogram and in the diversion of blood to the VRG for ages ranging from infant to adult appear in figure 7, 15. These graphs probably exaggerate the differences between ages because they are based on assumptions for perfusion in the very young—especially to the vessel rich group—which are a bit excessive. Therefore, they should be viewed as demonstrating the maximum differences which might result. The qualitative effect of age is the same for all anesthetics, but the effect is proportionately greater with anesthetics of higher solubility. For example, at 60 minutes the newborn methoxyflurane curve is more than double its adult counterpart, whereas

* We are not talking about an absolute increase in ventilation: ventilation of a baby obviously does not approach that of an adult. Rather, we are concerned with ventilation per kilogram which is greater in the young than in adults.

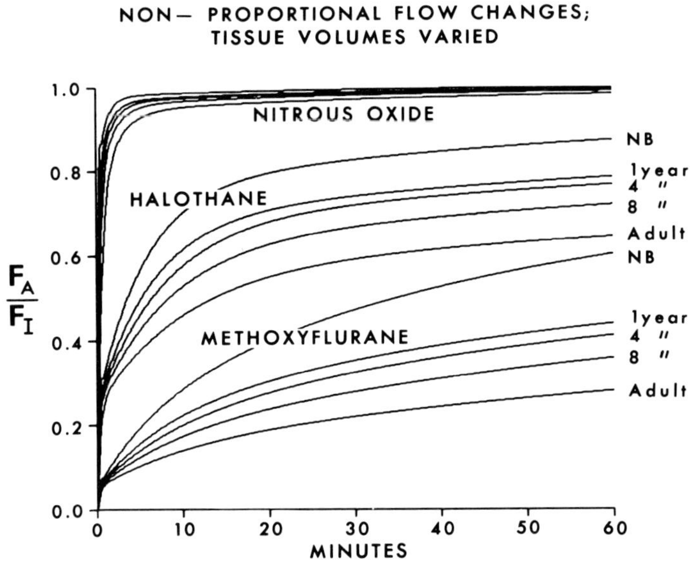

FIG. 7, 15. Figure 7, 15 like figure 7, 14 deals with the effect of proportionate increases in cardiac output and ventilation. However, in 7, 15, most of the increase in cardiac output per kilogram (4 fold in the newborn (NB), 3 fold in the 1 year old and 2 fold in the 4 year old) is directed to the VRG. This increases the impact of a given increase in cardiac output on the alveolar rate of rise. For example, the NB curves in 7, 15 have risen higher than the 18:21.6 curves in 7, 14, although in both cases the increase in cardiac output and ventilation is 4 fold. (Adapted with the permission from Eger *et al.*: Effect of age on the rate of increase of alveolar anesthetic concentration. Anesthesiology 35: 365–372, 1971.)

the newborn curve for halothane is only half again as great as the adult curve.

Figure 7, 15 suggests that anesthesia should be more rapidly induced in infants than adults, and indeed this is the usual clinical impression. A factor which works against this is the increase in MAC in the young (see fig. 1, 8). Unfortunately halothane is the only anesthetic for which the age dependent changes in MAC have been measured. If these data for halothane apply to all anesthetics, then the MAC increase should balance the accelerated alveolar rate of rise in the cases of halothane or methoxyflurane. The MAC increase actually is the dominant effect in the case of a poorly soluble agent such as nitrous oxide or cyclopropane. This ignores one other factor: the increased tissue perfusion in the young accelerates the rate of rise of the brain anesthetic partial pressure towards the partial pressure delivered from the alveoli (i.e., decreases the time constant). This, too accelerates the induction of anesthesia.

Effect of Increases in Flow Directed to the MG or FG

In contrast to the effect of increases in blood flow to the VRG, increased flow to the MG or FG may initially lower the rate of alveolar anesthetic rise (19). The lower rate of alveolar rise results from the greater extraction of anesthetic by these tissues. An extreme example illustrates this point: suppose that all anesthetic were removed from the blood traversing the MG or FG. An increase in flow to these tissues without concomitant increases in flow to the VRG then must lower the anesthetic partial pressure in central venous blood. As flow to the MG or FG increases further the mixed venous anesthetic partial pressure must approach zero. The result of such an increase is to disproportionately increase uptake (i.e., doubling cardiac output more than doubles uptake except for the first moment of anesthesia where the venous partial pressure begins at zero).

Since during anesthetic induction both muscle and fat (especially the latter) contain little or no anesthetic, they act as nearly infinite reservoirs. Note in figure 4, 7 that the anesthetic partial pressure difference between alveoli and muscle or fat is sustained for minutes to hours because of the large capacity of these tissues. Thus, a 3 to 15 fold increase in muscle blood flow may cause a *decrease* in alveolar rate of rise of halothane (fig. 7, 16). The effect does not persist since the capacity of muscle is not infinite and since the increase in muscle flow must cause a more rapid equilibration of the muscle anesthetic partial pressure with the arterial anesthetic partial pressure. The latter factor also explains why very high muscle blood flows (20 times normal) do not initially decrease the alveolar rate of rise. Such high flows cause the muscle anesthetic partial pressure to rise at a rate comparable to that achieved in the VRG.

Where may this concept apply in practice? Increased muscle activity that results from excitement during induction will produce an increase in muscle blood flow, cardiac output and ventilation. Increased muscle blood flow also will accompany parenteral infusion of a beta-sympathetic stimulant such as isoproterenol. Isoflurane anesthesia causes muscle flow to increase—and may thereby influence its own uptake (20). Finally, fasting may induce an increase in fat blood flow. Each of these increases in tissue blood flow may delay induction of anesthesia.

Summary

Changes in ventilation or circulation may profoundly alter the alveolar anesthetic rate of rise. Increases in ventilation without concomitant changes in cardiac output increase the alveolar rate of rise. The impact of a change in ventilation is greatest with the most soluble anesthetics. It would appear that induction should be accelerated by an increase in ventilation, particularly with more soluble anesthetics. However, the hypocapnea that accompanies hyperventilation may act in an opposite direction by lowering cerbral blood flow.

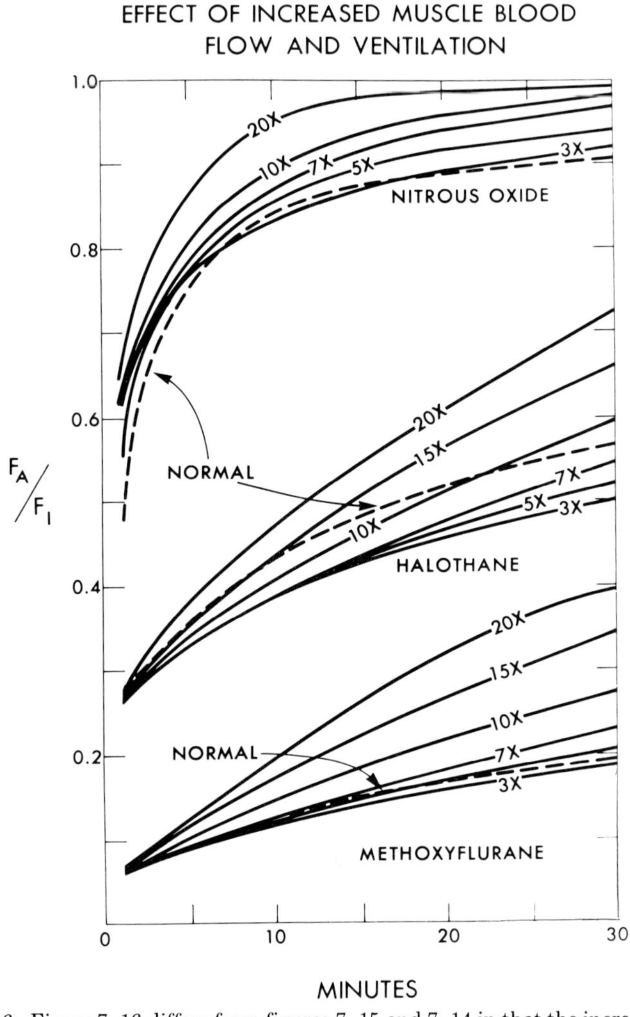

FIG. 7, 16. Figure 7, 16 differs from figures 7, 15 and 7, 14 in that the increase in cardiac output is directed only to muscle. The result is that the rate of alveolar rise may be slower than normal (normal indicated by the *dashed lines*). Thus, 3 to 15 fold increases in muscle blood flow (3× to 15×) actually may retard the rate of induction with halothane. These increases in blood flow to muscle produce the lower than normal curves because they increase the relative contribution of blood from muscle to the central venous pool. Since this contribution is relatively unsaturated, an increase in the contribution causes a disproportionate increase in uptake—and hence the slower rate of alveolar rise. (Reproduced with permission from Eger, E. I., II *et al.:* The effect of distribution of increased cardiac output on the pulmonary exchange of halothane, nitrous oxide, and methoxyflurane. Anesth. Analg., to be published.)

Anesthesia limits the height of alveolar anesthetic rise by depressing respiration. In steady state conditions, the depression of respiration restricts the input of anesthetic into the lungs to a subapnea producing level. However, during induction the delay in the cerebral perception of an alveolar concentration permits an "overshoot" of the apnea-producing alveolar concentration.

If ventilation is held constant, then raising the cardiac output tends to slow the rate of rise of the alveolar concentration, whereas lowering the output does the opposite. Again these effects relate to solubility, the changes being most pronounced with more soluble anesthetics. The effect of a reduced total cardiac output on induction depends on the participation of the cerebral blood flow in the total blood flow reduction. If the cerebral blood flow shares in the total reduction, then this retards the rate of rise of the anesthetic partial pressure in the brain and therefore opposes the effect of the accelerated alveolar rate of rise. However, if the cerebral blood flow is spared at the expense of flow to other tissues, then the perception by the brain of the accelerated alveolar rise will not be delayed and anesthetic induction should be more rapid than normal.

Certain anesthetics, in particular, halothane, depress cardiac output. This depression may exert a positive feed-back on the alveolar anesthetic rate of rise. That is, as the alveolar concentration increases, cardiac output falls, permitting a still more rapid rate of increase of the alveolar concentration. This suggests the greater safety of spontaneous respiration in the induction of an anesthetic which might depress circulation.

The patient in hemorrhagic shock suffers from a decrease in perfusion and often concomitant hyperventilation. Thus, great care must be taken to prevent an anesthetic overdose since both the change in ventilation and in circulation will tend to accelerate the alveolar anesthetic rate of rise. The difficulty in predicting how much the rate of rise should be also suggests that more soluble anesthetics should be avoided in the shock patient.

Parallel increases in ventilation and circulation exert opposing effects on anesthetic uptake. An accelerated rate of rise eventually results since the increased blood flow to tissues increases their rate of equilibration. However, the initial course of the alveolar rate of rise is determined by the distribution of the increased blood flow. If all tissues share proportionately then the alveolar concentration rises somewhat more rapidly than normal throughout induction but the difference usually is modest. If the VRG or any part thereof receives the major portion of the increased blood flow, then the alveolar concentration again is always greater than normal, but the difference may be considerable. Finally, if muscle or fat are the primary recipients of the increase in blood flow, then the initial rise in alveolar concentration may be slightly slower than normal.

QUESTIONS

1. Why does an increase in ventilation accelerate the alveolar anesthetic rate of rise? Why is the acceleration greater with more soluble anesthetics? Why is the accelerated alveolar rate of rise not necessarily reflected in the cerebral rate of rise? Why may induction with cyclopropane actually be slowed by hyperventilation?
2. Why does an increase in cardiac output hinder the alveolar anesthetic rate of rise? Why is the hinderance greater with more soluble anesthetics?
3. Using equation 12 from Chapter 4, calculate the independent effect of variations in ventilation and circulation on the F_A/F_I ratio for nitrous oxide, isoflurane, halothane and ether. First assume a cardiac output of 6 liters/minute: calculate F_A/F_I for alveolar ventilations of 2, 4, and 8 liters/minute. Second, assume an alveolar ventilation of 4 liters/minute: calculate F_A/F_I for cardiac outputs of 3, 6 and 12 liters/minute. What are the implications of the variations seen?
4. Again using equation 12 from Chapter 4, calculate the effect of concomitant variations in ventilation and circulation on alveolar concentrations of nitrous oxide, isoflurane, halothane and ether. Compare F_A/F_I ratios for an alveolar ventilation of 8 liters/minute and a cardiac output of 3 liters/minute with those ratios obtained previously when alveolar ventilation was 4 liters/minute and cardiac output 6 liters/minute. How does this apply to the patient in hemorrhagic shock? Second, calculate F_A/F_I for an alveolar ventilation of 8 liters/minute and a cardiac output of 12 liters/minute: again compare these ratios to those obtained previously for $\dot{V}_A$ equals 4 and Q equals 6 liters/minute. Do these answers imply that proportional changes in ventilation and circulation may exactly balance each other's effect on the alveolar concentration? Why, in fact is this not the case; what additional factor(s) disrupt(s) this balance?

REFERENCES

1. Eger, E. I., II: Applications of a mathematical model of gas uptake. In *Uptake and Distribution of Anesthetic Agents*, edited by E. M. Papper and R. J. Kitz, Ch. 8, pp. 88–103. McGraw-Hill, New York, 1963.
2. Severinghaus, J. W.: Role of lung factors. In *Uptake and Distribution of Anesthetic Agents*, edited by E. M. Papper and R. J. Kitz, Ch. 6, pp. 59–71. McGraw-Hill, New York, 1963.
3. Mapleson, W. W.: Quantitative Prediction of Anesthetic Concentrations. In *Uptake and Distribution of Anesthetic Agents*, edited by E. M. Papper and R. J. Kitz, Ch. 9, pp. 104–119. McGraw-Hill, New York, 1963.
4. MacKrell, T. N.: An electrical teaching model. In *Uptake and Distribution of Anesthetic Agents*, edited by E. M. Papper and R. J. Kitz, Ch. 17, pp. 215–223. McGraw-Hill, New York 1963.
5. Yamamura, H., Wakasugi, B., Okuma, Y., and Maki, K: The effects of ventilation on the absorption and elimination of inhalation anaesthetics. Anaesthesia 18: 427–438, 1963.
6. Yamamura, H.: The effect of ventilation and blood volume on the uptake and

elimination of inhalation anesthetic agents. In *Progress in Anaesthesiology*, pp. 394–399. Proceedings of the Fourth World Congress of Anaesthesiologists, Excerpta Medica International Congress Series 200, Amsterdam.

7. Munson, E. S., and Bowers, D. L.: Effects of hyperventilation on the rate of cerebral anesthetic equlibration. Anesthesiology 28: 377–381, 1967.
8. Munson, E. S., Larson, C. P., Jr., Babad, A. A., Regan, M. J., Buechel, D. R., and Eger, E. I., II: The effects of halothane fluroxene and cyclopropane on ventilation: a comparative study in man. Anesthesiology 27: 716–728, 1966.
9. Fourcade, H. E., Stevens, W. C., Larson, C. P., Jr., Cromwell, T. H., Bahlman, S. H., Hickey, R. F., Halsey, M. J., and Eger, E. I., II: Ventilatory effects of Forane—A new inhaled anesthetic. Anesthesiology 35: 26–31, 1971.
10. Munson, E. S., Eger, E. I., II, and Bowers, D. L.: Effects of anesthetic-depressed ventilation and cardiac output on anesthetic uptake. Anesthesiology 38: 251–259, 1973.)
11. Larson, C. P., Eger, E. I., II, Muallem, M., Buechel, D. R., Munson, E. S., and Eisele, J. H.: The effects of diethyl ether and methoxyflurane on ventilation: II. A comparative study in man. Anesthesiology 30: 174–184, 1969.
12. Munson, E. S., Eger, E. I., II, and Bowers, D. L.: The effects of changes in cardiac output and distribution on the rate of cerebral anesthetic equilibration: Calculations using a mathematical model. Anesthesiology 29: 533–537, 1968.
13. Rittman, W. W., and Swith, L. L.: Cerebral blood flow following severe hemorrhage. Surg. Gynec. Obstet. 123: 67–72, 1966.
14. McDowall, D. G.: Pharmacology of the cerebral circulation Int. Anesth. Clin. 7: 557–578, 1969.
15. Eger, E. I., II, Smith, N. T., Stoelting, R. K., Cullen, D. J., Kadis, L. B., and Whitcher, C. E.: Cardiovascular effects of halothane in man. Anesthesiology, 32: 396–409, 1970.
16. Ashman, M. N., Blesser, W. B., and Epstein, R. M.: A nonlinear model for the uptake and distribution of halothane in man. Anesthesiology. 33: 419–429, 1970.
17. Eger, E. I., II, Bahlman, S. H., and Munson, E. S.: Effect of age on the rate of increase of alveolar anesthetic concentration. Anesthesiology. 35: 365–372, 1971.
18. Salanitre, E., and Rackow, H.: The pulmonary exchange of nitrous oxide and halothane in infants and children. Anesthesiology 30: 388–394, 1969.
19. Eger, E. I., II, Bahlman, S. H., Halsey, M. J., and Sawyer, D. C.: The effect of distribution of increased cardiac output on the pulmonary exchange of halothane, nitrous oxide, and methoxyflurane. Anesth. Analg. To be published.
20. Cromwell, T. H., Eger, E. I., II, Stevens, W. C., and Dolan, W. M.: Forane uptake excretion and blood solubility in man. Anesthesiology 35: 401–408, 1971.

Chapter 8

Effect of Ventilation/ Perfusion Abnormalities

We have presumed that pulmonary perfusion and ventilation are perfectly matched. Thus, if the alveolar minute ventilation were 4 liters/minute and the cardiac output were 6 liters/minute, we assumed that the ratio of ventilation to perfusion would be 4:6 throughout the lung. Ventilation and perfusion need not be the same everywhere in the lung: for example, dependent lung segments receive a greater perfusion than superior segments. But in such cases we assumed that ventilation increased or decreased exactly in proportion to the increase or decrease in perfusion so that the ratio of ventilation to perfusion remained constant. Many diseases preclude such proportional changes: any condition which produces a right to left shunt (congenital cardiovascular defects, atelectasis, pneumonia) or an abnormal distribution of gas flow (emphysema) will cause disparities in ventilation/perfusion ratios between various parts of the lung.

Ventilation/perfusion abnormalities may alter anesthetic uptake in two ways: 1) they may raise the end-tidal anesthetic partial pressure and at the same time 2) they may lower the arterial anesthetic partial pressure. The alveolar (end-tidal) to arterial partial pressure difference that results indicates the presence of disparities in ventilation/perfusion ratios.

Arterial and alveolar anesthetic partial pressures are not always influenced to the same degree by ventilation/perfusion abnormalities. Since only a change in the arterial partial pressure affects the course of anesthesia, much of our subsequent discussion will describe the circumstances which influence or fail to influence the arterial anesthetic level.

Alveolar to Arterial Differences in Normal Man

The presence of pathology is not a necessary prerequisite for variations in ventilation/perfusion ratios (1, 2). Studies in young, healthy human volunteers demonstrate alveolar (end-tidal) to arterial anesthetic partial pressure differences for nitrous oxide (3), for halothane (4) and for isoflurane (5). Similarly, alveolar-arterial differences long have been known to exist for carbon dioxide and oxygen. These results indicate that variations in ventilation/perfusion ratios are present even within a normal lung. In addition, the results suggest that anesthesia itself increases such variations (2, 3).

Effects of Ventilation of Unperfused Alveoli (Dead Space Ventilation)

The differences between alveolar and arterial halothane partial pressures in the above volunteers (4) were small and could be related to the difference between the inspired and alveolar partial pressure (fig. 8, 1). This seems reasonable since a ventilated but nonperfused alveolus adds unaltered inspired gas to the end-tidal (alveolar) air. The more the

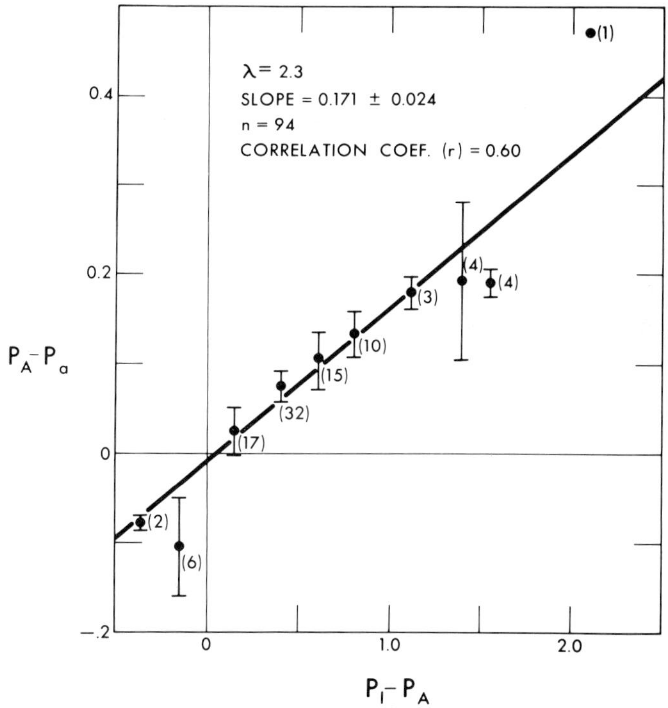

FIG. 8, 1. In human volunteers, the difference between alveolar (P_A) (end-tidal) and arterial (Pa) halothane partial pressures (*vertical axis*) relates directly to the difference between inspired (P_I) and alveolar partial pressures (*horizontal axis*). The relationship is such that P_A − Pa is about one-fifth of $P_I - P_A$. *Numbers* indicate number of samples at each point—*bars* indicate standard error of the mean. Pressure is in percent of 1 atmosphere. (Reproduced with permission from Eger, E. I., II, and Bahlman, S. H.: Is the end-tidal anesthetic partial pressure an accurate measure of the arterial anesthetic partial pressure? Anesthesiology 35: 301–303, 1971.)

inspired anesthetic concentration exceeds the alveolar concentration in perfused alveoli, the greater the effect of the contribution of the unperfused alveoli on the combined end-tidal gas. For example, suppose that the inspired anesthetic is 2 volumes percent and that four-fifths of the inspired gas reaches perfused alveoli. Suppose that uptake of half of the anesthetic leaves 1 volume percent in the alveoli (which is in equilibrium with the arterial anesthetic partial pressure if we assume no barrier to diffusion). Suppose that the remaining one-fifth of the inspired gas is directed to unperfused alveoli. On exhalation the gases from the perfused and unperfused alveoli mix, producing $0.8 \times 1 + 0.2 \times 2$ or 1.2 volumes percent in the end-tidal gas—a partial pressure 20 percent greater than that in arterial blood. Now consider how much greater the difference is if the anesthetic uptake and hence the inspired to end-tidal difference is larger. Suppose that the inspired anesthetic now is 5 volumes percent and that uptake removes four-fifths of this—again leaving 1 volume percent in perfused alveoli. If these perfused alveoli receive four-fifths of the ventilation then one-fifth of the inspired 5 volumes percent reaches unperfused alveoli. The resulting end-tidal concentration is $0.8 \times 1 + 0.2 \times 5$ or 1.8 volumes percent giving a partial pressure 80 percent greater than that in arterial blood. These examples suggest that the greater uptake associated with higher solubility produces a greater end-tidal to arterial partial pressure difference.

Should these end-tidal to arterial differences influence the rate of rise of the arterial anesthetic partial pressure—and hence the course of anesthesia? If we assume that arterial CO_2 remains normal with or without ventilation/perfusion abnormalities then ventilation of the perfused alveoli must be unchanged. This means that although additional ventilation is required to ventilate the unperfused alveoli (alveolar dead-space ventilation) it does not influence the effective ventilation and hence does not alter the arterial anesthetic rate of rise.

Effect of Perfusion of Unventilated Alveoli (Shunting)

If $PaCO_2$ is unchanged, ventilation of unperfused alveoli does not alter the course of anesthesia, but the reverse—the perfusion of unventilated alveoli—may have a considerable effect despite constancy of $PaCO_2$. If $PaCO_2$ is to continue unchanged, then perfusion of unventilated alveoli presumes an overventilation of the remaining perfused alveoli. This overventilation must raise the end-tidal concentration of anesthetic. On the other hand, no anesthetic is added to the blood perfusing unventilated alveoli, and such blood must lower the average arterial anesthetic partial pressure. Both of these ventilation/perfusion abnormalities (hyperventilation relative to perfusion and perfusion without ventilation) cause an end-tidal to arterial anesthetic partial pressure difference.

Although a difference appears with all anesthetics, not all anesthetics are affected in the same way. The arterial partial pressure of the more soluble anesthetics increases at a normal rate, but the alveolar partial pressure increases more rapidly than normal (fig. 8, 2). The reverse is true of poorly soluble anesthetics: the increase in alveolar concentration is only slightly faster than normal, while the increase in arterial anesthetic partial pressure is far slower (6). Since it is the arterial anesthetic partial pressure which raises the tissue partial pressures, this means that ventilation/perfusion abnormalities will delay the rate of induction of poorly soluble anesthetics but will have little effect on induction with highly soluble anesthetics. This does not mean that induction with, say, ether, will be accelerated; only that it will not be retarded.

Why this influence of solubility? Why do these ventilation/perfusion abnormalities scarcely affect the arterial rate of rise of ether while significantly affecting cyclopropane? To explain this difference imagine a patient without and then with ventilation/perfusion abnormalities. Without ventilation/perfusion abnormalities, his alveolar and arterial

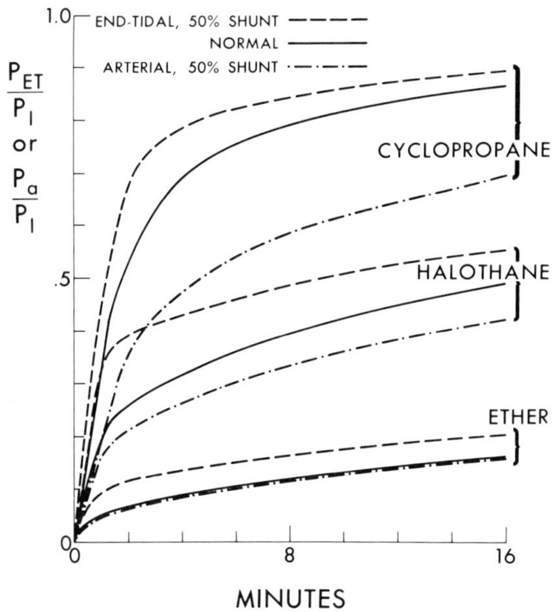

FIG. 8, 2. When no ventilation/perfusion abnormalities exist then the alveolar (P_A or P_{ET}) and arterial (P_a) anesthetic partial pressures increase together (*continuous lines*) toward the inspired partial pressure (P_I). When 50 percent of the cardiac output is shunted through the lungs then the rate of rise of the end-tidal partial pressure (*dashed lines*) is accelerated while the rate of rise of the arterial partial pressure (*dot-dashed lines*) is retarded. The greatest retardation is found with the least soluble anesthetic, cyclopropane.

anesthetic partial pressures increase at identical rates as indicated by the continuous lines in figure 8, 2. But suppose that anesthesia begins with thiopental, succinylcholine and intubation of the right main stem bronchus. The alveolar ventilation now goes to only one lung, thereby doubling its ventilation. The circulation remains equally divided between the ventilated and nonventilated lungs. The greater ventilation to the intubated side produces a more rapid alveolar anesthetic rate of rise (highest line for each anesthetic in fig. 8, 2). The acceleration is small for a poorly soluble anesthetic (cyclopropane) but relatively large for a highly soluble anesthetic (ether) (see fig. 7, 1 for the relative effects of ventilatory changes on alveolar rate of rise). Since the alveolar cyclopropane concentration is scarcely affected by the augmented ventilation, the cyclopropane partial pressure in the blood passing that lung also is scarcely changed from normal. This blood is then diluted by blood from the unventilated lung, blood to which no cyclopropane has been added in its passage through the lungs. Such dilution lowers the arterial cyclopropane partial pressure to well below normal (lowest of the cyclopropane curves). In contrast, the alveolar and hence the arterial ether concentration from the ventilated lung may be nearly twice normal. The dilution by an equal volume of ether-deficient blood from the unventilated lung cannot lower this to a concentration significantly below normal (lowest curve, fig. 8, 2).

The reason for the influence of solubility may be seen from another view. Since little of a poorly soluble agent is taken up, variations in ventilation cannot appreciably affect its uptake. The converse is true of highly soluble agents: almost all the agent which enters the lung is taken up, and doubling ventilation may double uptake. It follows that doubling ventilation cannot compensate for a decrease in the fraction of the cardiac output exposed to a poorly soluble agent but can compensate for such a decrease with a highly soluble agent.

The "boxes" in figure 8, 3 further illustrate this effect. Twelve volumes percent of an agent with a blood/gas partition coefficient of 0.5 is introduced into a lung where ventilation and perfusion are equal (*A*). Equilibration produces an arterial concentration of 4 volumes percent. If one bronchus is blocked, all ventilation is directed to the remaining lung perfused by half the cardiac output (*B*). Equilibrium then results in a 4.8 percent arterial anesthetic concentration which is diluted to 2.4 volumes percent by the blood from the unventilated lung (added empty square). Notice that this is 60 percent (100 times 2.4/4) of normal. When a highly soluble gas (blood/gas partition coefficient of 10) is used, (*C* and *D*) then equilibration without ventilation/perfusion abnormalities gives a blood concentration of 10.9 volumes percent (*C*). Halving the blood exposed to the same total ventilation (*D*) produces a blood concentration of 20

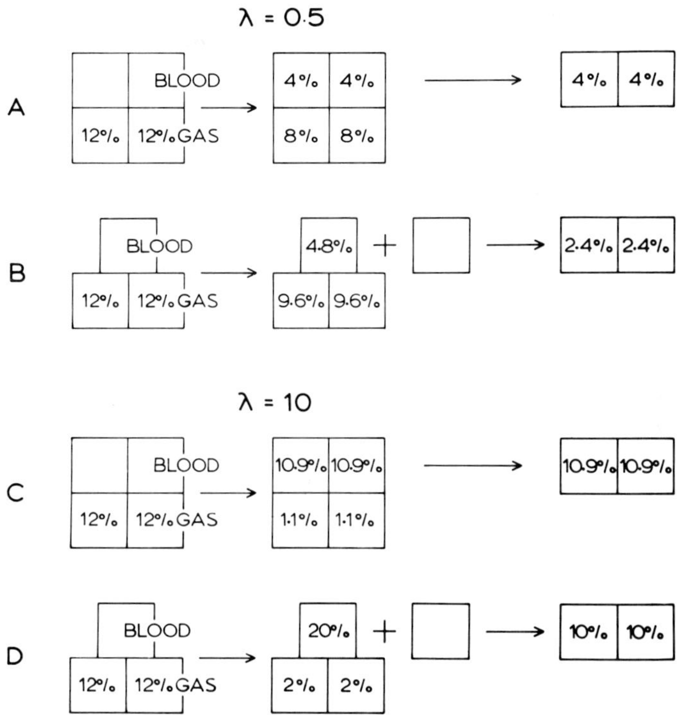

FIG. 8, 3. In all cases, 12 volumes percent of anesthetic are introduced into the lungs (*lower left boxes*). *A* and *C* illustrate the equilibrium which results between blood (*upper boxes*) and lung gas (*lower boxes*) in the absence of ventilation/perfusion abnormalities, while *B* and *D* illustrate the equilibrium which results when half of the cardiac output is unventilated. The *single empty boxes* in *B* and *D* indicate the unventilated venous blood. Note that the absence of anesthetic in the returning venous blood would only occur at the start of anesthesia. The final arterial concentration (*far right*) results from the combination of the ventilated and unventilated fractions of the cardiac output. The final concentration is greatly affected by ventilation/perfusion abnormalities when the blood/gas partition coefficient is 0.5 (*B* versus *A*) but little affected when the coefficient is 10 (*D* and *C*).

volumes percent—nearly twice normal—a concentration that is reduced to 10 volumes percent by recombination with the shunted blood. But 10 volumes percent is 92 percent of normal (100 times 10/10.9). Contrast this with the reduction to 60 percent of normal produced with the poorly soluble gas.

Stoelting and Longnecker (7) have verified the above predictions in dogs and in man. In dogs they measured the rate of rise of arterial cyclopropane, halothane and methoxyflurane in the presence and in the absence (control values) of a shunt produced by an endotracheal blocker. $PaCO_2$ was the same with and without the shunt. The rate of rise of the least soluble agent, cyclopropane, was considerably slowed by the presence of the shunt while the rate of rise of the most soluble agent, methoxyflurane, was unaffected (fig. 8, 4). The halothane rate of rise lay between the rates for cyclopropane and methoxyflurane. The effect of shunting on the rate of rise of arterial halothane also was measured in 3 humans before and after (control values) correction of tetralogy of Fallot. The rate of rise was slower in the presence of the tetralogy (fig. 8, 5).

Effect of Shunting of Blood Through the Body

Let us restore ventilation/perfusion ratios to normal and turn our attention from the lung to the body. Left to right shunts of blood occur in congenital cardiovascular defects or iatrogenically or pathologically produced arteriovenous fistulae. What is the effect of such shunts? We may consider several possibilities. If cardiac output remains constant then shunting blood must reduce tissue perfusion. The shunted blood cannot affect anesthetic uptake since it contains the same anesthetic partial pressure as that in the lungs. That is, when it returns to the lungs it cannot accept more anesthetic (unless the alveolar partial pressure has risen). Thus, shunting blood at a constant total cardiac output reduces the effective cardiac output in a manner identical to that illustrated in figure 6, 8: diverting two-thirds of a 6 liter/minute cardiac output

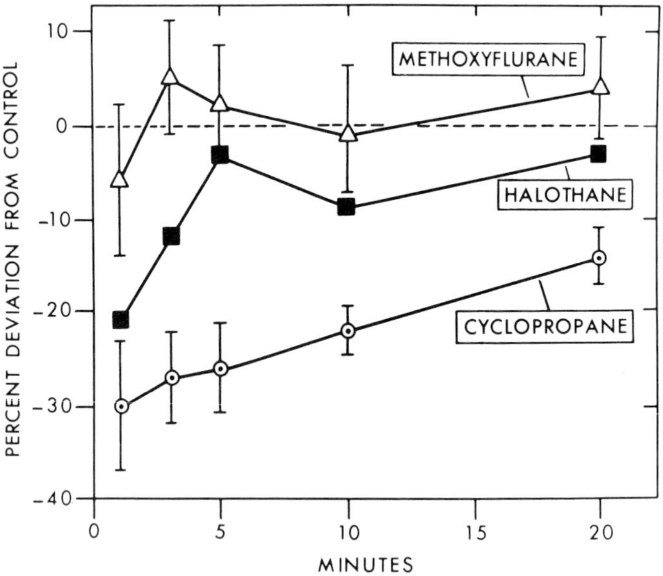

FIG. 8, 4. These graphs illustrate the percent deviation from a normal (control) arterial anesthetic rate of rise induced in dogs by introduction of an endobronchial blocker. Note the decreasing effect with increasing solubility. (Reproduced with permission from Stoelting, R. K., and Longnecker, D. E.: Effect of right-to-left shunt on rate of increase in arterial anesthetic concentration. Anesthesiology 36: 352–356, 1972.)

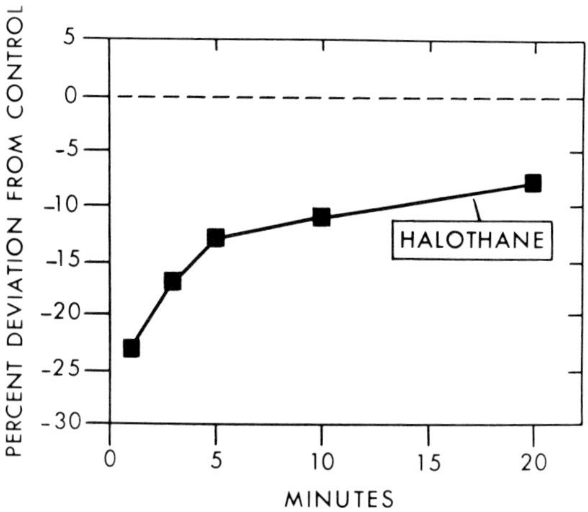

FIG. 8, 5. The arterial halothane rate of rise in 3 children was measured before and after (control) correction of Tetralogy of Fallot. The percent deviation of the "before" values from the "after" values is illustrated here. (Reproduced with permission from Stoelting, R. K., and Longnecker, D. E.: Effect of right-to-left shunt on rate of increase in arterial anesthetic concentration. Anesthesiology 36: 352–356, 1972.)

through a shunt reduces tissue perfusion to 2 liters/minute. The result is a more rapid rate of rise of the alveolar anesthetic partial pressure and a slower rate of rise in the tissues. This is readily seen at the extreme represented by diversion of all blood through the shunt: tissue uptake (and therefore, total uptake) must be zero and the alveolar rate of rise must be a function of the lung washin rate.

But significant tissue hypoperfusion is unlikely: the local control of vascular resistance assures maintenance of a tissue blood flow which satisfies local metabolic needs. If a left to right shunt is superimposed on a normal tissue perfusion, what happens to anesthetic uptake? The answer is: "Nothing." No anesthetic can be added to the fully equilibrated shunted blood. Since the shunted blood already has equilibrated with the alveolar anesthetic partial pressure it cannot further influence that pressure.

This is illustrated by the "boxes" in figure 8, 6 for an anesthetic with a blood/gas partition coefficient (λ) of 1. In the lower part of *A*, 10 volumes percent of anesthetic is inspired. In *B*, the 10 volumes percent equilibrate with an equal volume of blood (Q normal) to produce (*C*), an alveolar and blood concentration of 5 volumes percent. In the lower part of *D*, 10 volumes again are inspired. This is identical to *A*. However, in *D*, the blood comes from two sources: half from the tissues (Q normal, no anesthetic) and half from recirculation through a shunt (Q shunt). The latter blood contains the same concentration of anesthetic as it possessed when it left the lung. As we shall see, this equals 5 volumes percent. The

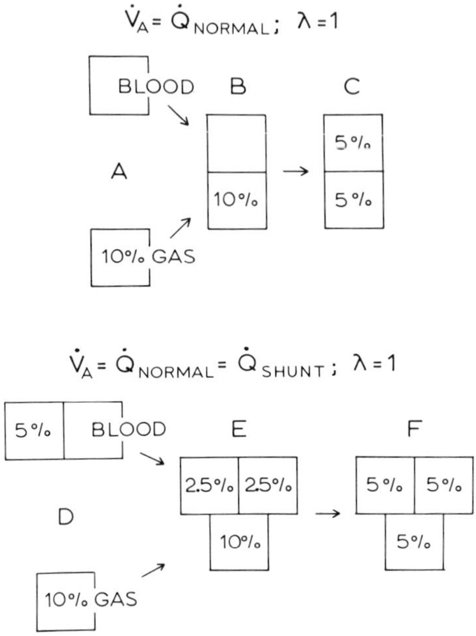

FIG. 8, 6. In the absence of any alteration in tissue blood flow (*unfilled boxes* in *A* and *D*) there is no effect of the addition of a left to right shunt (5% box in *D*) on the final alveolar or arterial anesthetic concentration. In this example, 10 volumes percent of an anesthetic is inspired (10% box in *A* and *D*) and equilibrates with blood (*B* and *E*). As required by a blood solubility of 1, equilibration produces an equal alveolar or arterial concentration of 5 volumes percent in both *C* and *F*.

flow through the tissues, flow through the shunt, and alveolar ventilation (V_A) all are equal. By the time the blood reaches the lungs (*E*), the anesthetic has distributed evenly to produce a concentration of 2½ volumes percent. Equilibration results in a 5 volumes percent concentration in both gas and blood. Note that this is identical to the concentration achieved in *C* without the shunt.

However, a left to right (body) shunt *can* influence uptake in the presence of a right to left (lung) shunt (8)! A body shunt antagonizes the reduction in arterial anesthetic partial pressure caused by the lung shunt. Why is this? How do two abnormalities combine to produce a more normal arterial anesthetic rate of rise? Addition of a body shunt to a normal tissue perfusion increases total cardiac output. Assume that a lung shunt diverts a constant *fraction* of the pulmonary blood flow away from ventilated lung. Thus, an increase in total cardiac output must increase the flow of blood through both ventilated and nonventilated portions of the lung. The increased flow through the ventilated lung contains blood returning from the tissues plus blood passing through the body (fig. 8, 7). Recirculation of unventilated blood through the body

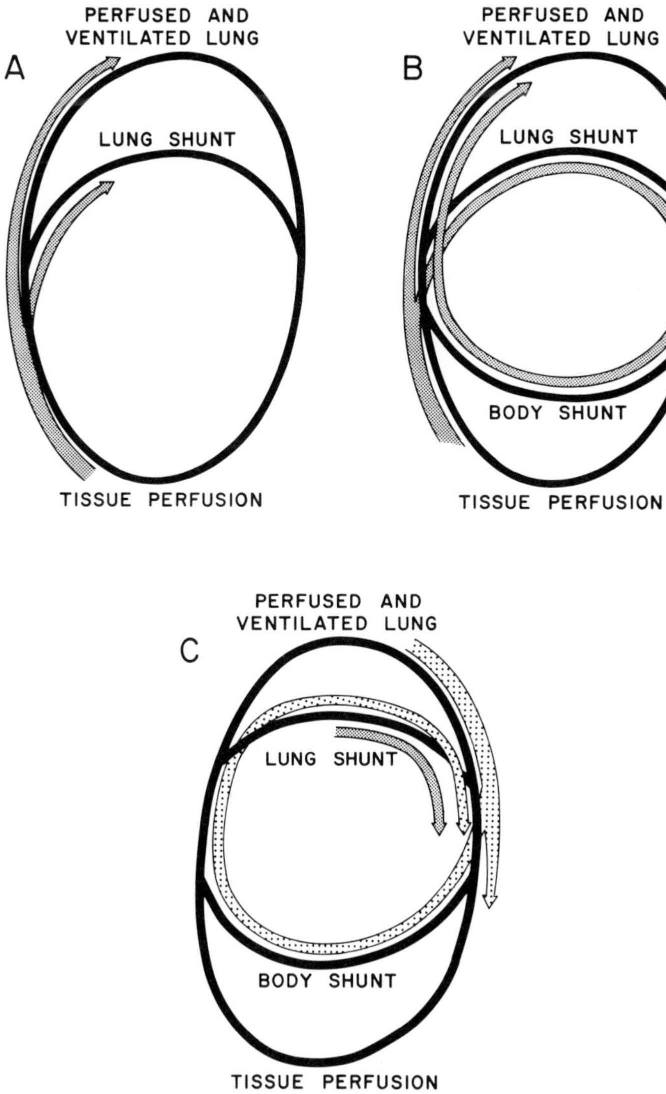

FIG. 8, 7. The *two heavy black lines* at the top of each drawing indicate the path blood flow might follow in the lungs: the uppermost to ventilated alveoli and the lower to a lung shunt. In *A*, all blood passes through the tissues (*the third, lowest path*). The blood which returns to the lungs from the tissues (*heavy stippled arrows*) will flow through ventilated lung or lung shunt. The blood from the tissues which fails to be ventilated before its return to the tissues is determined by the fraction of blood shunted through the lungs. In *B* and *C* a shunt path through the body has been added (*next to lowest path, black line*). As indicated in *B*, blood from the tissues which initially failed to pass ventilated lung may be so before its return to the tissues by recirculation through the body shunt. The result is that a greater fraction of blood returning to the body has been ventilated. The other side of the coin is shown in *C*. Blood leaving the lung (*light stippled arrows*) may either return to the tissues or recirculate through the body shunt and then through the lung shunt. The addition of this blood to the lung shunt blood dilutes the unventilated blood which passes through the lung shunt—that is, it increases the fraction of ventilated blood returning to the tissues. (Reproduced with permission from Saidman, L. J., and Eger, E. I., II: Influence of a left-to-right shunt on uptake in the presence of a shunt through the lungs. To be published.)

shunt therefore increases the delivery of blood from the tissues to the ventilated portion of the lungs. That is, the body shunt gives a portion of the unventilated blood (that passes through the lung shunt) a second (and third and more) passage through the lungs where it may equilibrate with the ventilated lung segment.

The fraction of the tissue blood flow which actually passes through ventilated lung (F_{VL}) is a function of both the fraction of cardiac output shunted through the lungs (S_L) and the fraction of cardiac output shunted through the body (S_B) (8). F_{VL} may be determined as:

$$F_{VL} = (1 - S_L)/(1 - S_B S_L)$$

The equation may be altered to give the apparent lung shunt, S_{Lapp}.

$$S_{Lapp} = 1 - F_{VL} = S_L\,(1 - S_B)/(1 - S_B S_L)$$

The apparent lung shunt indicates the effectiveness of the lung shunt in the presence of a body shunt. For example, if 20 percent of the cardiac output was shunted through the lungs (S_L equals 0.2) then a body shunt of 50 percent (S_B equals 0.5) would produce an apparent lung shunt of 0.11. That is, the effect of the lung shunt would be reduced from 20 percent to 11 percent. These relationships are indicated in figure 8, 8. When the body shunt is zero then the apparent and true lung shunts are

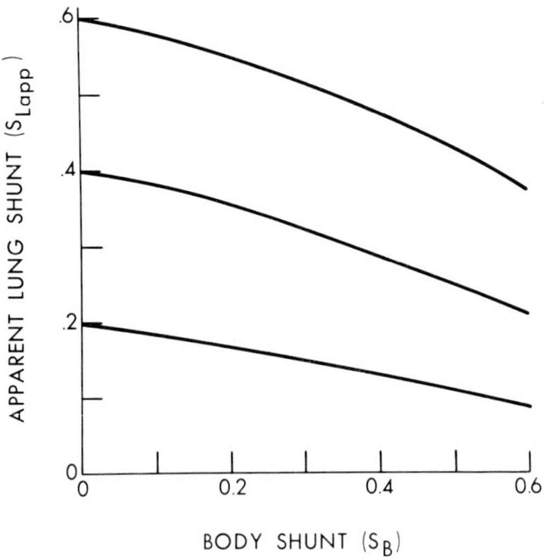

FIG. 8, 8. When the body shunt (S_B) is zero, the lung shunt (S_L) and apparent lung shunt (S_{Lapp}) are equal. The apparent lung shunt (but not S_L) is reduced by a body shunt. As the body shunt approaches 100 percent, the apparent lung shunt approaches zero. (Reproduced with permission from Saidman, L. J., and Eger, E. I., II: Influence of a left-to-right shunt on uptake in the presence of a shunt through the lungs. To be published.)

equal. As the body shunt increases then the apparent lung shunt falls. The effect of the body shunt is relatively greater on the smaller lung shunt. In the above example, the apparent lung shunt was nearly halved (0.2 to 0.11) by a body shunt of 50 percent. However, if the lung shunt (S_L) were 0.6, then a body shunt of 50 percent would reduce the apparent lung shunt by less than one-third (0.6 to 0.42). That is, a body shunt more effectively reduces the effect of a small lung shunt than a large one.

The effect of a body shunt is familiar in another form. A shunt through the lung reduces oxygenation of arterial blood. This condition can be improved without changing the lung shunt by increasing cardiac output. Presuming constancy of body metabolism, increasing cardiac output is directly analogous to adding a body shunt (and in fact, adding a body shunt without altering tissue perfusion will have the same effect on arterial oxygenation). The reason for the improvement in arterial oxygenation is illustrated in figure 8, 7*C*.

Where do body and lung shunts occur simultaneously? Congenital defects form one group. Perhaps septic shock with high output forms another. Fortunately such examples are infrequently encountered in anesthetic practice. However, it may be that combined body and lung shunts of a modest nature exist in us all. We have noted that ventilation/perfusion abnormalities are present in healthy volunteers (see above: "Alveolar to Arterial Differences in Normal Man"). Body shunting also may occur in normal man and furthermore may be augmented by anesthesia. For example, the increase in cutaneous blood flow that attends anesthesia is sufficient to arterialize peripheral venous

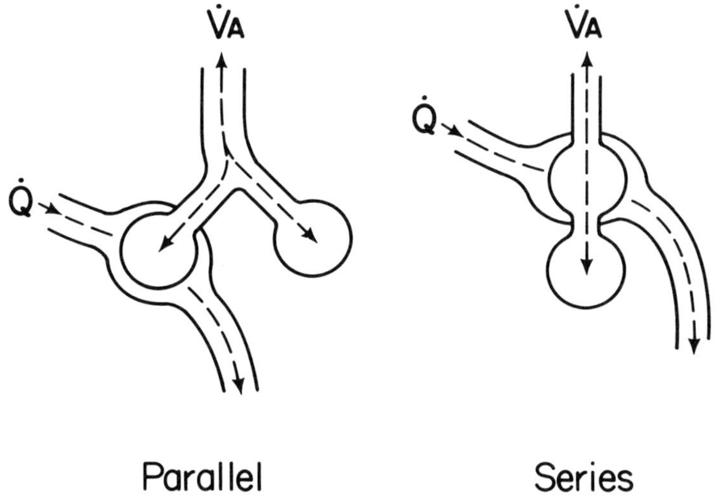

FIG. 8, 9. This figure illustrates the difference between one type of parallel and series ventilation/perfusion abnormalities. $\dot{Q}$ is cardiac output and $\dot{V}_A$ is alveolar ventilation.

blood (9). This increase in cutaneous blood flow is probably through shunts normally used to regulate heat loss. Here may be another example of anesthesia influencing its own uptake.

Other Causes of Effects of Ventilation/Perfusion Abnormalities

Ventilation/perfusion abnormalities may be caused in ways that differ from those noted above. We have assumed parallel ventilation/perfusion abnormalities but these abnormalities also may occur in series (fig. 8, 9). Peter Wagner (unpublished data) has calculated that such abnormalities should have little effect on inert gas exchange.

We have ignored the oscillatory nature of ventilatory exchange after noting (Chapter 4, fig. 4, 1) that tidal volumes in the physiological range produce lung washout or washin curves that are close to those produced by continuous flow through the lungs. However, the relationship of inspiration to peak pulmonary blood flow can affect the arterial anesthetic partial pressure (10). This effect, like the effect of in series abnormalities, is likely to be small.

Summary

Ventilation/perfusion abnormalities exist in normal man as well as in pathological states. Such abnormalities influence both the alveolar and arterial anesthetic rates of rise. Ventilation of unperfused alveoli has little effect on the rate of arterial anesthetic rise, although it may raise the end-tidal anesthetic concentration. Perfusion of unventilated alveoli may hinder the arterial rate of rise, particularly of less soluble anesthetics. Shunting of blood through the body is not likely to influence anesthetic uptake *except* in the presence of a lung shunt. A body shunt diminishes the impact of a lung shunt on uptake.

QUESTIONS

1. Why do ventilation/perfusion ratios vary in different parts of a normal lung? What pathological conditions may increase this variability?
2. What do ventilation/perfusion abnormalities do to the end-tidal anesthetic partial pressure? To the arterial anesthetic partial pressure?
3. What is the effect of perfusion of unventilated alveoli on the arterial anesthetic rate of rise? (Again assume that $PaCO_2$ is kept normal.)
5. Will perfusion of unventilated alveoli more affect induction with isoflurane or with methoxyflurane?
6. In the absence of a shunting of blood through the lung how may a left to right shunt affect induction of anesthesia?
7. Prove that even if the shunted blood in figure 8, 6 initially contained no anesthetic that it would soon reach 5 volumes percent (note that the shunted blood must come from the blood equilibrated in *F*; recycle this blood through

D and *E* to arrive at your answer). Prove the same thing when the shunted blood initially contains 10 volumes percent.

8. How does a left to right shunt (sustained normal tissue blood flow) reduce the effect of a shunt through the lung on induction of anesthesia?

REFERENCES

1. West, J. B., and Dollery, C. T.: Distribution of blood flow and the pressure-flow relations of the whole lung. J. Appl. Physiol. 20: 175–183, 1965.
2. Halands, G. H., Greene, R., Iliff, L. D., and Nunn, J. F.: Influence of anaesthesia on the regional distribution of perfusion and ventilation in the lung. Clin. Sci. 38: 451–460, 1970.
3. Eger, E. I., II, Babad, A. A., Regan, M. J., Larson, C. P., Jr., Shargel, R., and Severinghaus, J. W.: Delayed approach of arterial to alveolar nitrous oxide partial pressures in dog and man. Anesthesiology 27: 288–297, 1966.
4. Eger, E. I., II, and Bahlman, S. H.: Is the end-tidal anesthetic partial pressure an accurate measure of the arterial anesthetic partial pressure? Anesthesiology 35: 301–303, 1971.
5. Cromwell, T. H., Eger, E. I., II, Stevens, W. C., and Dolan, W. M.: Forane uptake excretion and blood solubility in man. Anesthesiology 35: 401–408, 1971.
6. Eger, E. I., II, and Severinghaus, J. W.: Effect of uneven pulmonary distribution of blood and gas on induction with inhalation anesthetics. Anesthesiology 25: 620–626, 1964.
7. Stoelting, R. K., and Longnecker, D. E.: Effect of right-to-left shunt on rate of increase in arterial anesthetic concentration. Anesthesiology, 36: 352–356, 1972.
8. Saidman, L. J., and Eger, E. I., II: Influence of a left-to-right shunt on uptake in the presence of a shunt through the lungs. To be published.
9. France, C. J., Eger, El II, and Bendixen, H. H.: The use of peripheral venous blood for pH and carbon dioxide tension determinations during general anesthesia. Anesthesiology 40: 311–314, 1974.
10. Suwa, K., and Bendixen, H. H.: Pulmonary gas exchange in a tidally ventilated single alveolus model. J. Appl. Physiol. 32: 834–841, 1972.

Chapter 9

Changes in Solubility

We have assumed that solubility of any one anesthetic in a particular solvent remains constant. But in fact, solubility may vary and such variations can affect anesthetic uptake. Three factors may alter solubility: 1) a change in solvent constituents; 2) a change in temperature; and 3) a deviation from Henry's Law.

Effect of Changes in Blood Constituents

Anesthetics usually are more attracted to lipids or proteins than water. Thus, a reduction in blood lipid or protein can decrease anesthetic solubility in blood. A lower serum albumin decreases halothane blood solubility (1). Anemia, through a reduction in hemoglobin and in the proteins and lipids forming red cells likewise may reduce blood solubility (1–4). However, the effect of anemia is surprisingly variable (fig. 9, 1). A reduction in hematocrit produced by dilution of red cells with plasma causes an increase in solubility of methoxyflurane, diethyl ether and perhaps halothane (3). The solubility increases because these anesthetics have a greater affinity for plasma proteins than for red blood cells. Were the hematocrit lowered by dilution with saline, both methoxyflurane and halothane—and perhaps ether—would show a lower blood solubility. Hyperlipemia invariably raises blood solubility (2, 5). Thus, the patient who has recently eaten has a higher blood/gas partition coefficient than the usual patient who has fasted for 12 or more hours.

An increase in blood solubility without any change in tissue solubility will slow the rate at which halothane increases in the alveoli (fig. 9, 2). Also depicted in figure 9, 2 is the rate of rise of the halothane partial pressure in the vessel rich group. Despite a 16 fold variation in the blood/gas partition coefficient, the anesthetic partial pressure in the vessel rich group rises at about the same rate for the first 10 to 30 minutes of anesthesia. After 10 to 30 minutes, the anesthetic levels diverge.

The similarity of the initial increases in vessel rich group anesthetic partial pressures results from changes in the tissue time constant which oppose the effect of the changes in alveolar rate of rise. A change in blood

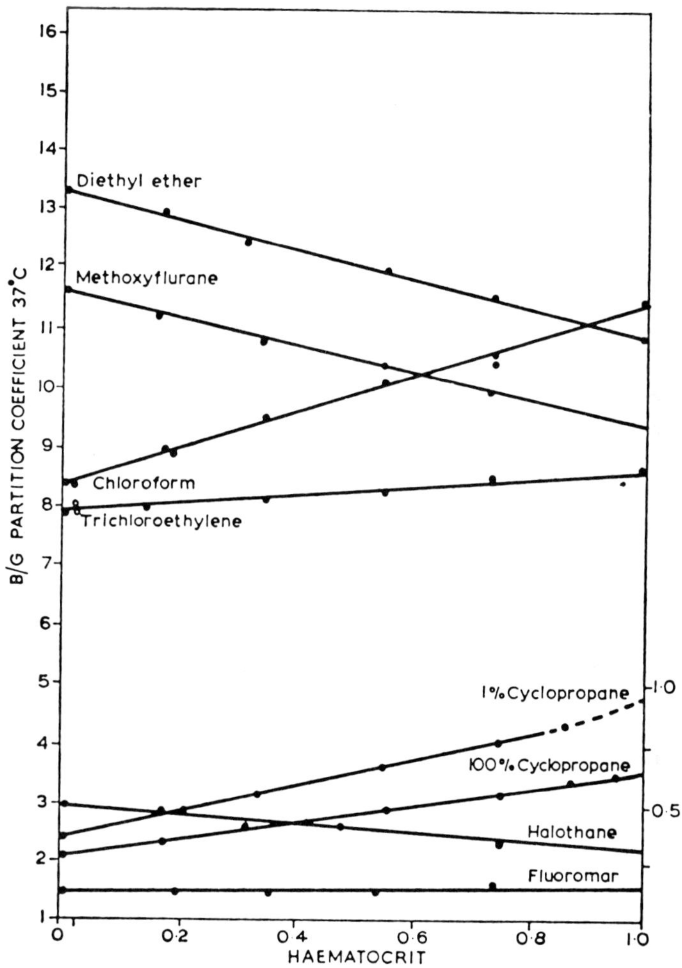

FIG. 9, 1. These graphs illustrate the effect of changes in hematocrit on blood/gas partition coefficients. Note that the ordinate scale for cyclopropane is to the right while that for the remaining anesthetics is to the left. (Reproduced with permission from Lowe, H. J., and Hagler, K: Determination of volatile organic anaesthetics in blood, gases, tissues and lipids: partition coefficients. In *Gas Chromatography in Biology and Medicine*, A Ciba Foundation Symposium, edited by Ruth Porter, pp. 86–112, J & A Churchill, Ltd., London, 1969.)

solubility alters the tissue time constant by altering the capacity of tissue relative to blood to hold anesthetics. Remember that the time constant is the time required for the flow through a container to equal the capacity of the container. If we double the solubility in blood relative to tissue (that is, halve the tissue/blood partition coefficient) then we halve the relative tissue capacity for that anesthetic. This doubling of blood solubility

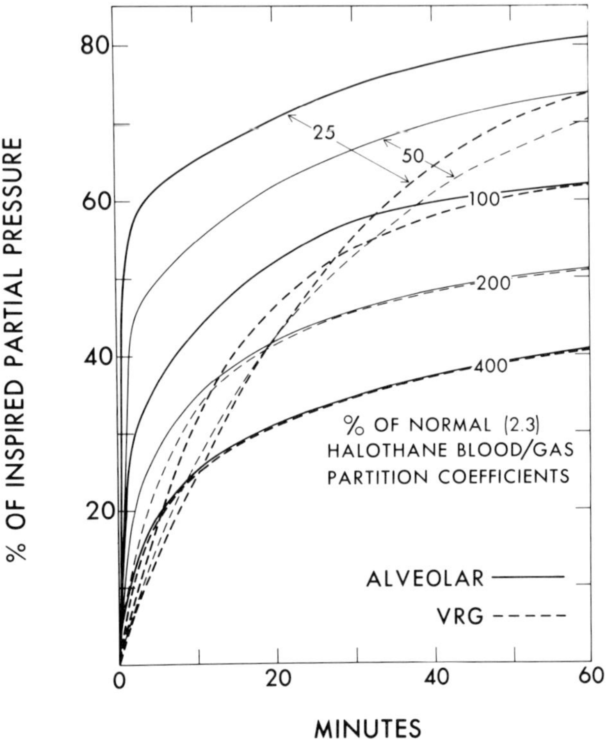

FIG. 9, 2. An increase in blood solubility slows the alveolar halothane rate of rise (*continuous lines*) while a decrease does the opposite. Although the vessel rich group rate of rise (*dashed lines*) eventually is similarly affected, the results in the first 10 to 30 minutes do not differ greatly from the 16 fold variation in blood solubility. All graphs are plotted as percent of the inspired halothane partial pressure. Tissue solubility is unchanged from normal.

slows the alveolar rate of rise but by halving the tissue time constant the higher blood solubility permits a more rapid approach of the tissue anesthetic partial pressure towards that in the alveoli. This figure suggests that the time required for induction with halothane may not be altered greatly by changes in blood solubility, although the depth achieved after 10 to 30 minutes may be considerably affected.

An increase in blood solubility may be simulated in the hydraulic model (Chapter 5, figs. 5, 4; 5, 5 and 5, 6) by changing the cross-sectional areas of the pipes leading from lung to tissues without changing the size of the tissue reservoirs: tripling the blood/gas partition coefficient triples the cross-section, while reducing the coefficient to one-third reduces the cross-section a like amount. Notice that the effect of a change in blood solubility is identical to the effect of a change in cardiac output (compare figs. 5, 6 and 5, 8). This is evident from the hydraulic models where the cross-section of the pipes conducting anesthetic to the tissues is the product of cardiac output times blood solubility. Thus, the impact of halving blood solubility is portrayed for both poorly soluble (cyclopropane) and highly soluble (methoxyflurane) agents as well as moderately soluble agents (halothane) by figure 7, 10. For cyclopropane the alveolar anesthetic rate of rise is scarcely affected by halving solubility (i.e., halving cardiac output) but the brain rate of rise is considerably slowed. With methoxyflurane the alveolar anesthetic rate of rise is sufficiently accelerated to exactly compensate for the decreased cerebral blood flow and thus the initial brain rate of rise is normal.

Effect of Changes in Tissue Constituents

Changes in tissue solubility may occur without change in blood solubility. For example, adiposity increases muscle solubility by the infiltration of muscle with fat. Note that this implies a greater muscle solubility in women than in men. The opposite may be true in the very young: the neonate has less fat than the adult and less infiltration of lean tissues with such fat. Changes in tissue solubility without concomitant changes in blood solubility may be simulated in the hydraulic model by altering only the capacity of the tissue reservoirs: a doubling of solubility doubles the cross-section of these reservoirs and a halving, halves them.

Like the effect of an increase in blood solubility, an increase in tissue solubility slows the alveolar anesthetic rate of rise (fig. 9, 3). However, as opposed to the effect of an increase in blood solubility, the increase in tissue solubility lengthens the time constant and thereby adds to the delay in the anesthetic partial pressure rise in the VRG and other tissues. This suggests that induction is particularly prolonged by an increase in tissue solubility if the increase extends to the brain. With or without a change in brain solubility, the eventual depth of anesthesia produced by a given inspired concentration is reduced by an increase in solubility in other tissues.

The effect of a change in tissue solubility on the alveolar or brain anesthetic rate of rise depends on the initial solubility. An increase in tissue solubility can only slightly reduce the alveolar rate of rise of a poorly soluble anesthetic: the blood/gas partition coefficient sets a limit on the effect of even an infinite increase in tissue solubility (see fig. 4, 6). Of course, the longer time constant associated with an increase in tissue solubility must delay the tissue rate of rise. If brain solubility is altered, this too will alter the time for anesthetic induction. The effect of the lengthened time constant is exaggerated in a highly soluble anesthetic by the concomitant decrease in the alveolar rate of rise.

Temperature Changes and Solubility

Body temperature often deviates from normal in the surgical patient. Fever may result from infections that must be drained. Mild hypo-

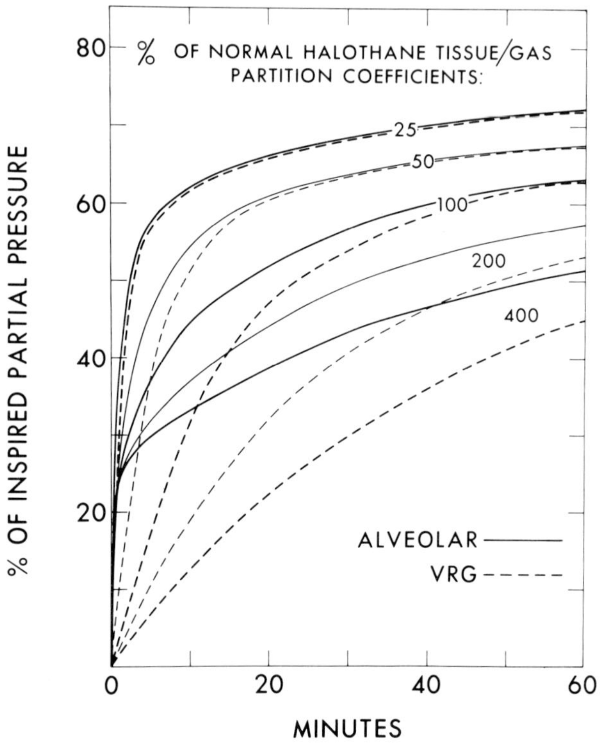

FIG. 9, 3. These graphs depict the changes in the alveolar (*continuous lines*) and vessel rich group (*dashed lines*) anesthetic partial pressures with changing tissue solubility. Tissue solubility at "100 percent of normal" is that of halothane. Changes in solubility from "100 percent" are distributed proportionately: if the solubility in muscle doubles, then solubility in fat and the vessel rich group likewise doubles. Halothane blood/gas partition coefficient remains at 2.3 at all levels of tissue solubility. Alveolar and brain anesthetic partial pressures are plotted as the percent of the inspired partially pressure.

thermia may accompany profound preoperative sedation or may occur in the infant with exposure to the frigid air of the operating suite. Intraoperative hypothermia is probably more common than normothermia. The cutaneous vasodilation, the infusion of cold fluids, and the reduced metabolism caused by most anesthetics all act to lower body temperature.

A decrease in temperature increases blood/gas (fig. 9, 4) (1, 3, 4, 6, 7) and tissue/gas (4) partition coefficients. A decrease in solubility with a decrease in temperature has not been observed in clinically used anesthetics but is known to occur with a few gases (for example, nitrogen) in media such as olive oil (8). Concomitant increases in blood and tissue solubility slow the development of alveolar and tissue anesthetic partial pressures. The issue is further complicated by the

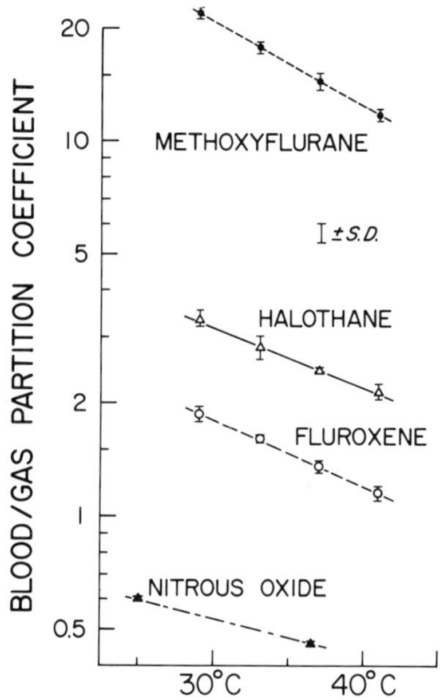

FIG. 9, 4. These graphs demonstrate the rises in blood solubility that accompany a decrease in temperature (6, 7).

decrease in metabolism that attends hypothermia: the resultant proportional reductions in ventilation and circulation also hinder the alveolar rate of rise (see Chapter 7). Moreover, by increasing the tissue time constants, the reduction in tissue blood flow that accompanies hypothermia further delays the rise in the tissue anesthetic partial pressure. All these factors delay the onset of (or recovery from) anesthesia during hypothermia.

One factor which opposes these effects on rate of induction is the lower MAC produced by hypothermia (fig. 1, 7). Although the alveolar anesthetic rate of rise is slower with hypothermia, the increase in anesthetic potency associated with hypothermia allows MAC to be reached about as quickly as during normothermia (9). At any given inspired concentration which is well in excess of MAC, the rate at which MAC is achieved in the alveoli is negligibly changed by alteration of body temperature. For example, when 8 percent fluroxene is inspired, MAC is attained in the alveoli (but not yet in the brain) in about 1 minute regardless of whether body temperature is 27° or 37°C (fig. 9, 5). At 6 percent inspired fluroxene, MAC is attained in 4 to 5 minutes at all temperatures. Although the alveolar attainment of MAC is achieved at about the same rate at all temperatures, hypothermia delays anesthetic transfer to brain by lowering cerebral perfusion.

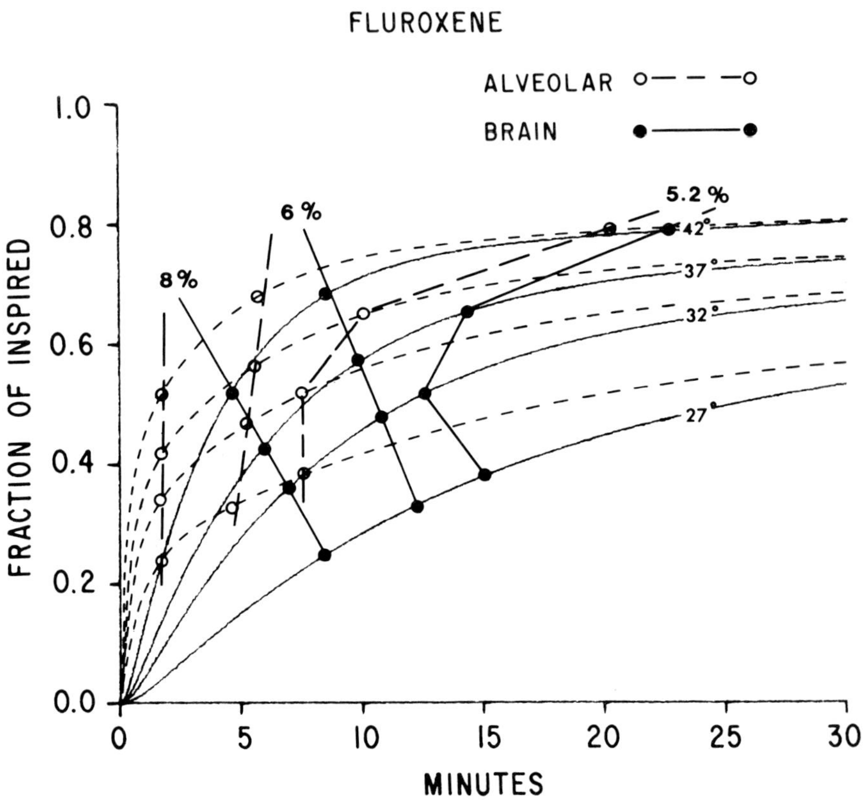

FIG. 9, 5. A reduction in temperature increases solubility and thereby slows both the alveolar (*dashed lines*) and the brain (*continuous lines*) fluroxene rates of rise toward the inspired fluroxene partial pressure. However, MAC also is reduced at lower body temperatures and hence the rate of attainment of MAC in the lung is unaffected (*open circles*) at an inspired concentration of 8 percent or at an inspired concentration of 6 percent (that is, a line drawn through the open circles is nearly vertical). At 5.2 percent the attainment of MAC is delayed at the higher temperature since the inspired fluroxene concentration is near MAC for that temperature. At 8 and 6 percent inspired fluroxene the brain (*filled circles*) reaches a partial pressure equivalent to MAC at a rate which decreases with decreasing temperature. The slower rate of rise with hypothermia is due to a lower brain blood flow. (Reproduced with permission from Munson, E. S., and Eger, E. I., II: The effects of hyperthermia and hypothermia on the rate of induction of anesthesia: calculations using a mathematical model. Anesthesiology 33: 515–519, 1970.)

The constancy of the rate at which MAC is attained in the alveoli is lost as the inspired concentration approaches the MAC of the higher temperature. At 5.2 percent inspired fluroxene, MAC is achieved twice as rapidly at 27° versus 42°C. Because MAC decreases with hypothermia, an inspired concentration which is below MAC at 37° may well be above it at 27°—and therefore capable of producing anesthesia at the lower but not at the higher temperature.

Henry's Law

Although unstated, our discussions presumed that Henry's Law applies to solubility. Henry's Law says that the amount of gas dissolved in a given volume of solvent (blood, tissue, etc.) is proportional to the partial pressure of the gas: if the partial pressure is doubled, the amount dissolved is doubled. However, Henry's Law is an "ideal law" which is only strictly applicable in dilute solutions of real gases. Evidence presented by Schoenborn (11) for xenon, and by Schoenborn (11) and others (3, 12, 13) for cyclopropane, all suggest that Henry's Law sometimes is disobeyed. A rise in cyclopropane partial pressure is associated with a fall in the blood/gas—and in particular in the hemoglobin/gas—partition coefficient (3, 12). That is, doubling cyclopropane partial pressure does not always double the volume of cyclopropane absorbed by blood. This may be explained by assuming that the cyclopropane binding sites on the hemoglobin molecule become saturated by increasing cyclopropane partial pressure. At very low partial pressures, cyclopropane molecules may occupy only a small fraction of the sites (fig. 9, 6*A*) and an increase in partial pressure results in a nearly proportional increase in the number of cyclopropane molecules attached to (dissolved in) those sites (fig. 9, 6*B*). However, at higher partial pressures (fig. 9, 6*C*) nearly all the sites are occupied—and further increases in partial pressure cannot effectively increase the attachment (solution) of cyclopropane (fig. 9, 6*D*). Thus, the cyclopropane concen-

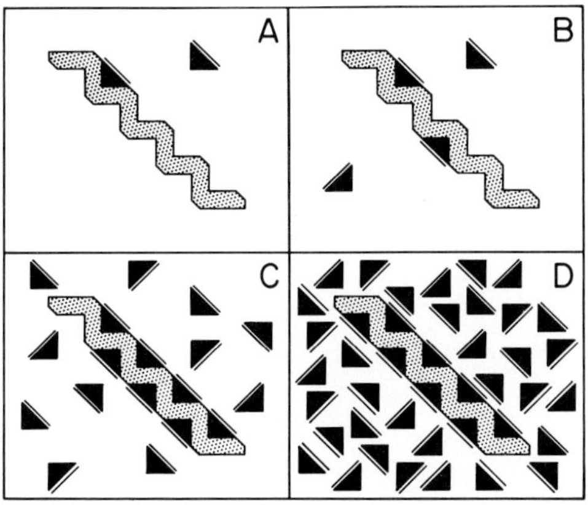

FIG. 9, 6. The worm-like figure represents a protein (such as hemoglobin) which possesses a number of sites attractive to an anesthetic (indicated by the *triangles*). The sites are the V-shaped depressions made by the undulations in the "worm." A low anesthetic partial pressure (*A*) causes the occupation of a single site; doubling the partial pressure (*B*) doubles the site occupancy. Up to this point Henry's Law is obeyed. However, further increases in partial pressure (*C* and *D*) cannot produce proportional increases in occupancy (Henry's Law is disobeyed) because of the limited number of available sites.

tration in hemoglobin may become fixed despite further increases in cyclopropane partial pressure. By definition, this means that the blood/gas partition coefficient must fall—and so it does (fig. 9, 7). This explains why the cyclopropane blood/gas partition coefficient in table 4, 1 is given as 0.44 to 0.6. Low concentrations (less than 1 percent) produce the greater coefficient while the smaller coefficient is found at 1 atmosphere total cyclopropane pressure. Still lower partition coefficients might be achieved at still higher pressures. Within the anesthetic range (10 to 30 percent of 1 atmosphere) the cyclopropane blood/gas partition coefficient lies near 0.6.

As noted previously, Schoenborn (11) has shown a similar effect for xenon in myoglobin and, in fact, has isolated the specific site of attachment of xenon to myoglobin. Lowe and Hagler (3) also found a greater muscle/gas partition coefficient for cyclopropane at lower cyclopropane partial pressures. No change in liver solubility was seen. Solubility changes with concentration changes have not been found for

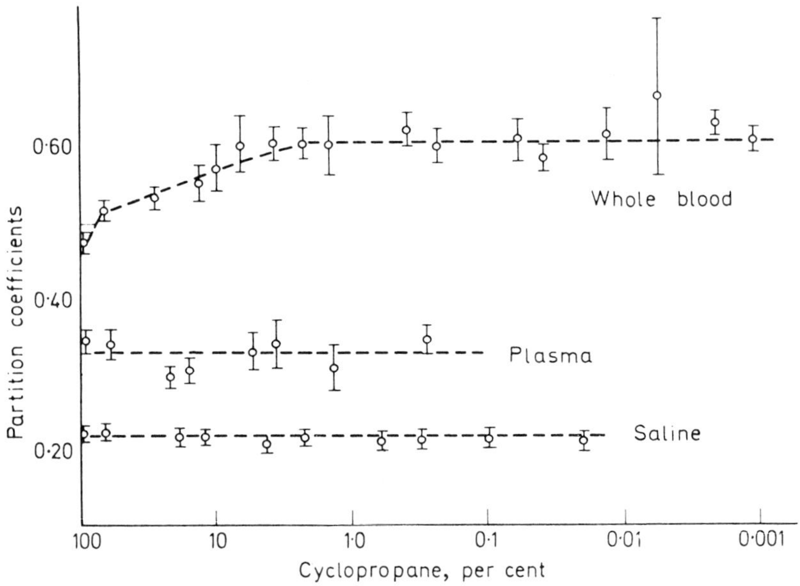

FIG. 9, 7. Cyclopropane saline/gas (*lowest graph*) and plasma/gas (*middle graph*) partition coefficients determined at various concentrations are constant over the entire range of concentrations examined (100 percent equals 1 atmosphere pressure) and therefore, follow Henry's Law. However, the blood/gas parition coefficient (*upper graph*) decreases at concentrations above 1 to 5 percent and does not follow Henry's Law. (Reproduced with permission from Gregory, G. A., and Eger, E. I., II: Inhalation anesthesia: pharmacokinetics. In *General Anaesthesia*, edited by T. C. Gray and J. F. Nunn, pp. 439–464, Butterworths, London, 1971.)

halothane or for nitrous oxide in blood. The applicability of Henry's Law to other anesthetics remains unknown.

The reverse of these findings, an increase in solubility with an increase in partial pressure, appears to occur with ether in water (14), or blood (3, 13) or with chloroform in oil (15). These cases may be explained by a change in the solvent with increasing anesthetic concentration. At higher concentrations the anesthetic forms an appreciable portion of the solvent phase and the anesthetic begins to dissolve in part in itself. Obviously these increases occur at partial pressures far beyond the anesthetic range.

These deviations from Henry's Law mean that a partition coefficient determined at one concentration may not apply at another. Thus, partition coefficients should be determined at the concentrations at which the anesthetic will be used. It also follows that the results of "tracer" studies of anesthetic uptake and distribution may suggest a significantly slower rate of alveolar anesthetic rise than actually occurs in practice.

Summary

Several factors may alter anesthetic solubility and hence alveolar and tissue anesthetic rates of rise. A reduction in alveolar rate of rise is produced by any factor which increases anesthetic solubility in either blood (hyperlipermia, increased blood proteins, decreased temperature) or tissues (increased lipid content, decreased temperature). The effect on tissue rate of rise depends on both the alveolar rate of rise and on the influence of the change in solubility on the tissue time constant. Henry's Law occasionally is not followed by some anesthetics at high anesthetic partial pressures. Partition coefficients of these agents will vary with their partial pressure.

QUESTIONS

1. A tissue has a blood flow of 100 ml/minute/100 ml of tissue. What is the time constant for that tissue for an anesthetic with a tissue/blood partition coefficient of 2? What happens to the time constant if the tissue/gas partition coefficient is halved without any change in the blood/gas partition coefficient? What happens if the blood/gas coefficient is halved without any change in the tissue/gas coefficient? What happens if both are halved?
2. What is the time constant for a tissue having a blood flow of 3 ml/100 ml of tissue/minute exposed to an anesthetic with a tissue/blood partition coefficient of 1? Say that hypothermia doubles both the tissue/gas and the blood/gas partition coefficients but halves the tissue blood flow: what is the time constant?
3. Why does a quartering of blood solubility not affect the alveolar rate of rise in

exactly the same way as a quartering of tissue solubility (compare figs. 9, 2 and 9, 3)?

4. How might uncontrolled diabetes affect blood solubility? What about cirrhosis and a resulting hypoprotenemia?
5. Use the law of mass action to derive Henry's Law and explain deviations from Henry's Law.
6. What changes in anesthetic requirement and in anesthetic uptake would accompany malignant hyperthermia: A) while respiration and circulation are sustained; and B) in the face of a failing circulation and respiration.

REFERENCES

1. Laasberg, L. J., and Hedley-Whyte, J.: Halothane solubility in blood and solutions of plasma proteins. Anesthesiology 32: 351–356, 1970.
2. Robbins, B. H.: Studies of cyclopropane I. The quantitative determination of cyclopropane in air, water, and blood by means of iodine pentoxide. J. Pharmacol. Exp. Ther. 58: 243, 1936.
3. Lowe, H. J., and Hagler, K.: Determination of volatile organic anesthetics in blood, gases, tissues and lipids: partition coefficients. In *Gas Chromatography in Biology and Medicine.* A Ciba Foundation Symposium. edited by Ruth Porter, pp. 86–112. J & A Churchill, Ltd., London, 1969.
4. Han, Y. H., and Helrich, M.: Effect of temperature on solubility of halothane in human blood and brain tissue homogenate. Anesth. Analg. 45: 775–780, 1966.
5. Kozam, R. L., Landau, S. M., Cubina, J. M., and Lukas, D. S.: Solubility of nitrous oxide in biologic fluid and myocardium. J. Appl. Physiol. 29: 593–597, 1970.
6. Stoelting, R. K., and Longshore, R. K.: Effect of temperature on solubility of fluroxene, halothane, and methoxyflurane blood/gas and cerebrospinal fluid/gas partition coefficients. Anesthesiology. 36: 503–505, 1972.
7. Saidman, L. J., Eger, E. I., II, Munson, E. S., and Severinghaus, J. W.: A method for determining solubility of anesthetics utilizing the Scholander apparatus. Anesthesiology 27: 180–184. 1966.
8. Altma, P. L., and Dittmer, D. S., editors: *Respiration and Circulation*, p. 19. Biological Handbook of the Federation of American Societies for Experimental Biology, Bethesda, Md., 1971.
9. Munson, E. S., and Eger, E. I., II: The effects of hyperthermia and hypothermia on the rate of induction of anesthesia: Calculations using a mathematical model. Anesthesiology 33: 515–519, 1970.
10. Schoenborn, B. P.: Binding of xenon to horse haemoglobin. Nature 208: 760–762, 1965.
11. Schoenborn, B. P.: Binding of cyclopropane to sperm whale myoglobin. Nature 214: 1120–1122, 1967.
12. Gregory, G. A., and Eger, E. I., II: Partition coefficients in blood and blood fractions at various concentrations of cyclopropane. Fed. Proc. 27: 705, 1968.
13. Cowles, A. L., Borgstedt, H. H., and Gillies, A. J.: Solubilities of ethylene, cyclopropane, halothane and diethyl ether in human and dog blood at low concentrations. Anesthesiology 35: 203–211, 1971.
14. Eger, E. I., II, Shargel, R., and Merkel, G.: Solubility of diethyl ether in water, blood and oil. Anesthesiology 24: 676–678, 1963.
15. Nunn, J. F.: The solubility of volatile anaesthetics in oil. Brit. J. Anaesth. 32: 346–352, 1960.

Chapter 10

Nitrous Oxide Transfer to Closed Gas Spaces

This chapter will discuss the impact of nitrous oxide transfer to closed internal gas spaces such as bowel gas. Because of its greater blood solubility, the volumes of nitrous oxide which can be carried to a closed gas space are many times the volumes of nitrogen, hydrogen or methane which can be carried away. For example, the blood/gas partition coefficient of nitrous oxide is 34 times that of nitrogen. Nitrogen is the major constituent of closed internal spaces except for methane and hydrogen which the intestine also may contain. The transfer of nitrous oxide to an internal gas space may considerably increase the enclosed volume or pressure. The nature of the change—whether volume or pressure—depends on the compliance of the wall surrounding the gas space. The entrance of nitrous oxide into a space enclosed by a highly compliant wall (intestinal gas, pneumoperitoneum, pneumothorax, air embolism) causes the gas space to expand. Entrance into an air space surrounded by a noncompliant wall (sinuses, middle ear, ventricle during a pneumoencephalogram) causes an increase in pressure.

Volume Changes in Spaces Surrounded by Highly Compliant Walls

The nitrous oxide concentration in the closed internal gas space may approach—but cannot exceed—the alveolar concentration. In this way, the alveolar concentration sets a limit to the increase in the gas space volume. If we assume that the nitrogen cannot leave (that it is totally insoluble), and that the walls of the space are infinitely compliant, then the volume reached at equilibrium is a multiple, *M*, of the original volume such that

$$M = 100/(100 - \%N_2O) \quad (1)$$

where % N_2O is the alveolar nitrous oxide concentration.* Thus, the

* By definition

$$M = (V_O + V_{N_2O})/V_O \quad (2)$$

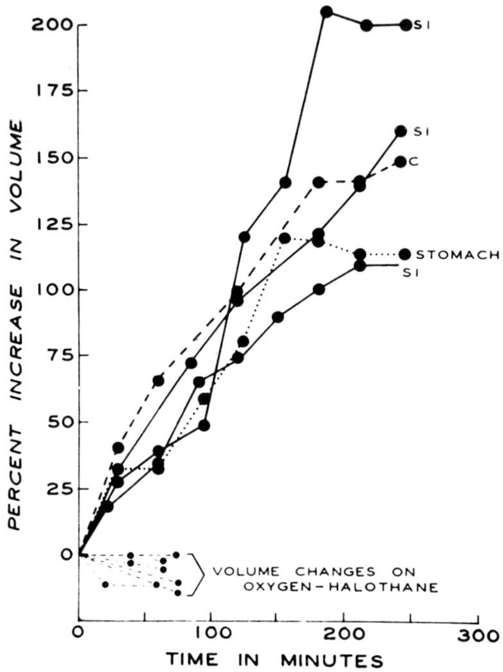

FIG. 10, 1. These graphs illustrate the increase in bowel gas volume produced by nitrous oxide administration (*large filled circles*). All parts of the bowel (colon, C; small intestine, SI; and stomach) show a similar change with time. Note that no volume increase occurs during halothane administered in oxygen (*small filled circles*). (Reproduced with permission from Eger, E. I., II, and Saidman, L. J.: Hazards of nitrous oxide anesthesia in bowel obstruction and pneumothorax. Anesthesiology 26: 61–66, 1965.)

original volume doubles at equilibrium if the alveolar nitrous oxide is 50 percent. If the alveolar concentration is 80 percent, then the final volume equals 5 times the original volume. The calculated volume increase becomes very large as the alveolar concentration approaches 100 percent.

The calculated limits are not reached in bowel gas spaces as measured in dogs (1). To determine the actual volume changes, intestinal loops were isolated and filled with air while the animals breathed halothane and oxygen. No change, or a decrease in volume occurred in the ensuing hour (fig. 10, 1). However, when 75 percent nitrous oxide was added to the respired gases, the intestinal gas volume increased 1.8 fold in 2 hours and 2.5 fold in 4 hours (fig. 10, 1). Note that although this is a considerable

---

where V_O is the original gas volume and V_{N_2O} is the volume of nitrous oxide added. Also, by definition

$$\%N_2O = 100\ V_{N_2O}/(V_O + V_{N_2O}) \qquad (3)$$

where $\%\ N_2O$ is the percent of nitrous oxide in the gas space at equilibrium. Solution of equation 3 for V_O and substitution for V_O in equation 2 gives equation 1.

increase in volume it is half the predicted 4 fold maximum increase.

The *in vivo* expansion of bowel gas is limited by two factors. First, some of the nitrogen escapes via the blood (2) and second, there is not sufficient time—even in a long procedure—to reach equilibrium. This is evidenced by the inequality of bowel and alveolar nitrous oxide concentrations even after 4 hours exposure to nitrous oxide (fig. 10, 2).

Expansion of bowel gas may hamper the surgeon's efforts in cases of intestinal distension. It may add to the requirement for muscle relaxation both to obtain exposure and to enable closure. In the immediate postoperative period, the added distension also may embarrass respiration by increasing intra-abdominal pressure. The question of whether or not to use nitrous oxide is of little importance if the procedure is short since the volume changes slowly. Of course, the problem can be avoided by omitting nitrous oxide. A compromise may be to limit the inspired

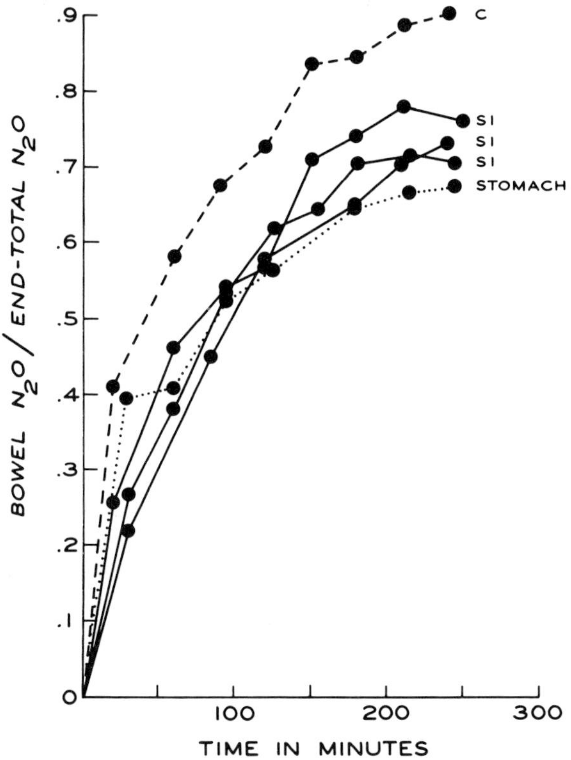

FIG. 10, 2. The bowel concentration of nitrous oxide does not equal the alveolar concentration even after breathing nitrous oxide for 4 hours. At this time the average bowel concentration is only 75 percent of that in the alveoli. (Reproduced with permission from Eger, E. I., II, and Saidman, L. J.: Hazards of nitrous oxide anesthesia in bowel obstruction and pneumothorax. Anesthesiology 26: 61–66, 1965.)

concentration of nitrous oxide to 50 percent—a concentration which at most, would double the intestinal gas space.

In patients not suffering from intestinal obstruction, no hazard usually accures to nitrous oxide administration since the volume of gas in the gut is normally about 100 ml (2, 3). Even tripling of such a volume would have little effect. However, apprehension in some patients may lead to air swallowing and a far higher than normal volume of intestinal gas prior to anesthesia. Administration of nitrous oxide to these patients may produce an unexpected abdominal distension (4). We have estimated normal changes in intra-abdominal volume from girth increases in volunteers who received 70 percent nitrous oxide (Stevens, W. C., unpublished data). In most of these volunteers, only small changes were found; but in about 1 out of 10 volunteers we found increases of 1 to 2 liters.

As suggested above, such expansion may have resulted from the effect of the nitrous oxide on an abnormally large volume of intestinal air produced by aerophagia. However, another untested possibility exists. Gases such as methane, hydrogen and hydrogen sulfide may be produced by the action of bacteria on bowel contents (2, 5). In humans who have fasted for 5 to 7 hours (previous diet not controlled) the average production of hydrogen and methane is 40 ml/hour with an upper range extending to 110 ml/hour (2). The high partial pressure of these gases in the intestine relative to blood permits their uptake by blood and elimination at the lungs. However, entrance of nitrous oxide in the intestinal gas space would dilute these gases and thereby diminish their partial pressure and uptake. The resulting retention of these gases might be an unlimited process. If the dilution by nitrous oxide caused the rate of elimination of intestinal gases to fall below their rate of production, then a continuous expansion of bowel gas would be expected. Of crucial importance to such a process would be the rate of intestinal gas production. This would be determined by the diet and perhaps also by anxiety (5). If 110 ml/hour were produced and entirely retained (this is the highest rate of production noted above) this would result in a maximum bowel gas expansion of slightly less than ½ liter/hour in the presence of an alveolar nitrous oxide concentration of 75 percent. We might note that in the studies done in dogs (figs. 10, 1 and 10, 2), the intestine was flushed until clear prior to the start of the experiment.

In contrast to the slow changes in bowel gas volume produced by nitrous oxide, the changes produced in a pneumothorax occur quickly, and in addition are larger (1). In dogs, the inspiration of 75 percent nitrous oxide doubled a 300 ml pneumothorax in 10 minutes, tripled it in 45 and caused a quadrupling in 2 hours (fig. 10, 3). The reason for the more rapid change is not certain. The most likely (but unproven) explanation is that the thin lung and pleural membranes which separate

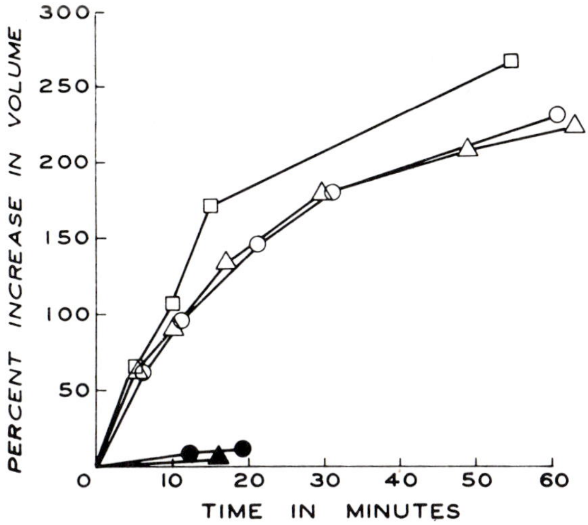

FIG. 10, 3. Intrapleural gas volume increases rapidly in the presence of 75 percent inspired nitrous oxide plus halothane in oxygen (*open circles*, *squares* and *triangles*) but shows little change when only halothane in oxygen is respired (*filled triangle* and *circles*). (Reproduced with permission from Eger, E. I., II, and Saidman, L. J.: Hazards of nitrous oxide anesthesia in bowel obstruction and pneumothorax. Anesthesiology 26: 61–66, 1965.)

the alveolar gas from the intrapleural space permit a greater transfer of nitrous oxide than can be achieved by the blood which perfuses the intestinal mucosa.

Presence of a significant closed pneumothorax constitutes an absolute contraindication to the use of nitrous oxide. Hunter (6) has reported that the use of nitrous oxide in such cases is often associated with circulatory and possible, respiratory embarrassment. Noncommunicating blebs, or blebs which permit ingress but not egress of gas may present a similar hazard. Blebs may confer two additional hazards. Administration of nitrous oxide in the presence of a bleb may produce a pneumothorax where one did not exist previously (7). A still greater danger is that the expanding gas may rupture into blood vessels lining the bleb wall and cause an air embolus. Such a catastrophe has been observed in decompression sickness which produced an analogous expansion of a bleb (8).

Intraperitoneal gas has been used in the past for treatment of tuberculosis and more recently for laparoscopy and in the preoperative preparation of patients with large abdominal wall defects (9). Johnson (10) reported a near catastrophe in such a patient anesthetized with nitrous oxide. Twenty minutes following induction and endotracheal intubation the blood pressure began to fall and reached unmeasurable levels 8 minutes later. These changes were associated with a progressive abdominal distension and reduction in ventilatory compliance. Incision of the peritoneum and the escape of gas resulted in an immediate restoration of blood pressure and increase in compliance. The procedure continued uneventfully thereafter. Perhaps nitrous oxide also is contraindicated in such cases until the abdominal cavity is entered.

The expansion of an air embolus by the entrance of nitrous oxide from blood was predicted by Nunn (11). An experiment by Munson and Merrick (12) suggests that the expansion approaches the theoretical limit described earlier. They demonstrated that 0.55 ml/kg of air was required to produce a fatal air embolus in rabbits breathing oxygen, but only 0.16 ml/kg in rabbits breathing 72 to 76 percent nitrous oxide (fig. 10, 4). An inspired concentration of 72 to 76 percent nitrous oxide would produce an alveolar concentration of 70 percent after dilution with water vapor. The M (equation 1) calculated from this would indicate a 3.3 fold increase in volume. Such a volume change would equalize the absolute volumes of gas required to produce death with (3.3 times 0.16 equals 0.52 ml/kg) and without (0.55 ml/kg) nitrous oxide.

Do patients in hazard of air embolism (such as patients undergoing posterior fossa craniotomies in the sitting position) benefit more from the omission or from the inclusion of nitrous oxide in their anesthetic? The presence of nitrous oxide would exaggerate the circulatory effect of a given volume of intravenous air. However, such exaggeration would give

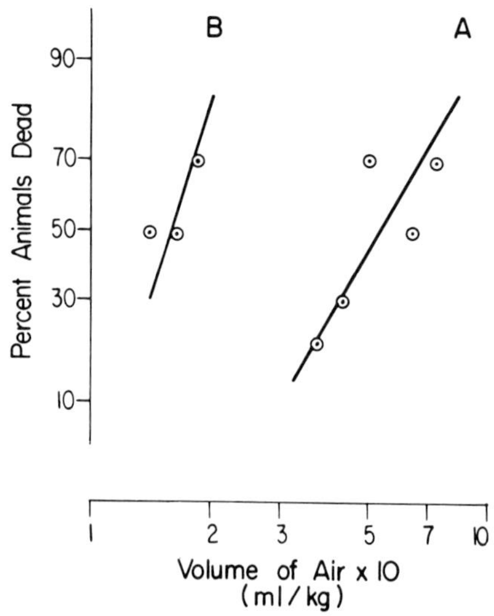

FIG. 10, 4. The volume of intravenous air required to kill 50 percent of rabbits (LD_{50}) anesthetized with halothane (*A*) is 3.4 times as great as the volume required when anesthesia is accomplished with halothane plus 75 percent nitrous oxide (*B*). The respective LD_{50} values are 0.55 versus 0.16 ml of air/kg. (Reproduced with permission from Munson, E. S., and Merrick, H. C.: Effect of nitrous oxide on venous air embolism. Anesthesiology 27: 783–787, 1966.)

an earlier warning to the presence of embolization. In addition, the prior administration of nitrous oxide would assist in the treatment of embolization, in that the subsequent elimination of the nitrous oxide would rapidly reduce the size and effect of the embolus (13). This treatment might be important not only to the management of cardiovascular depression due to air in the heart, but also to the treatment of emboli that may reach the left side of the circulation and hence heart or brain. Such nitrous oxide-containing emboli could be rapidly reduced in size by conversion of the respired gas to 100 percent oxygen. Air emboli lacking nitrous oxide could not be similarly reduced.

Pressure Changes in Spaces Surrounded by Noncompliant Walls

When the walls surrounding an internal gas space are rigid, the entrance of nitrous oxide cannot expand the space but instead must produce an increase in pressure. As in spaces surrounded by highly compliant walls, the nitrous oxide partial pressure may approach but not exceed the alveolar nitrous oxide pressure. Unlike the geometric increase in volume effected in a highly compliant space, the limit of the theoretical pressure change in a poorly compliant space bears a rectilinear (i.e., straight line) relationship to the alveolar nitrous oxide partial pressure. The maximum theoretical increase produced by an alveolar nitrous oxide partial pressure of half of an atmosphere would be half an atmosphere. Seventy percent alveolar nitrous oxide at sea level might produce a 0.7 atmosphere or 532 torr increase in pressure! Obviously such pressures would not be tolerable nor in practice can they be achieved. But they do suggest the magnitude of the pressure problem that may be incurred with the use of nitrous oxide.

A few natural cavities such as the air sinuses and the middle ear are surrounded by rigid or poorly compliant walls. Waun *et al.* (14) found that middle ear mechanics may be impaired and a hearing deficit result following nitrous oxide administration. A deficit was particularly likely if edema of the Eustachian tube was present secondary either to disease or to operation near the entrance of the tube to the nasopharynx. Thomsen *et al.* (15) measured middle ear pressure in a volunteer who breathed 40, 60 and 80 percent nitrous oxide via a face mask. The pressure rose 22 to 35 cm of water before discontinuance of the experiment (fig. 10, 5). Otolaryngologists have noted another manifestation of the same phenomenon. The apposition of tympanic membrane grafts (tympanoplasty) tends to be disrupted by gas bubbles from the middle ear when nitrous oxide is administered. The phenomenon is not present in the absence of nitrous oxide.

The hearing deficit that follows nitrous oxide anesthesia may relate to a decrease in middle ear pressure rather than an increase! It is usually not necessary for an individual to initiate any action to reduce an

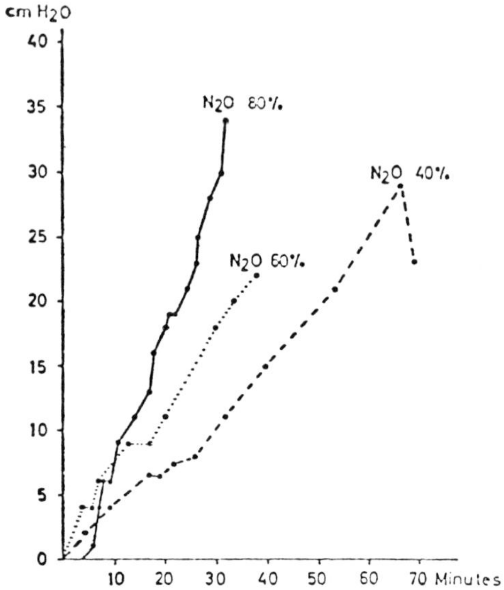

FIG. 10, 5. Nitrous oxide inhalation increases middle ear pressure in man. The rate of increase is directly related to the inspired nitrous oxide concentration. (Reproduced with permission from Thomsen, K. A., Terkildsen, K., and Arnfred, I.: Middle ear pressure variations during anesthesia. Arch. Otolaryng. 82: 609–611, 1965.)

elevated middle ear pressure; only rarely will the egress of gas be prevented once the middle ear pressure exceeds 20 to 25 cm water (16). Thus, the use of nitrous oxide may cause a rise in middle ear pressure which is relieved spontaneously. However, after the termination of anesthesia, the removal of nitrous oxide from the middle ear may result in a negative pressure. Unlike an increase in pressure, a negative pressure may not be relieved spontaneously because of the ball valve-like action of the Eustachian tube. Opening of the tube to permit ingress of gas may require a voluntary effort. Such opening may be inhibited by a residual anesthetic effect or by disease of the tube. Since this negative pressure may persist, it may result in exudation of serum or blood into the middle ear producing a condition similar to acute catarrhal otitis media (14). Perhaps nitrous oxide should be avoided when the Eustachian tube is obstructed or when surgery may produce trauma and edema to the nasal opening of the tube. The same thoughts also may apply to the sinuses although there are no reports of difficulties in this area.

Pneumoencephalography requires the injection of gas into a space surrounded by poorly compliant walls. Nitrous oxide administration following air injection into the lumbar or cisternal space may result in marked subarachnoid pressure increases (17). In dogs anesthetized with pentobarbital plus halothane in oxygen, 5 to 10 ml of cerebrospinal fluid were removed and replaced with an equal volume of air injected into the cisternal space. Subsequent addition of 75 percent nitrous oxide to the

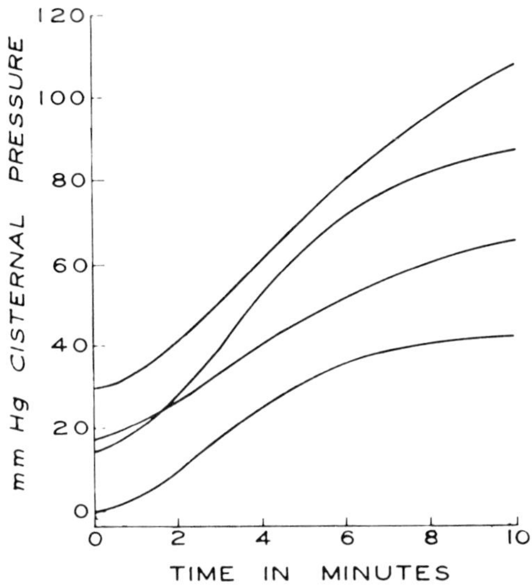

FIG. 10, 6. Four dogs were anesthetized with pentobarbital plus halothane in oxygen. Removal of cerebrospinal fluid and replacement with air injected into the cisternal subarachnoid space produced transient pressure changes which returned to near normal within a few minutes. At zero time, 75 percent nitrous oxide was added to the respired gases and the subsequent rise in cisternal pressure measured. (Reproduced with permission from Saidman, L. J., and Eger, E. I., II: Change in cerebrospinal fluid pressure during pneumoencephalography under nitrous oxide anesthesia. Anesthesiology 26: 67–72, 1965.)

respired mixture raised the cisternal pressure an average of 60 torr within 10 minutes (fig. 10, 6). No further rise occurred after this time. The results obtained in dogs were duplicated in man, differing only in that the site of injection and pressure measurement was in the lumbar rather than the cisternal subarachnoid space. Although these pressure changes are far less than the theoretical maximum pressure attainable, they may be of considerable physiological significance: such pressures may approach the mean perfusion pressure and thereby may compromise cerebral blood flow (18–20).

The failure to reach the maximum theoretical pressure may be explained by: 1) absorption of some nitrogen; 2) compression of some vascular channels (i.e., a volume rather than a pressure change); and 3) loss of cerebrospinal fluid and air through the arachnoid granulations. Loss of fluid and air through the arachnoid granulations is suggested by some tracings in which a curious phenomenon was observed. Attainment of a peak cisternal pressure was followed by a sudden fall in pressure. Following this the cisternal pressure rose again, and again suddenly fell. This "sawtooth" rise and fall repeated itself several times (fig. 10, 7). If the decreases in pressure reflect the escape of bubbles through the arachnoid granulations, this suggests a second hazard to the use of nitrous oxide during air encephalography—that of air embolism. It is noteworthy that air embolism is one of the major causes of death during pneumoencephalography (20).

Although thousands of pneumoencephalograms have been obtained with apparent safety during nitrous oxide anesthesia, the preceding data suggest the avoidance of nitrous oxide during or immediately (24 to 48 hours) following this procedure, particularly if cerebrospinal fluid pressure is elevated or if a space-occupying lesion is suspected. It may be reasonable to use nitrous oxide for anesthesia if nitrous oxide also is used as the contrast gas. The concomitant use for anesthesia and for contrast should result in no net gas transfer to the closed gas space; in fact, the reverse should occur since the injected nitrous oxide partial pressure (1 atmosphere at sea level) would exceed the partial pressure in the respired gases. This technique also has the advantage of permitting rapid removal of the contrast gas at the end of the procedure, which in turn, reduces the nausea and headache caused by pneumoencephalography. The use of anesthetic gases as the contrast material has been suggested by reports (21, 22) which imply the safety of their use for this purpose. However, at least one report has cautioned that the rapid absorption of nitrous oxide following anesthesia may lead to hazardous distortion of the brain (23).

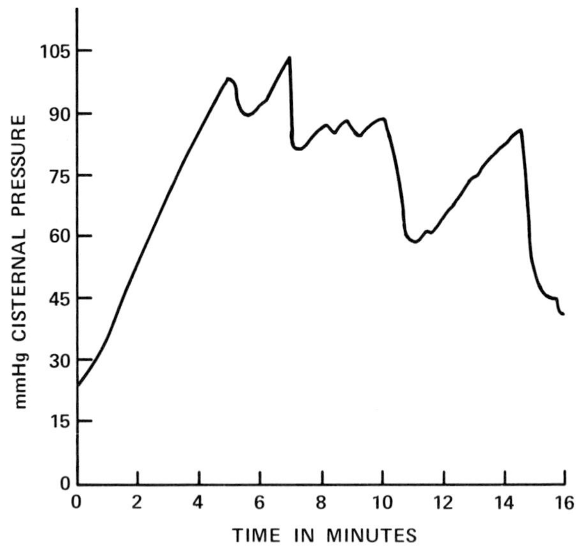

FIG. 10, 7. A dog was prepared in a manner identical to that used to prepare the 4 dogs described in figure 10, 6. The administration of 75 percent nitrous oxide produced the same initial rise in cisternal pressure. This rise, however, was followed by a "sawtooth" fall and rise as seen above. The decreases in pressure are thought to be due to the escape of bubbles of gas through the arachnoid granulations. (Reproduced with permission from Saidman, L. J., and Eger, E. I., II: Change in cerebrospinal fluid pressure during pneumoencephalography under nitrous oxide anesthesia. Anesthesiology 26: 67–72, 1965.)

Summary

The volume of pressure within closed gas spaces containing poorly soluble gases (nitrogen, hydrogen, methane) may be increased by administration of nitrous oxide. The volume is increased if the walls of the space are highly compliant. Highly compliant spaces are found in both of the major body cavities including bowel spaces, pulmonary blebs, pneumothorax or pneumoperitoneum. Intravascular air also represents a space with highly compliant walls. Volume increases in such spaces may compromise respiration or circulation.

Spaces with poorly compliant walls include those occurring naturally (sinuses and middle ear) as well as those created by physicians during pneumoencephalography. The entrance of nitrous oxide will increase the pressure within these spaces. Thus, nitrous oxide administration during pneumoencephalography may increase intracranial pressure, and in addition may add to the hazard of air embolism.

QUESTIONS

1. How might you modify your usual anesthetic technique in the management of the patient with gaseous bowel distention? If you believed there was a special indication for the use of nitrous oxide, what precautions and limitations might you impose on its use?
2. You are giving 60 percent alveolar nitrous oxide in San Francisco. What maximum volume change might this produce in a highly compliant internal gas space? What would be the maximum theoretical pressure change in a poorly compliant space? You have moved to Leadville, Colorado (elevation 10,000 feet, barometric pressure 520 torr) and again, you are administering 60 percent nitrous oxide. Are your answers to the above questions altered by your move?
3. A diet of baked beans has conferred an intestinal gas production of 200 ml/hour in a patient who is to have an emergency orthopedic procedure. Anesthesia is maintained with an alveolar nitrous oxide concentration of 80 percent. What maximum rate of bowel gas expansion might you predict from these data?
4. Seventy-five percent carbon dioxide in oxygen has been used to expand the intraperitoneal space during laparoscopy. The solubility of carbon dioxide in blood is similar to that of nitrous oxide. What would happen to the intraperitoneal gas space volume following injection of carbon dioxide if the anesthetic administered were halothane in oxygen? Halothane plus 75 percent nitrous oxide in oxygen?
5. Defend the position that nitrous oxide should be used in cases where air embolism may occur.
6. Why might you avoid the use of nitrous oxide in a patient with sinusitis? If nitrous oxide were used in such a patient would you expect the sinus gas

space to be increased or decreased during anesthesia? What volume change would you expect in the postanesthesia period?

7. Under what conditions might it be safe to use nitrous oxide anesthesia during pneumoencephalography?

REFERENCES

1. Eger, E. I., II, and Saidman, L. J.: Hazards of nitrous oxide anesthesia in bowel obstruction and pneumothorax. Anesthesiology 26: 61–66, 1965.
2. Levitt, M. D.: Volume and composition of human intestinal gas determined by means of an intestinal washout technic. New Eng. J. Med. 284: 1394–1398, 1971.
3. Bendill, G. N., Marshall, R., Dubois, A. B., and Harris, J. H.: Measurement of the volume of gas in the gastro-intestinal tract. Values in normal subjects and ambulatory patients. J. Clin. Invest. 35: 336–345, 1956.
4. Foldes, F. F., Kepes, E. R., and Ship, A. G.: Severe gastrointestinal distention during nitrous oxide and oxygen anesthesia. J. A. M. A. 194: 1146–1148, 1965.
5. Calloway, D. H., and Murphy, E. L.: The use of expired air to measure intestinal gas formation. Ann. N. Y. Acad. Sci. 150: 82–95, 1968.
6. Hunter, A. R.: Problems of anaesthesia in artificial pneumothorax, Proc. Roy. Soc. Med. 48: 765, 1955.
7. Gold, M. I., and Joseph, S. I.: Bilateral tension pneumothorax following induction of anesthesia in two patients with chronic obstructive airway disease. Anesthesiology. 38: 93–97, 1973.
8. Walder, D. N.: A possible explanation for some cases of severe decompression sickness in compressed air workers. In *The Regulation of Human Respiration*, edited by D. J. C. Cunningham, and Lloyd, B. B. Blackwell Scientific Publications, Oxford.
9. Connolly, D. P., and Perri, R. F.: Giant hernias managed by pneumoperitoneum. J. A. M. A. 209: 71–75, 1969.
10. Johnson, W. C.: Pneumoperitoneum for ventral hernia repair: Anesthesia Complication. J. A. M. A. 271: 968, 1971.
11. Nunn, J. F.: Controlled respiration in neurosurgical anaesthesia (letter to the editor). Anaesthesia 14: 413–414, 1959.
12. Munson, E. S., and Merrick, H. C.: Effect of nitrous oxide on venous air embolism. Anesthesiology 27: 783–787, 1966.
13. Munson, E. S.: Effect of nitrous oxide on the pulmonary circulation during venous air embolism. Anesth. Analg. 50: 785–792, 1971.
14. Waun, J. E., Sweitzer, R. S., and Hamilton, W. K.: Effect of nitrous oxide in middle ear mechanics and hearing acuity. Anesthesiology 28: 846–850, 1967.
15. Thomsen, K. A., Terkildsen, K., and Arnfred, I.: Middle ear pressure variations during anesthesia. Arch. Otolaryng. 82: 609–611, 1965.
16. Fruin, R. L.: Aero-otitis media in infants. J. Aviation Med. 21: 150–169, 1950.
17. Saidman, L. J., and Eger, E. I., II: Change in cerebrospinal fluid pressure during pneumoencephalography under nitrous oxide anesthesia. Anesthesiology 26: 67–72, 1965.
18. Kjallquist, A., Siesjo, B. K., and Zwetnow, N.: Effects of increased intracranial pressure on cerebral blood flow and on cerebrospinal fluid HCO_3, pH, lactate and pyruvate in dogs. Acta Physiol. Scand. 75: 345–352, 1969.
19. Kjallquist, A., Siesjo, B. K., and Zwetnow, N.: Effects of increased intracranial pressure on cerebral blood flow and on cerebral venous PO_2, PCO_2, pH lactate and pyruvate in dogs. Acta Physiol. Scand. 75: 267–275, 1969.

20. Jacoby, J., Jones, J. R., Ziegler, J., *et al.*: Pneumoencephalography and air embolism: simulated anesthetic death. Anesthesiology 20: 336–340, 1959.
21. Aird, R. B.: Experimental encephalography with anesthetic gases. Arch. Surg. 32: 193, 1936.
22. Newman, H. W.: Encephalography with ethylene. J. A. M. A. 108: 461, 1937.
23. Collan, R., and Iivanainen, M.: Cardiac arrest caused by rapid elimination of nitrous oxide from cerebral ventricles after encephalography. Canad. Anaesth. Soc. J. 16: 519–524, 1969.

Chapter 11

Metabolism of Anesthetics

Until recently we believed that most anesthetics remained inviolate in their journey through the body. Fifty years ago, Haggard (1) suggested he could retrieve most of the ether taken up by dogs. Similarly, in 1959 Duncan and Raventos (2) indicated that halothane was eliminated unchanged via the lungs. Van Dyke *et al.* (3) shattered the illusion of anesthetic inertness by demonstrating the biotransformation of ether, chloroform, methoxyflurane and halothane in animals. Fluroxene, too was found to be metabolized (4). Stier *et al.* (5) extended these observations to man by demonstrating the appearance of bromine in urine following halothane anesthesia. Rehder *et al.* (6) later reported that up to 20 percent of the halothane taken up by man was metabolized. A similar percent of fluroxene was found to be degraded (7). Holaday *et al.* (8) topped these findings with their discovery of a 50 percent degradation of methoxflurane in man.

Impact of Metabolism on Arterial Anesthetic Rate of Rise

Of what import is metabolism to anesthetic uptake and distribution? To predict the effect of metabolism requires some assumptions as to site and definition of metabolism. Let us assume that the liver is the principle site of metabolism of anesthetics (an assumption which agrees with all reports). Further, let us define metabolism as *the fraction of anesthetic which is transformed as it traverses the liver.* For example, alteration of half the anesthetic passing through the liver (in the liver blood flow) by definition would be 50 percent metabolism. Note that this is not metabolism in the sense of milliliters of anesthetic transformed per unit time. Such a definition would mean that metabolism would be a function of both the fractional hepatic extraction (as in our definition) and the concentration of anesthetic seen by the liver. Nor does this definition indicate the fraction of anesthetic within the body which is transformed per unit time. This latter fraction is a function not only of hepatic metabolism but also of the accessibility of the anesthetic: if the anesthetic is sequestered in the tissues then the liver cannot metabolize it.

Our definition of metabolism may be simulated with the hydraulic model (Chapter 5). Simulation requires that the hepatic blood flow pipe and liver reservoir be separated from the vessel rich group. Further, an open ended pipe which allows the spillage of fluid (i.e., anesthetic) must exit from the side of the liver reservoir at the level of the "blood flow" pipe. The escape of fluid through this pipe simulates metabolism. Metabolism defines the size of exiting pipe. For 50 percent metabolism, the cross-section of the pipe equals the cross-section of the hepatic blood flow pipe; for 75 percent metabolism the cross-section is 3 times the size of the flow pipe. The cross-section of the exiting (metabolic) pipe may be calculated as $\%M \times F/(100 - \%M)$ where $\%M$ is the percent metabolized and F is the cross-section of the blood flow pipe to the liver.

This sort of simulation suggests that metabolism can significantly alter the alveolar anesthetic partial pressure (fig. 11, 1). The effect increases with time. After 1 minute of anesthesia, alveolar concentrations are nearly identical with either 0 or 100 percent metabolism, but after this, they diverge. When metabolism extracts all of the anesthetic passing the liver the curves rise modestly for the next 10 to 20 minutes and then remain remarkably constant. This constancy reflects a relative constancy of total uptake as opposed to the decreasing uptake and rising alveolar concentration obtained when no agent is metabolized. Note that the divergence is relatively greater for the more soluble methoxyflurane.

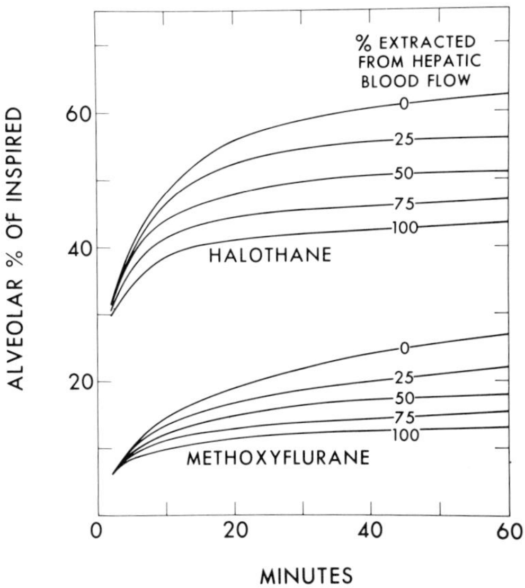

FIG. 11, 1. The alveolar anesthetic rate of rise is decreased as the percent of halothane or methoxyflurane removed from liver blood flow (metabolized) is increased. The effect of metabolism on anesthetic dose is greatest with the more soluble agent, methoxyflurane.

For example, at 60 minutes, lack of methoxyflurane metabolism produces an alveolar concentration twice as great as that found with 100 percent metabolism while the 100 percent metabolism curve for halothane is three-fourths the height of the zero metabolism curve. The greater effect achieved with the more soluble anesthetic reflects the greater relative extraction produced by a given metabolism. At the same partial pressure, a unit volume of blood carries more of the soluble agent: thus, the same percent extraction removes a greater amount of soluble agent. This greater uptake by the liver is reflected at the lungs.

The *in vivo* importance of metabolism to anesthetic uptake is largely unexplored. There are suggestions that factors which stimulate metabolism make induction of anesthesia more difficult. Berman *et al.* (9) measured the uptake of halothane and of methoxflurane in rats pretreated with phenobarbital. Phenobarbital is known to stimulate induction of the enzymes which metabolize these agents. For both anesthetics, uptake was increased over saline treated controls; 53 percent in the case of halothane and 36 percent in the case of methoxyflurane. Elimination studies suggested that a greater tissue distribution could not explain the additional uptake in the phenobarbital treated rats since less agent was eliminated by both the treated group anesthetized with halothane (19 percent less) and the treated group anesthetized with methoxyflurane (21 percent less). Finally, the blood levels of methoxyflurane in the phenobarbital pretreated rats rose at a significantly slower rate on induction and fell more rapidly on recovery (fig. 11, 2). Anesthesia was induced at approximately the same methoxyflurane blood level in control and pretreated rats. However, the slower rise associated with pretreatment resulted in a longer induction period in the pretreated animals. During recovery the pretreated animals awakened first—but at approximately the methoxyflurane blood level which permitted awakening in the control rats.

These results suggest that induction of anesthesia may be prolonged in patients ingesting drugs which cause enzymatic induction (for example, barbiturates or dilantin). Less obvious stimulators of enzyme induction may be cigarette smoke (10–12) or atmospheric pollutants (12). An increased metabolism of pentazocine or thiopental in smokers or urban dwellers (as opposed to nonsmokers or rural dwellers) is suggested by the larger dose of these drugs which is required for anesthesia (12). However, the increased drug requirement associated with smoke or atmospheric pollutants apparently does not apply to halothane or nitrous oxide (12). The effect on other anesthetics has not been tested.

Anesthetics may induce the enzymes which cause their own destruction. Exposure of rats to 0.03 percent methoxyflurane for 7 hours a day for 10 days roughly doubles their metabolism of that agent (13). There is

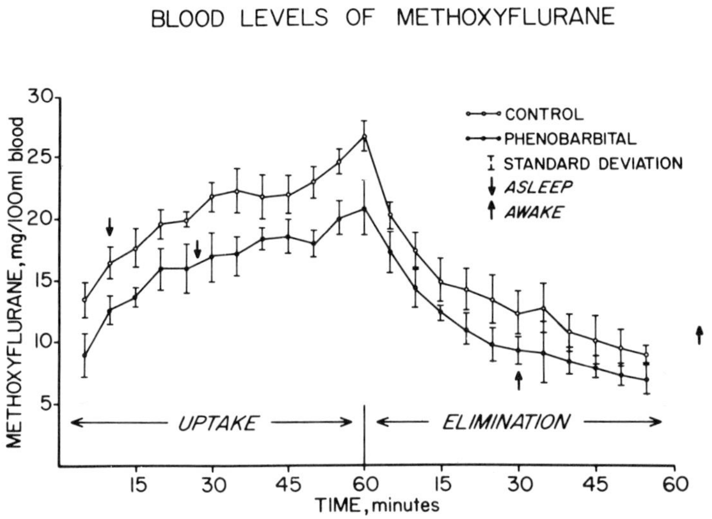

FIG. 11, 2. Pretreatment of rats with phenobarbital slows the rate of rise of blood levels of methoxyflurane (*filled circles*) compared to saline treated controls (*open circles*) during 60 minutes of "uptake." On recovery, the fall in blood levels is more rapid in the pretreated rats (see "elimination"). The *arrows* indicate the time at which a change from wakefulness to sleep occurred during "uptake" and sleep to wakefulness during "elimination." (Reproduced with permission from Berman, M. L., Lowe, H. J., Hagler, K. J., and Bochantin, J.: Uptake and elimination of methoxyflurane as influenced by enzyme induction in the rat. Anesthesiology 38: 352–357, 1973.)

indirect evidence for a similar stimulation of halothane metabolism in man: anesthetists excrete more metabolic products following exposure to halothane than nonanesthetists exposed to the same halothane challenge (14). These studies suggest that prior exposure to an anesthetic may alter the uptake of that anesthetic during a subsequent exposure. However, not all anesthetics may be similarly affected: prior treatment with fluroxene fails to enhance the metabolism of that agent (4).

The Effect of Anesthetic Partial Pressure on Anesthetic Metabolism

The report by Sawyer and co-workers (15, 16) both simplifies and complicates this picture. In miniature swine, they measured the concentration of halothane entering and leaving the liver and from this calculated the fraction removed (that is, metabolized). They discovered that this fraction varied inversely with the alveolar halothane partial pressure (fig. 11, 3). Nearly complete metabolism occurred at very low partial pressures, but at alveolar concentrations near or above MAC there was no measurable metabolism. It may well be that halothane was extracted by the liver at the higher concentrations, but that their techniques were too crude to detect such extractions. A continued

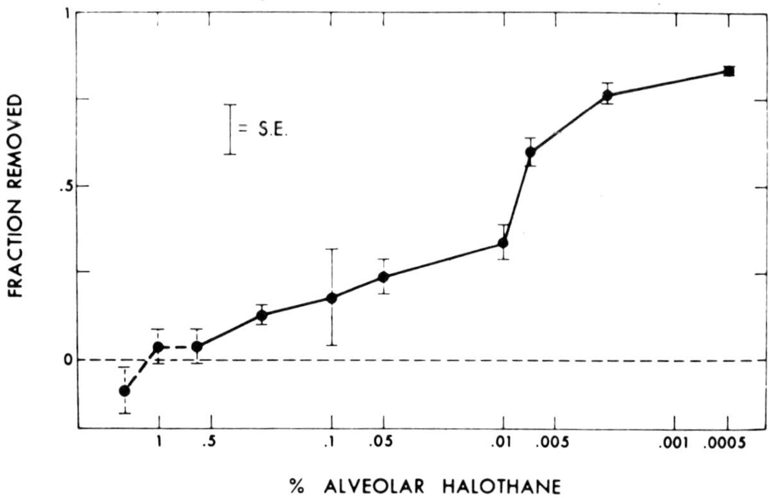

FIG. 11, 3. The fraction of halothane removed from the blood passing through the liver of miniature swine increases from 0 at concentrations of greater than 0.5 percent to 0.8 (80 percent removal) at concentrations of approximately 1/1000 MAC. *Dashed line* indicates values not significantly different from 0. (Reproduced with permission from Sawyer, D. C., Eger, E. I., II, Bahlman, S. H., et al: Concentration dependence of hepatic halothane metabolism. Anesthesiology 34: 230–235, 1971.)

extraction would be expected with enzyme saturation. Enzyme saturation occurs when the amount of substrate (anesthetic) present is sufficient to produce a maximum enzymatic degradation. Degradation thus cannot be further increased by addition of more substrate. Such a condition also implies that the number of molecules metabolized per minute is independent of increases in anesthetic concentration.

Similar results were obtained for fluroxene: hepatic clearance was unmeasurable near MAC but reached 80 percent at concentrations between 0.01 and 0.003 MAC (16). The results are consistent with the finding by Blake *et al.* (4) that concomitant fluroxene anesthesia inhibits the metabolism of tracer amounts of radioactive fluroxene in the dog. If these results apply to man, than during general anesthesia metabolism is too small to influence anesthetic uptake and the alveolar concentration. It is of interest that metabolism is nearly complete at the concentrations breathed by anesthetists (17).

The relationship of metabolism to alveolar concentration has two implications. First, results of studies of uptake at subanesthetic levels may differ considerably from results obtained at anesthetizing concentrations. "Tracer" studies of uptake may underestimate the rate of rise of alveolar concentration during general anesthesia. For example, compare the rate of rise to halothane or methoxyflurane when no anesthetic is extracted from the hepatic flow to the rate of rise when 75 percent is extracted (fig. 11, 1). Tracer studies of anesthetic uptake should be viewed with suspicion unless it can be shown that metabolism is not dependent on concentration. Second, these findings plus our understanding of solubility explain why 50 percent (8) of the methoxyflurane can be recovered as metabolites while only 20 percent (6) of the halothane which is taken up appears as metabolites. The high solubility of methoxyflurane causes it to persist at subanesthetic levels long after anesthesia has been discontinued. Thus, the same methoxyflurane may repeatedly pass through the liver at a concentration which readily permits biotransformation. The lower solubility of halothane results in a more rapid elimination of the intact halothane molecules via the lungs; the liver has fewer chances to attack these molecules at a concentration which allows a large fraction of them to be altered. This reasoning applies to all anesthetics: lower solubility confers more rapid elimination and hence a briefer residence at the low anesthetic partial pressures which permit high metabolic rates. This may be of importance to the toxic effects of anesthetics. If metabolites of anesthetics are all equally toxic, then the least soluble agent should produce the least injury.

Do Sawyer's results in miniature swine apply to man? Is there a relationship in man between anesthetic partial pressure and fractional metabolism of anesthetics such that metabolism does not appreciably affect uptake at anesthetic concentrations? Or is man more like the rat in Berman's study (fig. 11, 2) where stimulated metabolism at anesthetic partial pressures significantly altered anesthetic uptake? Perhaps there is no simple answer. It may be that all agents follow the pattern suggested by Sawyer's work but that the partial pressure at which metabolism is reduced differs between anesthetics or differs in the same anesthetic with prior exposure to agents causing enzyme induction. For example, phenobarbital pretreatment might cause the curve illustrated in figure 11, 3 to shift to the left. If the shift were large enough, there would be an appreciable extraction of halothane at anesthetizing partial pressures. There is indirect evidence which qualitatively supports the applicability of Sawyer's findings to man. First, halothane anesthesia in man decreases the metabolism of tracer amounts of radioactive halothane (14). Second, excretion of urinary metabolites of methoxyflurane in man is sustained at relatively constant levels for up to 40 hours following the cessation of methoxyflurane anesthesia (8). That is, the reduction in the methoxyflurane partial pressure that must occur with time does not reduce the absolute amount of agent metabolized. This would be consonant with the concept of enzyme saturation noted earlier.

Are there agents which are not metabolized? Sawyer (16) found no metabolism of nitrous oxide. Halsey *et al.* (18), using Sawyer's technique measured hepatic extraction only at very low alveolar concentrations

(18). They confirmed Sawyer's finding for halothane and in addition, found a large metabolism of methoxyflurane. They could not detect metabolism of cyclopropane or isoflurane. Metabolism of enflurane was small. Chase *et al.* (19) similarly found that enflurane biotransformation in man is far smaller than the biotransformation of methoxyflurane, fluroxene or halothane.

Summary

The metabolism of inhaled anesthetics may significantly increase anesthetic uptake and thereby slow the induction of anesthesia. The effect is likely to be greater with more soluble anesthetics. However, halothane and fluroxene biotransformation by the liver may be limited so that increasing their partial pressure beyond a certain point may not result in a proportional increase in biotransformation. If this limiting partial pressure is well below the anesthetic range, metabolism would not significantly alter uptake and induction. The limiting partial pressure may be raised by drugs or other agents which induce the enzymes causing the biodegradation of anesthetics. It may approach the anesthetic range for agents such as methoxyflurane.

QUESTIONS

1. Why does metabolism of a soluble anesthetic exert more of an effect on alveolar anesthetic concentration than metabolism of a poorly soluble anesthetic?
2. A small fraction of the total amount of enflurane (Ēthrane) taken up is metabolized. How would you explain why this fraction is far smaller than the fraction for methoxyflurane? Why is it smaller than the halothane fraction?
3. Why would an increase in the fraction of methoxyflurane extracted by the liver be more likely to cause toxicity than a similar increase in the fraction of halothane extracted?
4. Why does the fraction of anesthetic extracted from the hepatic blood flow decrease as the anesthetic partial pressure is raised?
5. Assume that two agents are nearly completely metabolized at subanesthetic partial pressures. Suppose these agents are administered concomitantly, the first at an anesthetic concentration and the second at a low, subanesthetic concentration. Under these circumstances, what fraction of each might be metabolized?

REFERENCES

1. Haggard, H. W.: The absorption, distribution and elimination of ethyl ether. I. The amount of ether absorbed in relation to the concentration inhaled and its fate in the body. J. Biol. Chem. 59: 737–751, 1924.
2. Duncan, W. A. M., and Raventos, J.: The pharmacokinetics of halothane (Fluothane) anesthesia. Brit. J. Anaesth. 31: 302–314, 1959.

3. Van Dyke, R. A., Chenoweth, M. B., and Van Poznak, A.: The metabolism of volatile anesthetics. I. Biochem. Pharmacol. 13: 1239–1247, 1964.
4. Blake, D. A., Rozman, R. S., Cascorbi, H. F., and Krantz, J. C., Jr.: Anesthesia LXXIV: Biotransformation of fluroxene. I. Metabolism in mice and dogs *in vivo*. Biochem. Pharmacol. 14: 1237–1248, 1967.
5. Stier, A., Alter, H., Hessler, O., and Rehder, K.: Urinary excretion of bromide in halothane anesthesia. Anesth. Analg. 43: 723–728, 1964.
6. Rehder, K., Forbes, J., Alter, H., et al: Halothane. Biotransformation in man: a quantitative study. Anesthesiology 28: 711–715, 1967.
7. Blake, D. A., and Cascorbi, H. F.: A note on the biotransformation of fluroxene in two volunteers. Anesthesiology 32: 560, 1970.
8. Holaday, D. A., Rudofsky, S., and Treuhaft, P. S.: Metabolic degradation of methoxyflurane in man. Anesthesiology 33: 579–593, 1970.
9. Berman, M. L., Lowe, H. J., Hagler, K. J., and Bochantin, J.: Uptake and elimination of methoxyflurane as influenced by enzyme induction in the rat. Anesthesiology 38: 352–357, 1973.
10. Beckett, A. H., and Triggs, E. J.: Enzyme induction in man caused by smoking. Nature 216: 587, 1967.
11. Welch, R. M., Harrison, Y. E., Conney, A. H., et al: Cigarette smoking: stimulatory effect on metabolism of 3–4 Benzpyrene by enzymes in human placenta. Science 160: 541–542, 1968.
12. Keeri-Szanto, M., and Pomeroy, J. A.: *Atmospheric Pollution, Enzyme Induction and Intravenous Anaesthetic Requirements: A Causal Correlation?* pp. 139–140. Abstracts of Scientific Papers, American Society of Anesthesiologists 1970 Annual Meeting.
13. Van Dyke, R. A.: Metabolism of volatile anesthetics. III. Induction of microsomal dechlorinating and ether-cleaving enzymes. J. Pharmacol. Exp. Ther. 154: 364–369, 1966.
14. Cascorbi, H. F., Blake, D. A., and Helrich, M.: Differences in the biotransformation of halothane in man. Anesthesiology 32: 119–123, 1970.
15. Sawyer, D. C., Eger, E. I., II, Bahlman, S. H., et al: Concentration dependence of hepatic halothane metabolism. Anesthesiology 34: 230–235, 1971.
16. Sawyer, D. C., Eger, E. I., II, Bahlman, S. H., *et al.*; Metabolism of inhalation anesthetics. In *Cellular Biology and Toxicity of Anesthetics*, edited by B. R. Fink, pp. 238–247. Williams & Wilkins Co., Baltimore, 1972.
17. Whitcher, C. E., Cohen, E. N., and Trudell, J. R.: Chronic exposure to anesthetic gases in the operating room. Anesthesiology 35: 348–353, 1971.
18. Halsey, M. J., Sawyer, D. C., Eger, E. I., II, Bahlman, S. H., and Impelman, D. J. K.: Hepatic metabolism of halothane, methoxyflurane, cyclopropane, Ēthrane and Forane in miniature swine. Anesthesiology 35: 43–47, 1971.
19. Chase, R. E., Holaday, D. A., Fiserona-Bergerona, V., *et al.*: The biotransformation of Ēthrane in man. Anesthesiology 35: 262–267, 1971.

Chapter 12

Effect of Anesthetic Circuit on Alveolar Rate of Rise

Thus far we have examined the approach of an alveolar anesthetic concentration towards a fixed inspired concentration. This constancy of the inspired concentration disappears in a rebreathing anesthetic circuit.* In a rebreathing system, the inspired concentration may vary and only the concentration flowing into the circuit from the machine remains constant.

In this chapter, we will examine the factors which determine the rate of rise of the alveolar anesthetic concentration towards a constant *inflowing* concentration. The factors that govern this relationship include all those previously discussed plus several new ones. All of these new factors slow the rate of rise of the alveolar concentration by slowing the rate of rise of the inspired concentration.

The Time Constant of the Anesthetic Circuit

The gas volume within an anesthetic circuit dilutes the inflowing anesthetic. The inflow must wash out the circuit in order to develop an inspired anesthetic concentration. Two factors govern the rate of washout: the gas volume and the inflow rate. The normal system volume includes corrugated tubes (0.5 to 0.7 liters each), carbon dioxide absorber (2 liters), fittings and valves (1 liter), and rebreathing bag (3 liters) or a total volume of about 7 liters. An inflow rate of 5 liters/minute gives a time constant of 1.4 minutes (i.e., 7 liters/(5 liters/minute)) and produces a reasonably rapid rise in inspired anesthetic concentration. A 1 liter/minute inflow gives a time constant of 7 minutes. By restricting the rate of rise of the inspired concentration, low inflow rates may delay the development of anesthesia (fig. 12, 1). This hindrance to the development of an adequate inspired concentration may be overcome with a potent agent by raising the inflowing concentration. However, the hazard of hypoxia limits the usefulness of such a maneuver with nitrous oxide.

* By circuit, we mean a circle absorption system. Other systems will be discussed in the next chapter.

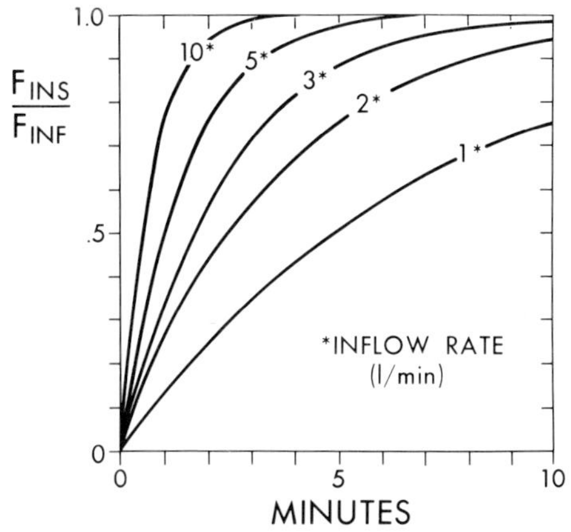

FIG. 12, 1. An increase of the inflow rate into a circle system increases the rate of rise of the concentration within the system (F_{INS}) toward the inflowing (F_{INF}) concentration. The inflow rate is indicated on the individual curves. Not indicated is that the circle system volume is 7 liters; that the gases flowing into the system are immediately mixed with those already within the system, and that there is no anesthetic uptake from the system.

The rapid establishment of the maximum safe inspired concentration of nitrous oxide requires a high (5 to 10 liters/minute) initial inflow rate.

Anesthetic Uptake by Rubber and Other Circuit Components

Another barrier to the development of an inspired concentration is the uptake of anesthetic by circuit components, principally rubber (1–3). The effect of this uptake was demonstrated by the following experiment. Two corrugated rubber hoses and a 5 liter rubber bag were connected in a circle and the gases within this system were mixed with a gas circulator. A 3 liter/minute flow of nitrous oxide or halothane or methoxyflurane was directed into this system and the anesthetic concentrations flowing into and within the system were measured. The rise in concentration of these agents in the circle towards the inflowing concentration is shown in figure 12, 2. Nitrous oxide increased most rapidly, and at a rate which would be predicted if nitrous oxide were not taken up by rubber. Halothane concentration rose less rapidly and methoxyflurane least rapidly. Even after 30 minutes, loss of methoxyflurane to rubber equalled 22 percent of the amount delivered. Such uptake obviously hinders the development of an anesthetizing inspired concentration.

This difficulty can be surmounted by increasing the inflow rate. Since the amount extracted by the rubber is relatively constant, an increased delivery reduces the fraction removed (i.e., enlarges the denominator without changing the numerator). This effect, and the converse effect achieved by reducing the inflow, are shown in figure 12, 3. Unfortunately, the use of high flows is wasteful and perhaps hazardous. How else can we

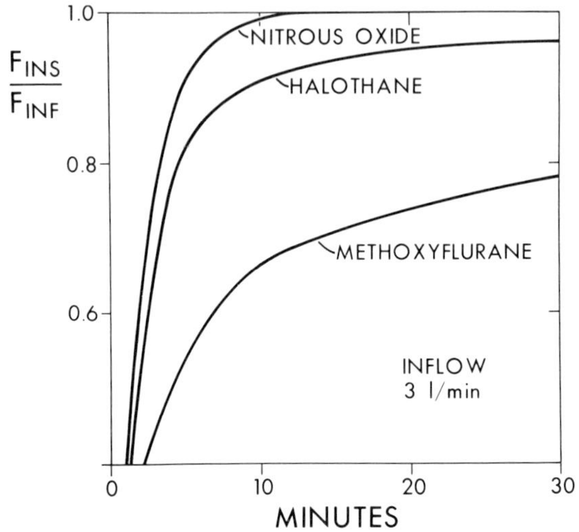

FIG. 12, 2. This figure describes the effect of rubber uptake on the rate of rise of nitrous oxide, halothane and methoxyflurane within a 6.2 liter anesthetic system. The system is composed of a 5 liter rubber bag, 2 corrugated rubber hoses and a gas circulator (no patient). F_{INS} is the concentration within the system (i.e., the concentration which would be inspired) while F_{INF} is the concentration in the 3 liter/minute inflow. Uptake is greatest with the most rubber-soluble agent, methoxyflurane, and hence its rate of rise is most impeded (2).

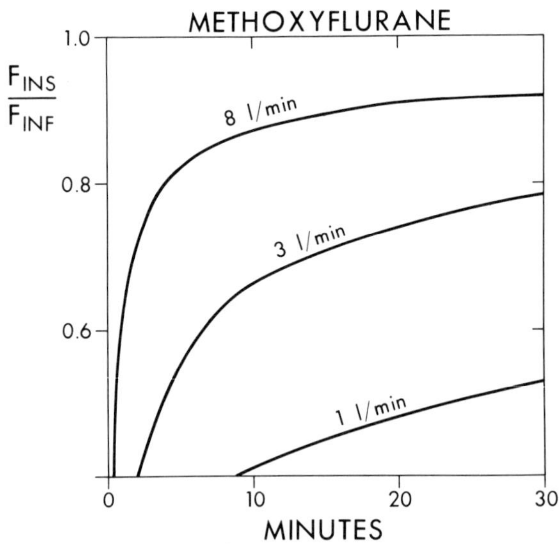

FIG. 12, 3. This figure again demonstrates the impact of rubber uptake on anesthetic concentration within a circle system. In contrast to figure 12, 2, the anesthetic (methoxyflurane) is the same for all curves but the inflow is 1, 3 or 8 liters/minute. An increase in inflow reduces the effect of methoxyflurane uptake (2).

avoid this problem? One way is to choose an anesthetic which is poorly soluble in rubber (see table 12, 1). Hopefully, most new anesthetics will not be as rubber soluble as methoxyflurane or trichloroethylene. The new anesthetics enflurane and isoflurane apparently fit this description.

Soda lime also may absorb anesthetic. Initial studies suggested a halothane soda lime/gas partition coefficient of about 1 (1). Later studies suggested that halothane solubility in soda lime might vary; that solubility increases logarithmically with decreasing water content of the soda lime (4). Finally, the dye which indicates exhaustion of the absorbant also may take up anesthetic (5). Unfortunately, the data available are too limited to precisely define the effects of indicating soda lime on the inspired concentration of anesthetic.

The Effect of Inflow Rate, Uptake and Ventilation on the Inspired Concentration

For the moment let us ignore the effect of rubber uptake and of system washout. In the absence of these factors, what determines the inspired anesthetic concentration in a rebreathing circuit? The inspired gas has two origins: the inflow (which contains a constant anesthetic concentration) and rebreathed gas. The rebreathed gas has a concentration lower than that inspired by virtue of uptake of anesthetic from the lung. The addition of this anesthetic depleted gas to the inflowing gas must produce an inspired concentration which is less than the concentration in the inflow.

The reduction in inspired concentration depends on the extent of rebreathing and on the amount of anesthetic taken up (6–8). The extent

TABLE 12, 1*

Agent	Rubber/Gas Partition Coefficient at 23°C
Nitrous oxide	1.2
Cyclopropane	6.6
Fluroxene	20
Divinyl ether	45
Diethyl ether	58
Isoflurane	62
Enflurane	74
Halothane	120
Chloroform	300
Methoxyflurane	630
Trichloroethylene	830

* All values are from Titel, J. H., and Lowe, H. S.: Rubber/gas partition coefficients. Anesthesiology 29: 1215–1216, 1968, except for the isoflurane and enflurane data which are from Lowe, H. S., personal communication.

of rebreathing is determined by the relationship between inflow rate and alveolar ventilation: an increase in inflow rate reduces rebreathing while an increase in alveolar ventilation does the opposite. The interaction of these factors may be described by the following equation:*

$$F_{INS}/F_{INF} = \dot{V}_{INF}/(\dot{V}_{INF} + \dot{V}_A (1 - R)) \tag{5}$$

Equation 5 indicates that the approach of the inspired to inflowing concentrations (F_{INS}/F_{INF}) depends on a relationship between the inflow rate ($\dot{V}_{INF}$), alveolar minute ventilation ($\dot{V}_A$) and the fraction of gas extracted from the respired gases (1 − R). R is the ratio of the alveolar to the inspired anesthetic concentrations. If the inflow rate is high relative to ventilation or if uptake is low (R approaches 1), then the inspired concentration will be close to the inflowing concentration. However, if ventilation is large relative to the inflow and if much of the inspired anesthetic is taken up, then the inspired concentration will be far below that in the inflowing gas. The extremes obtainable are intuitively obvious: a high inflow rate puts the inspired concentration close to the inflowing concentration. If ventilation far exceeds the inflow rate, the expired gas concentration makes up most of the inspired concentration.

Let us look at some specific examples (fig. 12, 4). Assume a normal alveolar ventilation of 4 liters/minute. At an inflow of 4 liters/minute, the inspired concentration may be as little as 55 percent of that inspired if 80 percent (R = 0.2) of the anesthetic breathed is taken up. This might be

---

* The volume of anesthetic entering the system per minute equals the concentration delivered (F_{INF}) times the inflow rate ($\dot{V}_{INF}$). This also must equal the amount lost to the patient by uptake ($\dot{V}_U$) plus the amount lost through the overflow (pop-off) valve (the whole equals the sum of its parts). The amount lost through the overflow equals the concentration in the exiting gas times the total volume ejected. If all the gases entering the system are mixed immediately with the gases within the system, then the concentration in the ejected gas also is that inspired (F_{INS}). If the volume of anesthetic and oxygen taken up by the patient is small compared to the volume flowing in, then the volume flowing out must nearly equal the inflowing volume. From these assumptions:

$$F_{INF} \cdot \dot{V}_{INF} = F_{INS} \cdot \dot{V}_{INF} + \dot{V}_U \tag{1}$$

which is a restatement of the assertion that the amount of anesthetic delivered to the system ($F_{INF} \cdot \dot{V}_{INF}$) equals the amount lost through the overflow ($F_{INS} \cdot \dot{V}_{INF}$) plus the amount taken up by the patient ($\dot{V}_U$). Let

$$R = \frac{F_A}{F_{INS}} \tag{2}$$

where F_A is the alveolar concentration and F_{INS} the inspired concentration. If $\dot{V}_A$ is the alveolar minute ventilation and $\dot{V}_D$ the dead space minute ventilation, then:

$$\dot{V}_E = \dot{V}_A + \dot{V}_D \tag{3}$$

The amount of anesthetic taken up must equal the amount inspired minus the amount exhaled.

$$\dot{V}_U = F_{INS}\dot{V}_E - (F_A\dot{V}_A + F_{INS}\dot{V}_D) \tag{4}$$

Substituting 2 and 3 into 4, and 4 into 1 and rearranging gives equation 5 (see text).

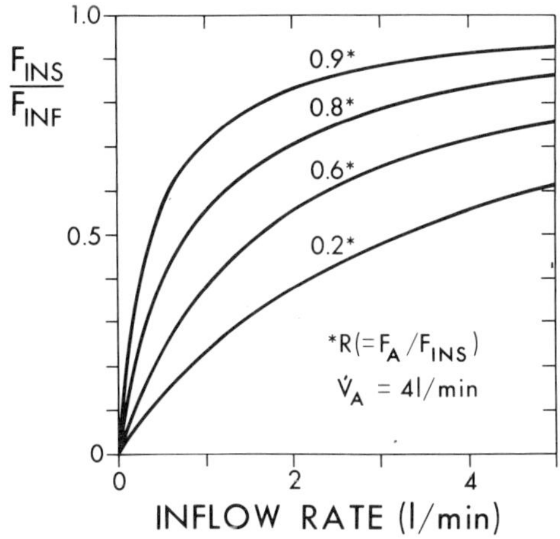

FIG. 12, 4. Rebreathing reduces the inspired (F_{INS}) concentration of anesthetic below that delivered in the inflow (F_{INF}). The extent of rebreathing is inversely related to the inflow rate. The impact of the rebreathed gas on the inspired concentration depends on how much anesthetic has been removed (taken up) from the respired gas. The effect of uptake appears in the R value which is the ratio of alveolar (F_A) to inspired anesthetic concentrations: the greater the uptake the smaller the R. Note that there is no time scale; that is, these curves describe "steady state" conditions as indicated by equation 5.

expected with methoxyflurane. If 40 to 10 percent (R = 0.6 to 0.9) of the anesthetic is removed (halothane, enflurane, isoflurane or fluroxene) then the inspired concentration still is only 70 to 90 percent of inspired. Thus, at a 4 liter/minute inflow rate, the inspired concentration may not equal the concentration delivered from the machine even with anesthetics that are only modestly soluble. This discrepancy becomes far greater at lower inflow rates: at a 1 liter/minute inflow even when uptake causes the removal of only 20 percent of the respired gases, the concentration inspired is reduced to nearly half of that in the inflowing gas. How difficult it is at these inflow rates to predict the inspired and therefore the alveolar concentration!

The Effect of Inflow Rate and Uptake on the Alveolar Anesthetic Concentration

Let us now add the factors of system and lung washout and allow for the rising ratio of alveolar to inspired concentration that accompanies an increase in duration of anesthesia. What is the impact of inflow rate and of ventilation on the *alveolar* concentration. Regardless of inflow rate, alveolar ventilation sets an upper limit to the rate of alveolar anesthetic rise. This is not surprising since an infinite inflow rate simply converts the circle system to a nonrebreathing system, and as noted in Chapter 3, the rate of alveolar anesthetic rise in a nonrebreathing system is governed

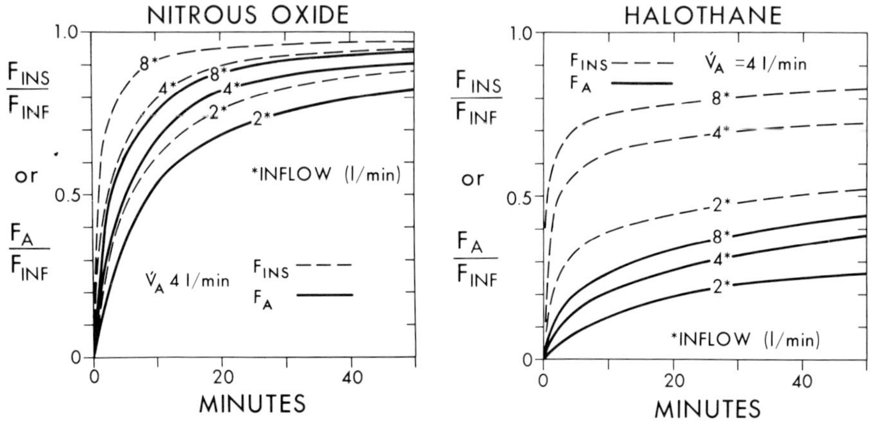

FIGS. 12, 5; 12, 6 and 12, 7. The rate of rise of the inspired (*dashed lines*, F_{INS}) and consequently the rate of rise of the alveolar (*continuous lines*, F_A) anesthetic concentration toward the inflowing concentration (F_{INF}) is influenced by inflow rate and by anesthetic solubility. Nitrous oxide (fig. 12, 5) is less soluble than halothane (12, 6) which in turn is less soluble than methoxyflurane (12, 7); as a result the inspired (and alveolar) rate of rise of methoxyflurane is slower than halothane while halothane rises more slowly than nitrous oxide. For all three anesthetics, an increase in inflow rate decreases rebreathing and thereby raises the inspired and alveolar concentrations. The effect of inflow rate on anesthetic dose increases with increasing solubility. Alveolar ventilation in all cases is 4 liters/minute.

by ventilation. Similarly, a finite inflow rate limits the rate of alveolar rise no matter what the ventilation. The limiting effects of *both* inflow and ventilation come about because their effects are imposed independently *and* in series. Perhaps the importance of their in series relationship is best appreciated as inflow and ventilation approach zero. At zero inflow, the alveolar concentration cannot rise regardless of ventilation; at zero ventilation, the alveolar concentration cannot rise regardless of inflow.

The effect of differences in inflow and uptake on the rise of the alveolar and inspired concentrations is shown in figures 12, 5; 12, 6 and 12, 7. Alveolar ventilation is constant at 4 liters/minute. By diminishing rebreathing, a high inflow rate raises the inspired concentration (dashed lines). The importance of a high inflow rate decreases as solubility and hence uptake diminishes. When uptake is zero, the inhaled and exhaled anesthetic concentrations are equal (except for an initial dilution by gas in the lung), and therefore rebreathing cannot influence the inspired concentration. The rate of rise of inspired concentration is then primarily governed by the washin rate produced by flow and circuit volume and secondarily, by the smaller dilution by gases in the lung. Since this washin occurs quickly the alveolar rate of rise also must be relatively rapid with poorly soluble agents over a wide range of inflow rates. Even

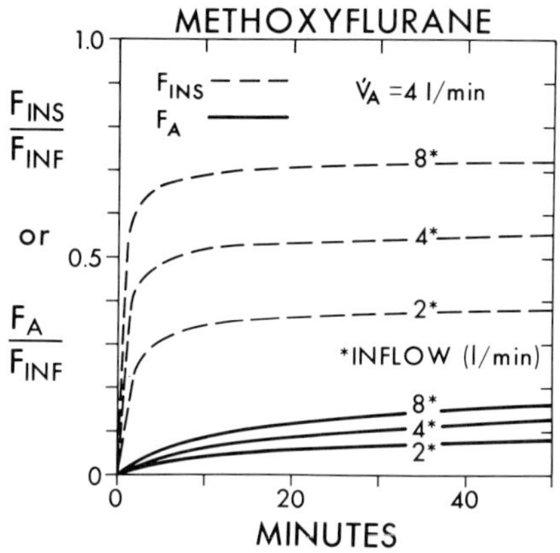

FIG. 7

so, a significant difference exists between the inspired nitrous oxide concentrations generated by various inflows for several minutes after the start of anesthesia when uptake is at its greatest rate (fig. 12, 5). For example, at 10 minutes the inspired concentration is 60 percent of the inflowing when the inflow rate is 2 liters/minute but is 90 percent when the inflow is 8 liters/minute. The effect this will have on induction is obvious. With time (and decreasing uptake) the difference becomes negligible. For example, at 50 minutes, the inspired concentration produced by a 2 liter/minute inflow is nearly 90 percent of that inspired (fig. 12, 5). With a highly soluble agent such as methoxyflurane the inflow rate is of importance at all times. At 50 minutes a 2 liter/minute inflow produces an inspired methoxyflurane concentration which is only 38 percent of the inflowing concentration (fig. 12, 7). An increase in inflow can considerably increase the inspired and hence the alveolar methoxyflurane concentration. The clinical importance of this effect is immediately apparent: once anesthesia is established, changes in inflow rate will not significantly alter the depth of anesthesia of a poorly soluble agent but may alter the depth of a moderately or highly soluble agent.

Saturation of tissues with anesthetic decreases anesthetic uptake. Since a decrease in uptake raises the inspired concentration, it follows that with a given anesthetic and inflow rate, the inspired concentration will rise with increased duration of administration. This implies that higher inflows may be required to sustain an inspired concentration during the high uptake which accompanies induction of anesthesia, but may be wasteful during maintenance where a lower uptake allows the inspired to approach the inflowing concentration nearly as well with low inflow rates. This thought applies in particular to the poorly soluble agents.

Effect of Ventilation and Uptake on the Alveolar Anesthetic Concentration

Let us now hold the inflow rate constant at 4 liters/minute while we vary alveolar ventilation. An increase in ventilation accelerates the rate of alveolar rise (figs. 12, 8; 12, 9 and 12, 10). The alveolar concentration of a more soluble agent such as halothane (fig. 12, 9) or methoxyflurane (fig. 12, 10) is altered more by ventilatory changes than the concentration of a

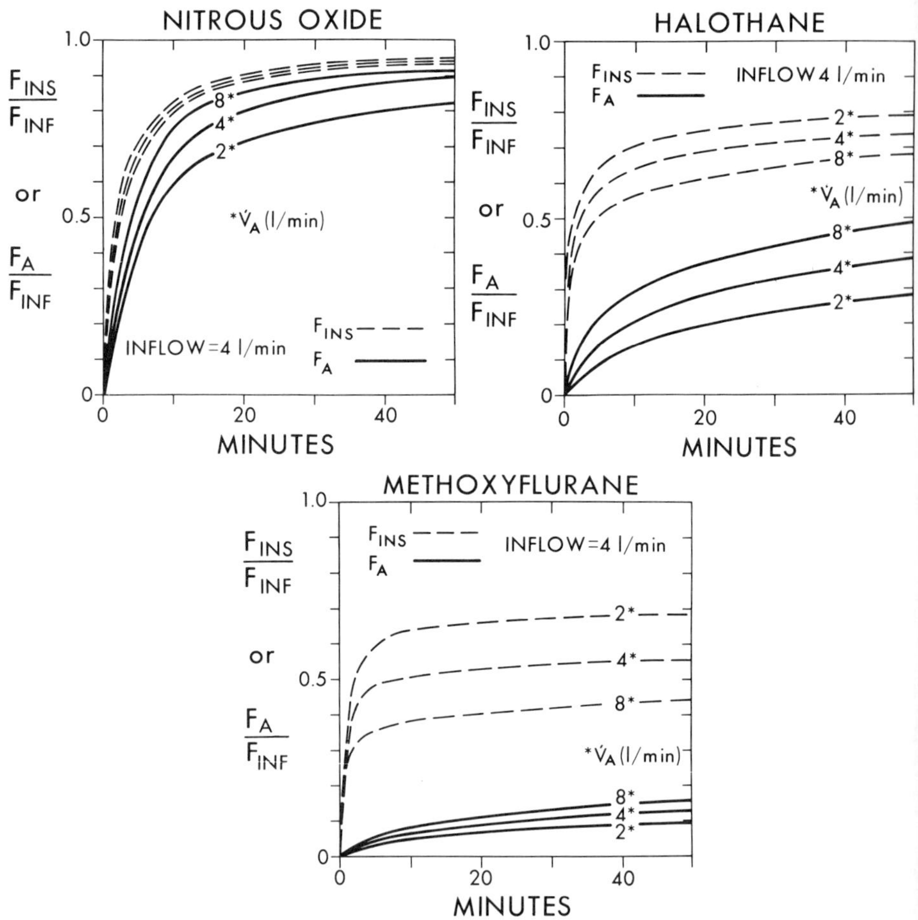

FIGS. 12, 8; 12, 9 and 12, 10. These figures are similar to the preceding 3 figures except that now the inflow is held constant at 4 liters/minute while alveolar ventilation ($\dot{V}_A$) is varied. Note that an increase in ventilation raises the alveolar concentration (*continuous lines*) but that the resultant lowering of the inspired concentration (*dashed lines*) limits the alveolar rise. The effect on the inspired concentration is most prominent with the most soluble anesthetic.

poorly soluble agent such as nitrous oxide (fig. 12, 8). However, these alterations in alveolar concentration achieved with a rebreathing circuit are less than those achieved with a nonrebreathing system. Compare the spread of the alveolar rates of rise in these figures with those displayed in fig. 7, 1. The difference is most striking with the most soluble agents. With a rebreathing system the alveolar methoxyflurane concentration is not even doubled when ventilation is increased from 2 to 8 liters/minutes (fig. 12, 10). In contrast, with a nonrebreathing system, alveolar ether is more than tripled by the same increase in ventilation (fig. 7, 1). The cause of this difference is found in the effect of an increased ventilation on the inspired anesthetic concentration. As ventilation increases, the rebreathed gases contribute more to the inspired concentration which accordingly falls. In the case of the highly soluble agents, this fall is great enough to limit the rise in alveolar concentration.

This limitation to the effect of an increase in ventilation is augmented by lower inflow rates. At a 1 liter/minute inflow, an 8 fold difference in ventilation has a relatively small effect on the alveolar concentration of methoxyflurane (fig. 12, 11). The impact of an increase in ventilation on the inspired and hence the alveolar concentration is evident. One clinical implication that emerges is that the use of a low flow system may produce a more stable alveolar anesthetic concentration in the face of variations in ventilation. Contrast the changes found in figure 12, 11 with those in figure 7, 1 or 12, 10. However, the constancy of this condition does depend on the constancy of cardiac output: variations in cardiac

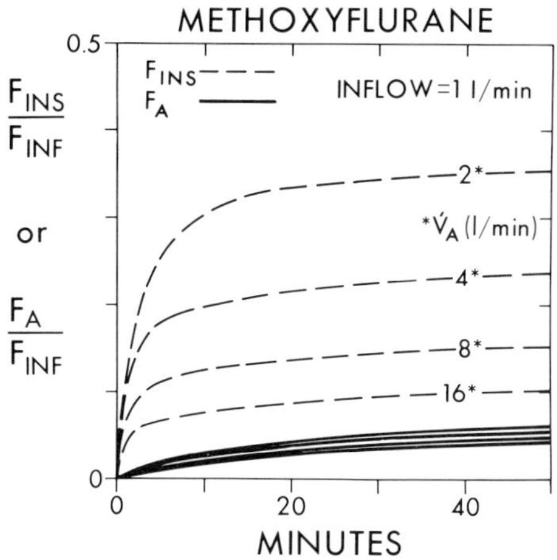

FIG. 12, 11. This figure differs from figure 12, 10 in that the inflow is reduced to 1 liter/minute. The effect is to increase the impact of an increase in alveolar ventilation on the inspired methoxyflurane concentration. The result is a greater stability of the alveolar concentration. Note that the vertical scale runs from 0 to 0.5 rather than 1.0.

output will cause considerable variations in uptake and hence alveolar concentration.

Effect of Changes in Uptake

In a nonrebreathing system, an increase in uptake (say by an increase in solubility or cardiac output) lowers the alveolar concentration relative to the concentration being inspired. In a rebreathing system, the alveolar concentration is lowered still more by an increase in uptake because of the consequent reduction in the inspired concentration. In a nonrebreathing system if an increase in uptake is accompanied by a proportional increase in ventilation there may be little change (fig. 7, 16) or even an increase (figs. 7, 14 or 7, 15) in the alveolar concentration. As noted in Chapter 7, the augmented ventilation and (if the increased uptake is caused by an increase in cardiac output) accelerated tissue

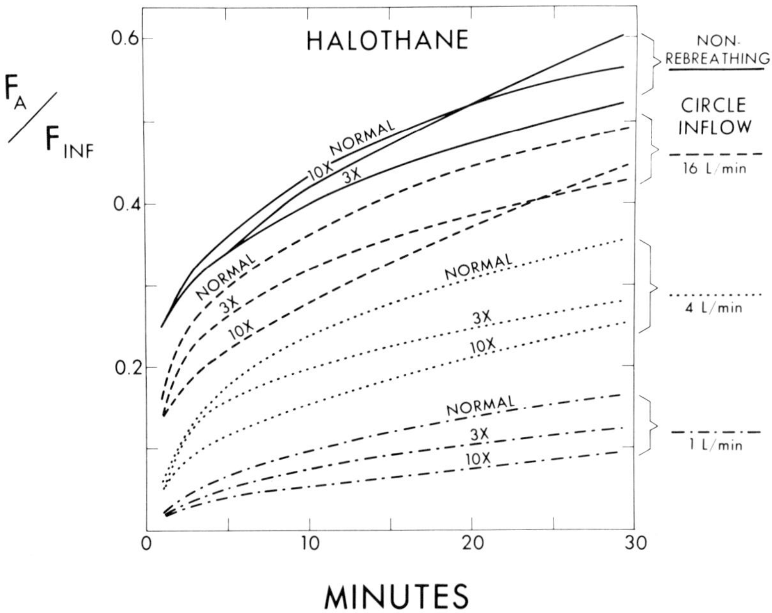

FIG. 12, 12. A 3 (3 ×) to 10 (10 ×) fold increase in muscle blood flow has little effect on the alveolar rate of rise of halothane in a nonrebreathing system (alveolar ventilation increased in proportion to the attendant increase in total cardiac output). However, in a rebreathing circuit an increase in muscle blood flow exerts an increasing influence on the alveolar rate of rise as inflow rate decreases. At a 1 liter/minute inflow, the alveolar halothane concentration with a 10 fold increase in blood flow is about half the concentration at normal flows, over the 10 to 30 minute interval: at a 16 liter/minute inflow the difference is less than a quarter. (Reproduced with permission from Eger, E. I., II, Bahlman, S. H., Halsey, M. J., and Sawyer, D. C.: The effect of distribution of increased cardiac output on the pulmonary exchange of halothane, nitrous oxide and methoxyflurane. Anesth. Analg. 52: 625–632, 1973.)

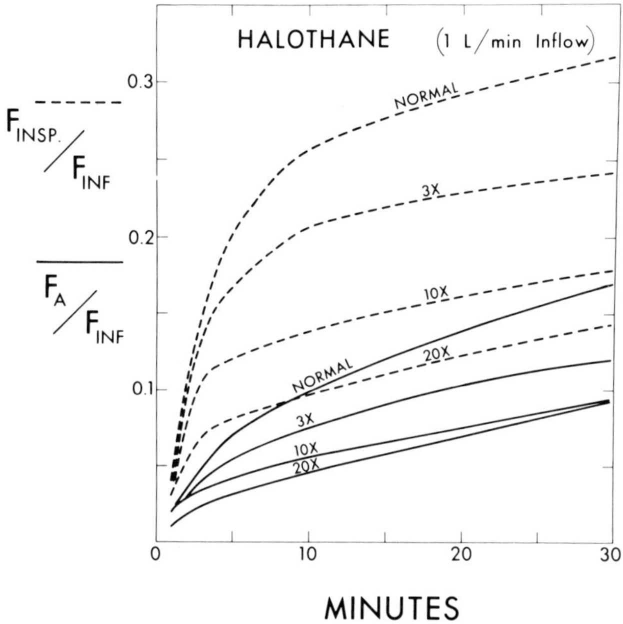

FIG. 12, 13. As seen in figure 12, 12 an increase in halothane uptake due to an increase in muscle blood flow may hinder the alveolar rate of rise of halothane. The figure shows that this effect is achieved in a rebreathing circuit by reducing the inspired concentration. Inflow is 1 liter/minute. (Reproduced with permission from Eger, E. I., II, Bahlman, S. H., Halsey, M. J., and Sawyer, D. C.: The effect of distribution of increased cardiac output on the pulmonary exchange of halothane, nitrous oxide and methoxyflurane. Anesth. Analg. 52: 625–632, 1973.)

equilibration oppose the tendency of the increased uptake to lower the alveolar concentration. However, the impact of an increased ventilation is weakened by rebreathing (especially see figs. 12, 10 and 12, 11). The result is that in a rebreathing system an increase in uptake reduces the alveolar concentration despite an augmented ventilation. This is seen for the increased uptake that results from greater muscle blood flow (fig. 12, 12) (9). Despite a proportional rise in ventilation the result of an increase in muscle blood flow and uptake is to reduce the anesthetic alveolar concentration. A greater reduction is seen with a lower inflow rate. The increase in rebreathing reduces the inspired and hence the alveolar concentrations (fig. 12, 13).

We learned that children were more readily induced than adults because the alveolar and brain rates of rise were more rapid in the young patient (Chapter 7). (We also learned that the concomitant rise in MAC would compensate for this). There are other benefits from smallness. Even if the alveolar approach to the inspired concentration in the young were the same as in adults, the smaller total ventilation of the child would reduce rebreathing. Thus, for a given inflow rate, induction should be accelerated in a child. Similarly, a small adult should be "easier" to induce and maintain than a large one; a fat person "easier" than a muscular one of the same weight; an old adult "easier" than a young adult.

Summary

The insertion of an anesthetic circuit between the patient and the source of anesthetic agent creates additional hindrances to the alveolar rate of anesthetic rise. The additional gas volume must be washed out: the rate of washout depends on the relationship of inflow rate to the volume of the anesthetic circuit. The rubber or soda lime in the anesthetic circuit may further hinder the development of an inspired anesthetic partial pressure by absorbing anesthetic agent.

Anesthetic uptake influences the alveolar concentration in two ways. First, as noted in previous chapters, uptake prevents the alveolar anesthetic concentration from reaching the concentration in the inspired gas. Second, uptake lowers the anesthetic concentration in the rebreathed gases and hence lowers the inspired concentration. Any factor which increases rebreathing (such as a decrease in inflow rate or an increase in ventilation) or increases uptake (such as an increase in solubility or in cardiac output) will lower the inspired anesthetic concentration. This in turn, will be reflected in a slower rate of alveolar anesthetic rise.

QUESTIONS

1. Graph the relationship between the oil/gas partition coefficients (table 4, 1) and the rubber/gas partition coefficients (table 12, 1). A new inhaled anesthetic has an oil/gas partition coefficient of 800. What would you predict the rubber/gas partition coefficient to be? Would the rubber in an anesthetic circuit significantly affect the inspired concentration of this agent? How might we reduce the effect of rubber uptake?
2. What hazards accrue to the use of high inflow rates?
3. Given that an anesthetic has an alveolar concentration which is half that inspired ($F_A/F_I = 0.5$). At an inflow rate of 4 liters/minute, an alveolar ventilation of 4 liters/minute, and an inflowing concentration of 1 percent, what is the inspired concentration (presume washout of system and lung has been completed and rubber uptake is of no moment)? What would the inspired concentration be if $F_A/F_I = 0.1$?
4. Which is more important to the alveolar rate of rise: inflow rate or alveolar ventilation?
5. At a low inflow rate (1 liter/minute) why do changes in ventilation, 2 to 8 liters/minute, have little effect on the alveolar methoxyflurane concentration?

6. At a low ventilation (1 liter/minute) why do changes in inflow from 2 to 8 liters/minute have little effect on the alveolar concentration?
7. How might hypothermia or hyperthermia alter the inspired concentration in a rebreathing circuit?

REFERENCES

1. Eger, E. I., II, Larson, C. P., Jr., and Severinghaus, J. W.: The solubility of halothane in rubber, soda lime and various plastics. Anesthesiology 23: 365–383, 1962.
2. Eger, E. I., II, and Brandstater, B.: Solubility of methoxyflurane in rubber. Anesthesiology 24: 679–683, 1963.
3. Titel, J. H., and Lowe, H. J.: Rubber-gas partition coefficients. Anesthesiology 29: 1215–1216, 1968.
4. Titel, J. H., Lowe, H. J., Elam, J. O., and Grosholz, J. R.: Quantitative closed-circuit halothane anesthesia. Anesth. Analg. 47: 560–569, 1968.
5. Nichols, R., and Topping, A.: Absorption of ethylene by self-indicating soda lime. Nature 211: 217, 1966.
6. Mapleson, W. W.: The concentration of anaesthetics in closed circuits with special reference to halothane. I. Theoretical study. Brit. J. Anaesth. 7: 298–309, 1960.
7. Galloon, S.: The concentration of anaesthetics in closed circuits with special reference to halothane. II. Laboratory and theatre investigations. Brit. J. Anaesth. 7: 310–232, 1960.
8. Mushin, W. W., and Galloon, S.: The concentration of anaesthetics in closed circuits with special reference to halothane. III. Clinical aspects. Brit. J. Anaesth. 7: 324–333, 1960.
9. Eger, E. I., II, Bahlman, S. H., Halsey, M. J., and Sawyer, D. C.: The effect of distribution of increased cardiac output on the pulmonary exchange of halothane, nitrous oxide and methoxyflurane. Anesth. Analg. 52: 625–632, 1973.

Chapter 13

Anesthetic Systems: Construction and Function

An anesthetic system is a device for presenting an anesthetic mixture to a patient. It may be as simple as a gauze mask moistened with ether or as complex as a circle-absorption system. Hundreds of different devices have been constructed—and abandoned for better models. Although much of their development resulted from trial and error rather than prospective plan, the forms that evolved have a lovely logic. The logic of these systems is the subject of this chapter.

A Classification of Anesthetic Systems

All anesthetic systems may be classified by 1) the presence or absence of a reservoir; and 2) whether they permit rebreathing (1). Open systems neither have a reservoir nor permit rebreathing. Semiopen systems have a reservoir but prevent rebreathing. Semiclosed systems also have a reservoir but differ from the semiopen system by allowing partial rebreathing. A semiclosed system becomes closed when all exhaled gases except carbon dioxide are rebreathed. The borders between these groups may be fuzzy: for example, a semiclosed system such as a circle absorption system may become a semiopen system at high inflow rates. Still, this grouping is the simplest general classification available and one which sorts systems by the two characteristics which dictate how they function.

Open Systems

The once great popularity of the open drop, insufflation, and the Ayre's T piece techniques has waned. Although these devices are simple (no moving parts!), inexpensive and impose little resistance to breathing, their many disadvantages outweigh their advantages and make them less satisfactory than more modern techniques. They are wasteful of anesthetic. The dilution of inspired anesthetic by ambient air makes the use of impotent agents such as nitrous oxide ineffectual. Lack of a reservoir hinders the assessment of the depth of respiration. Lack of a reservoir also precludes assisted or controlled respiration with insufflation or open drop techniques. Respiration may be controlled (but not assisted) with the Ayre's T piece by occluding the open end of the T. However, prolonged occlusion may lead to overinflation and rupture of the lungs by the thousands of torr pressure which can be delivered via the inflow line pressures (2). Overinflation is more likely to occur with this system because there is little or no "feel" to the pressure developed.

Perhaps the greatest defect of the open system is that it produces an unstable anesthetic state. Peak inspiratory flow rates during anesthesia may range from 15 to 50 liters/minute in children and adults and 5 to 10 liters/minute in infants (3). Since these flows exceed the inflow rate from the machine, they must cause the dilution of inflowing gas with ambient air (fig. 13, 1). An increase in ventilation reduces the inspired concentration. Thus, lightening of anesthesia with its attendant stimulation of ventilation (3) should further lighten anesthesia. The opposite also is true. Deepening anesthesia depresses both the peak inspiratory flow rate (3) and total minute ventilation and thereby increases the inspired concentration and depth of anesthesia. Fortunately, depression of respiration limits the rise in alveolar concentration, and apnea usually (but not always—see Chapter 7) supervenes before lethal concentrations are obtained in the lungs. The tendency for light anesthesia to progress to lighter anesthesia and deep to deeper is characteristic of the open systems. It makes their use a challenge since it requires observation of the patient rather than percentages from a vaporizer. This art of perceiving depth of anesthesia in the complex setting of surgery belongs to few anesthetists. Most of us find it far easier to work with the more

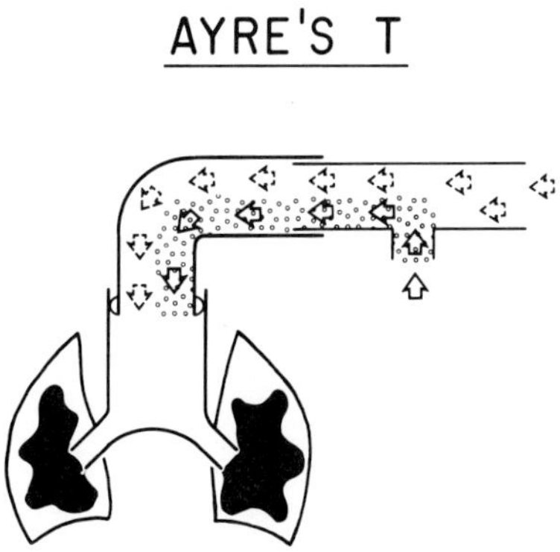

FIG. 13, 1. This diagram illustrates the dilution of inflowing anesthetic (*light stippled area*, *arrows* outlined with *continuous lines*) by ambient air (*clear area*, *arrows* formed by *dashed lines*) that occurs on inspiration using Ayre's T. In this diagram, the Ayre's T is connected to an *in situ* endotracheal tube. *Black area* in lungs indicates alveolar gas.

complicated systems to be described. These systems protect against the oscillations of depth associated with the open systems. However, perhaps it would be well to continue our acquaintance with the open systems. Some procedures such as bronchoscopy or laryngoscopy may require their use, and a national or regional disaster might make them the only available systems. They are still a common system in underdeveloped countries where more expensive devices are economically less feasible.

Semiopen Systems

Semiopen systems may be classified by the number of valves they possess. The Rees modification of Ayres T piece (fig. 13, 2) has no valves (4), the Magill attachment (fig. 13, 3) has one while the various nonrebreathing valves have two. These devices avoid many of the disadvantages of the open systems. They allow the effective use of impotent agents such as nitrous oxide. Respiration may be assessed from the oscillations of the reservoir bag, and compression of the bag may be used to assist or control respiration. But best of all, they produce a more stable anesthetic state: an increase in ventilation cannot dilute the inspired concentration with ambient air, nor can a decrease in ventilation raise the inspired concentration.

However, these systems exact a price for their advantages over the open systems. They are more expensive and cumbersome. They can be more wasteful of anesthetic. Heat loss and drying are great. Nor are their virtues perfect. The assessment of ventilation is hampered by the high inflow rates required to prevent rebreathing. Rebreathing (with its attendant rise in CO_2 and fall in inspired anesthetic concentration) occurs with the Rees and Magill devices if inflow is too low. Too low an inflow produces obstruction with most non-rebreathing valves and in the remainder, causes dilution of inspired gas with ambient air. Thus the use of each semiopen system demands certain precautions regarding inflow rate and the management of ventilation. Let us see what these are.

The Rees T. An inflow of twice the minute volume is prescribed to prevent rebreathing in the Rees T (5). During the first and middle portions of expiration, alveolar (black area, white arrows) and fresh inflowing (clear area, black arrows) gases mix in the reservoir attached to the T (fig. 13, 2*A*). This portion of the inflow is wasted (except that it dilutes any expired gas that may be rebreathed). Figure 13, 2 *B*, *C* and *D* show how the high inflow rate prevents the exhaled fresh gas mix from re-entering the alveoli. At the end of expiration, the inflow sweeps the alveolar gas from the T and adjacent reservoir (fig. 13, 2*B*). The initial portion of inspiration comes from this fresh gas reserve plus the fresh gas which is continuously injected in the inflow (fig. 13, 2*C*). The latter part of inspiration may contain some (diluted) alveolar gas, but this is of no

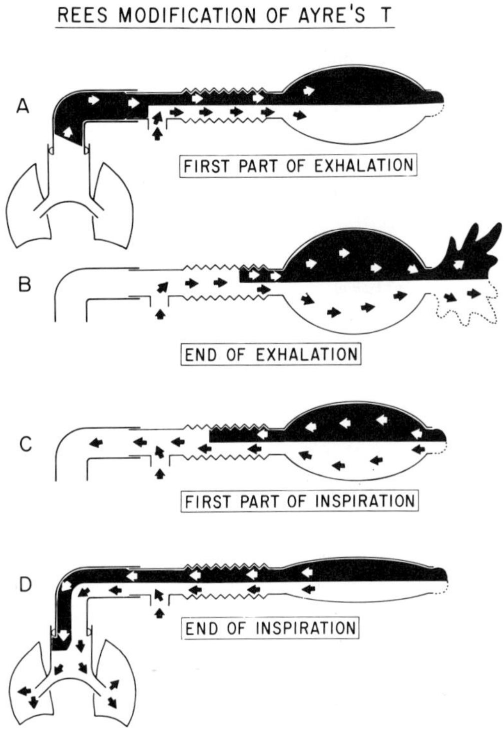

FIG. 13, 2. The Rees modification of Ayre's T adds to the "T" a tube reservoir plus a rebreathing bag which also acts as a reservoir. This device may be connected to a mask or (as in this illustration) to an endotracheal tube. This *black area*, with *white arrows* represents alveolar gas (containing CO_2 and partially depleted of anesthetic) while the *clear area* with *black arrows* represents fresh gas. The *arrows* point in the direction of gas flow.

concern since it lodges in the dead-space (fig. 13, 2*D*). Note that the fresh inflow at the end of the inspiration and through most of exhalation is wasted.

Theoretical analyses (5) and mechanical models (6) indicate that an inflow rate of twice (actually 1.8 times) the minute volume indeed is sufficient to prevent rebreathing. We have confirmed this prediction in studies of patients. Ventilation and alveolar CO_2 remained unchanged at inflow rates 2 times greater than the normal minute volume (Eger, E. I., II: unpublished data). In fact no change in CO_2 or ventilation occurred until we lowered the inflow to less than 1.5 times the minute volume obtained during nonrebreathing.

These predictions and studies assumed that ventilation is sinusoidol. Deviation from this usual ventilatory pattern may radically change the inflow required to prevent rebreathing. For example, the inflow requirement is drastically increased during apneustic breathing where expiration is immediately followed by a rapid and sustained inspiration. Most of the inflow is wasted since it enters the system during the time of sustained inspiration. The brief period between expiration and inspiration allows little time for inflow to "washout" the exhaled gas from the T and reservoir. Moreover, the high inspiratory flow rate prevents the relatively low inflow rate from significantly diluting the previously exhaled gas during inspiration. An inflow rate far in excess of twice the minute volume would be required to prevent rebreathing with an apneustic ventilatory pattern.

Conversely, an inflow rate well below twice the minute ventilation prevents rebreathing if a prolonged end-expiratory pause follows a rapid inspiration and expiration. The inflow is efficiently used since it clears the alveolar gas from the reservoir during the end-expiratory pause. The succeeding inspiration draws on this fresh gas reservoir. The inflow rate required to prevent rebreathing may approach the alveolar minute ventilation.

As noted above, rebreathing usually is prevented by an inflow twice the normal minute volume of ventilation. Rebreathing occurs if ventilation is increased (by assistance or control) without altering the inflow rate. However, the increase in ventilation more than balances the rise in inspired CO_2 and alveolar CO_2 is lowered. The lower limit to which CO_2 may be reduced is slightly less than half normal (it would be exactly half normal if the inflow were twice the normal *alveolar* ventilation).

The Rees T finds many uses and appears in many forms. It frequently is employed in pediatric anesthesia since it imposes little resistance to breathing (no valves) and is least cumbersome of the semiopen systems. The "bag and mask" is a variant of the Rees T. The inflow rate required to eliminate rebreathing in this system is the same as that required for the Rees T (Eger, E. I., II: unpublished data). Finally, the "to-and'fro" system is a Rees T, modified by the addition of a carbon dioxide absorber.

The Magill Attachment. The insertion of the inflow at the tail of the reservoir bag and the addition of a valve distinguishes the Magill attachment from the Rees T (fig. 13, 3). These differences permit a far lower inflow rate to prevent rebreathing by preferentially exhausting alveolar gas through the overflow and by conserving inflow and dead-space (i.e., fresh) gas. This may be understood by examining the distribution of alveolar, dead-space and inflowing gas in the course of one respiratory cycle. At the end of inspiration, assume that the system and dead-space contain only fresh gas. The reservoir bag is flattened (fig. 13, 3*A*). On exhalation assume that the unused (fresh) dead-space gas (stippled area with black arrows) followed by the alveolar gas (black area with white arrows) flows towards the reservoir bag which concomitantly

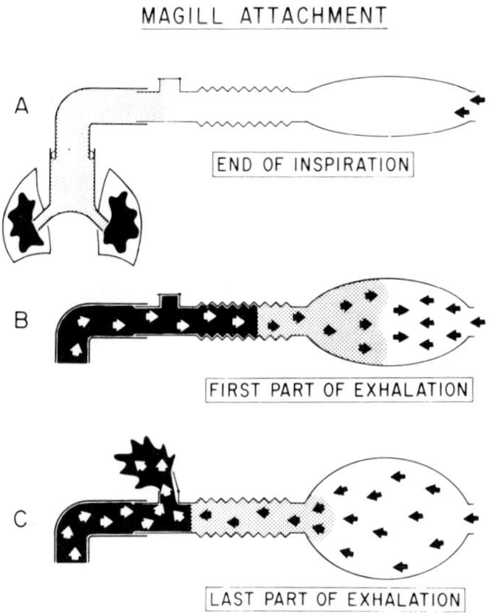

FIG. 13, 3. The symbols used to illustrate the Magill attachment are the same as those used in the previous diagram. Again, the *black area* with *white arrows* represents alveolar gas; the *clear area* with *black arrows* represents fresh gas; and the *stippled area* with *black arrows* represents gas which has resided in the dead-space and has not exchanged gases in the alveoli. The areas in *A* which have no arrows indicate no gas flow; the *arrows* otherwise indicate the direction of flow.

is filled by the inflow (clear area with black arrows) (*B*). No gas is ejected until the reservoir bag fills and the pressure in the system rises. At this point, the overflow valve opens and the remainder of exhalation—containing only alveolar gas—exhausts through the now open valve (*C*). In addition, the continuing inflow now reverses the flow of exhaled gases. The alveolar gas which initially had passed the overflow valve now returns and exits. Note that no dead-space or fresh gas can be ejected unless all the alveolar gas is ejected. Thus, the inflow rate required to eject all the alveolar gas need only equal the alveolar minute ventilation. It had been thought that this theoretical limit could not be achieved in practice because of the mixing of the dead-space and alveolar gas in the reservoir (5). However, the studies of Kain and Nunn (7) have proven otherwise: an inflow equalling the alveolar minute ventilation completely prevents rebreathing.

Unlike the Rees T, the pattern of spontaneous respiration (apneustic or prolonged end-expiratory pause) does not affect the required inflow rate. However, controlled respiration preferentially may increase the inflow rate required to prevent rebreathing. The egress of gas during inspiration (i.e., the time of greatest pressure in the system) rather than at end-expiration causes the loss of fresh as opposed to alveolar gas. The loss of fresh gas can be prevented by using a valve which closes with rapid increase in system pressure (Steen or Georgia valves). This prevents the loss of gas during inspiration and causes the overflow again to occur during the latter part of expiration. The Magill apparatus is used infrequently as such in the United States. However, we shall meet it in disguise in our analysis of circle absorption systems.

Nonrebreathing Valves. Nonrebreathing valves such as the Ruben, Fink, Sierra and Stephen-Slater entirely prevent rebreathing (if the valves are competent). However, they demand that inflow match or exceed minute ventilation. Respiration may become obstructed if minute ventilation exceeds the inflow. The Steen valve prevents obstruction by permitting the ingress of ambient air. Although this is preferable to obstruction it dilutes the inspired anesthetic and introduces the disadvantages of the open systems.

Semiclosed and Closed Systems

Absorption of carbon dioxide gives semiclosed systems a great economic advantage over semiopen systems. It permits the use of low inflow rates, and rebreathing without elevating inspired CO_2. In addition, low inflow rates allow a more accurate assessment of respiration and they reduce the contamination of the operating suite with these toxic vapors we call anesthetics. Finally, rebreathing humidifies the respired gas and thereby delays or prevents the drying of the respiratory mucosa.

Part of the price paid for these advantages is the increased complexity, cost and cumbersomeness of semiclosed devices. As noted in Chapter 12, another drawback is a reduction in the inspired anesthetic concentration. The remainder of this chapter will discuss the rationale behind the construction and arrangement of the individual components of semiclosed systems. The arrangement of system components is of interest since the arrangement may significantly affect the inspired anesthetic concentration.

The To-and-Fro System. Two semiclosed systems exist; the to-and-fro and the circle absorption systems. Although cheaper, simpler and easier to sterilize, the to-and-fro system is obsolete. It is far more cumbersome than the circle system since elimination of CO_2 requires that the soda lime canister be next to the mask or endotracheal tube. Moreover, its CO_2 absorption system is inefficient. Unlike the circle absorption system, partial exhaustion of the to-and-fro absorber permits rebreathing. The last gases expired enter the exhausted absorbant and are rebreathed without removal of CO_2 (fig. 13, 4). This defect can be remedied by increasing the flow rate to twice the minute volume (i.e., by changing to a Rees T). But then why start with an absorption system?

At commonly used inflow rates the arrangement of to-and-fro components permits considerable rebreathing of expired gases other than CO_2. Moreover, the alveolar gases are the last to leave the lungs and therefore are the first gases rebreathed. Since it is the first part of inspiration which reaches the alveoli, such rebreathing reduces the effective inspired (and alveolar) anesthetic concentrations. The magnitude of the reduction is a function of the uptake of the anesthetic. The inspired anesthetic concentration may be greatly reduced with very soluble agents but little affected with poorly soluble agents. The to-and-fro absorption system originally was designed for use with cyclopropane. Since cyclopropane is poorly soluble, rebreathing had little effect on its inspired concentration. This would not be true of more modern, more soluble anesthetics such as halothane or isoflurane. The inspired concentrations of these agents would be considerably reduced.

The Circle Absorption System. Despite its complexity, fallibility and

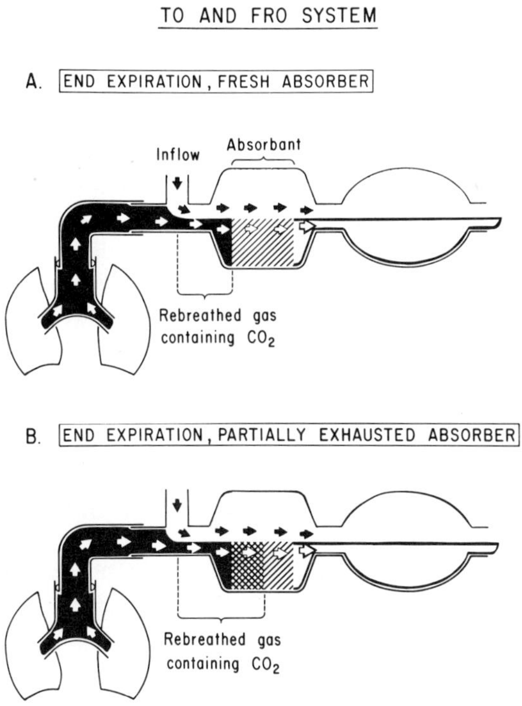

FIG. 13, 4. This figure illustrates the to-and-fro absorber system before (*A*) and after (*B*) partial exhaustion of the absorbant. The rebreathed gas containing CO_2 increases as the absorbant becomes exhausted. However, even with fresh absorbant, rebreathing of expired gas (albeit without CO_2) must occur at low inflow rates. Such rebreathing will lower the inspired anesthetic concentration.

expense, the circle absorption system is the most widely used modern anesthetic system. It has displaced the to-and-fro system both because it is functionally less cumbersome, and because it is far more efficient in removal of carbon dioxide. As we shall see, it also can be surprisingly efficient in the maintenance of inspired anesthetic concentrations.

Components of the Circle System. The components of the circle system must meet certain specifications to function well and safely. The nonwetting characteristics of inspiratory and expiratory valves allows them to open and close without sticking. Their lightness adds little resistance to breathing. Similarly, the large internal diameter of all system components makes resistance to breathing negligible. The large cross-sectional area of modern canisters makes resistance to flow through the absorption system small despite the presence of the absorbant. The most economical use of these canisters requires that they be divided in half. This division allows the absorbant in one half to be completely used before being discarded. The wrinkles in corrugated tubing prevent kinking from causing obstruction. At the same time, they lend flexibility to the connection of patient and absorber. The reservoir bag must be 2 to 5 liters for adults and proportionately smaller for children. Such a size permits full inflation of the lungs (one inspiratory capacity) and yet does not present too large a volume to grasp. The bag must be highly compliant from zero to full capacity but of low compliance at greater volumes (fig. 13, 5). At normally used volumes the high compliance permits little change in system pressure with ventilation and hence adds little to the work of breathing. At full capacity the low compliance prevents the bag from giving way in uncovered areas when it is squeezed to control or assist ventilation. This allows gas to be forced into the patient rather than into other parts of the bag. However, some compliance must remain after the reservoir bag has filled. Too low a compliance may result in excessive airway pressures during oxygen flush or high flows into the circuit (8).

Prevention of CO_2 Rebreathing. Three rules must be followed to prevent rebreathing of exhaled CO_2: 1) a valve must be interposed between reservoir bag and patient on both the inspiratory and expiratory sides; 2) and inflow must not enter the system between the expiratory valve and the patient; and 3) the overflow (pop-off) valve must not be placed between the patient and the inspiratory valve. Figure 13, 6 shows several examples in which one of these rules was violated: rebreathing of CO_2 will occur in each. If the 3 rules are followed, any arrangement of inflow, overflow and inspiratory-expiratory valve placement will prevent rebreathing of CO_2 (fig. 13, 7).

Conservation of Fresh Gases: Arrangement H. Although the arrangements described by figure 13, 7 prevent rebreathing of CO_2, they all

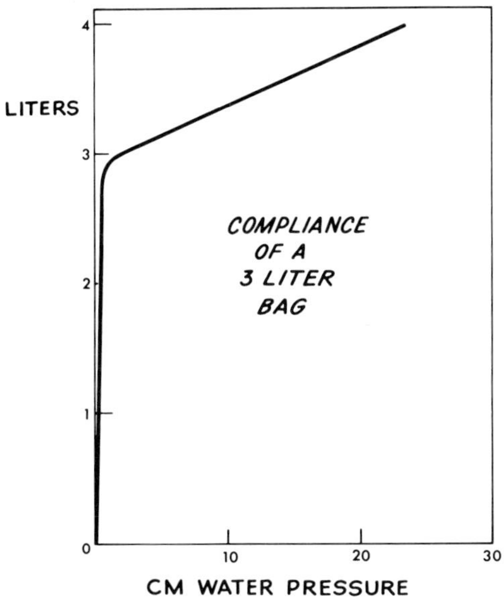

FIG. 13, 5. The compliance of a 3 liter bag is very high over volumes from 0 to 3 liters, but is low at volumes above 3 liters.

permit rebreathing of other exhaled gases. The extent of rebreathing of other gases depends on the particular arrangement and the inflow rate. The more efficient systems conserve fresh inflowing and dead-space gases and preferentially eliminate alveolar gas (9). For example, when the overflow valve is near the patient (fig. 13, 7 *B*, *D*, *H*, *G*) primarily alveolar gas is lost. Let us see how this occurs in arrangement H, the most efficient of all the systems. At end inspiration, the dead-space is filled with fresh gas (stippled area with black arrows, fig. 13, 8*A*). As expiration begins, dead-space gas followed by alveolar gas (black area with white arrows) flows down the expiratory limb, driving the gas before it into the reservoir bag (fig. 13, 8*B*). The inflow gas (clear area with black arrows) similarly fills the reservoir, but from the opposite direction. When the reservoir bag is full, the rising pressure in the system opens the overflow valve (fig. 13, 8*C*). The remainder of the exhalation, containing alveolar gas, now exits through the overflow valve. The inflow, no longer can enter the filled bag and instead moves into the expiratory limb, reversing the flow there and driving back the previously exhaled gas. This gas, too, exits through the overflow valve. Since the gas nearest the overflow is alveolar gas, this exists first. Only after all alveolar gas has been ejected can the dead-space gas leave the system. Notice that the function of arrangement H is nearly identical to that of the Magill attachment (fig. 13, 3). As with the Magill attachment, alveolar gas is preferentially ejected regardless of the pattern of spontaneous respiration. Unlike the

CIRCLE SYSTEMS PERMITTING REBREATHING

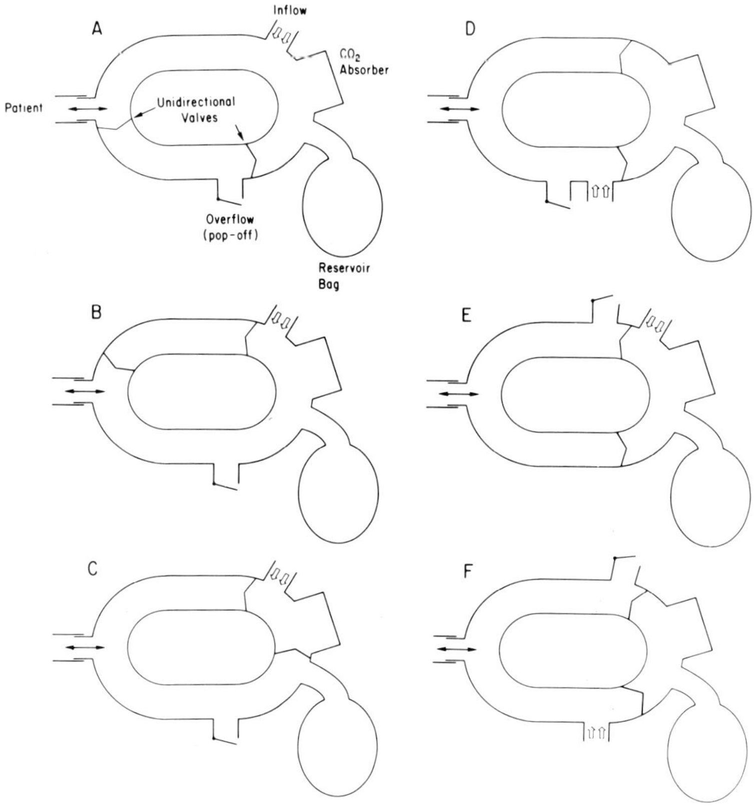

FIG. 13, 6. Each of these arrangements violated one or more of the three rules which must be followed to prevent rebreathing of exhaled CO_2.

Magill apparatus, the preferential ejection of alveolar gas persists when ventilation is controlled. This is not necessarily true of arrangements B, D and G. Controlled ventilation with B, D and G ejects fresh gases if the overflow valve opens with the increase in system pressure imposed during inspiration. Preferential ejection of alveolar gas can be retained if the overflow closes (for example with a Steen valve) during inspiration.

The effect of arrangement H on the inspired concentration may be calculated* from the following equation:

$$F_{INS}/F_{INF} = \dot{V}_{INF}/(\dot{V}_A - R(\dot{V}_A - \dot{V}_{INF})) \tag{5}$$

---

* Assume that all gas ejected through the overflow is alveolar gas and that the volume of gas ejected per minute equals the inflow gas rate, $\dot{V}_{INF}$
Then

$$\dot{V}_{AR} = \dot{V}_A - \dot{V}_{INF} \tag{1}$$

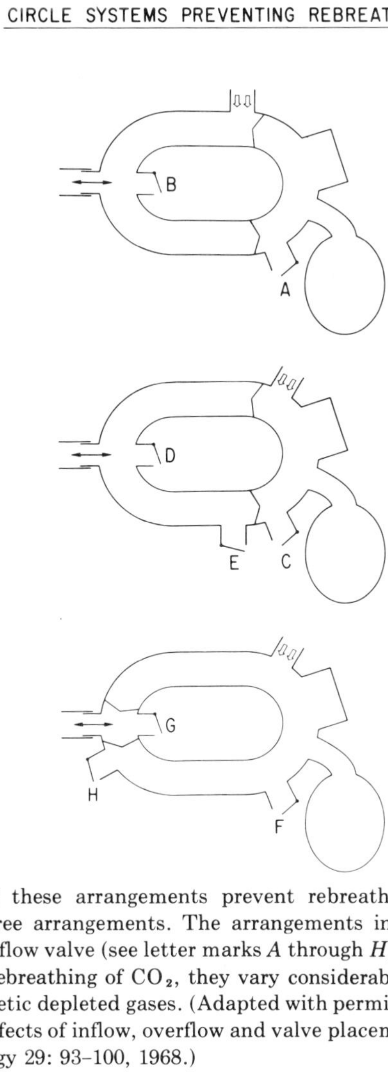

FIG. 13, 7. All of these arrangements prevent rebreathing of CO_2. Each drawing illustrates two or three arrangements. The arrangements in each drawing differ in the placement of the overflow valve (see letter marks *A* through *H*). Although all arrangements completely prevent rebreathing of CO_2, they vary considerably in their ability to prevent rebreathing of anesthetic depleted gases. (Adapted with permission from Eger, E. I., II, and Ethans, C. T.: The effects of inflow, overflow and valve placement on economy of the circle system. Anesthesiology 29: 93–100, 1968.)

Where $\dot{V}_{AR}$ is the volume of alveolar gas rebreathed (not ejected) per minute and $\dot{V}_A$ is the alveolar minute volume.

$$\dot{V}_D = \dot{V}_E - \dot{V}_A \qquad (2)$$

where $\dot{V}_E$ is the total minute ventilation and $\dot{V}_D$ is dead-space minute ventilation. All dead-space gas is rebreathed. The concentration of anesthetic in the inflow is F_{INF}. The alveolar concentration, F_A, is some fraction, R, of the inspired concentration, F_{INS}. That is,

$$F_A = R \cdot F_{INS} \qquad (3)$$

The volume of anesthetic inspired equals the sum of the volumes of anesthetic in the different gases (rebreathed alveolar, dead-space and fresh inflowing) that make up the inspired gas. Thus,

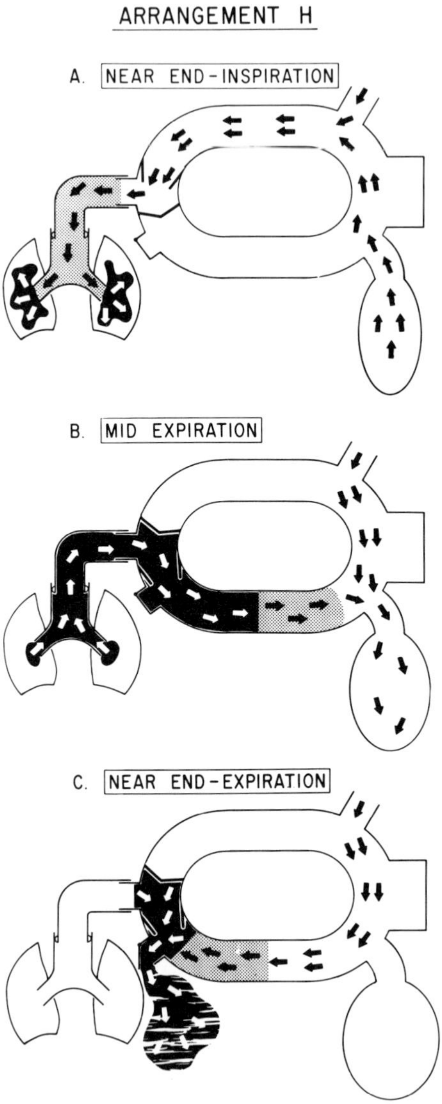

FIG. 13, 8. In this illustration of arrangement H (see fig. 13, 7), the symbols again define the source of gases and direction of flow: *clear areas* with *black arrows* are fresh gas, *black areas* with *white arrows* are alveolar gas, *stippled areas* with *black arrows* are dead-space gas. *Arrows* indicate the direction of flow; their omission indicates no gas movement.

$$\dot{V}_E \cdot F_{INS} = \dot{V}_{AR} \cdot F_A + \dot{V}_D \cdot F_{INS} + \dot{V}_{INF} \cdot F_{INF} \quad (4)$$

Substituting 1, 2 and 3 into 4,

$$\dot{V}_E \cdot F_{INS} = (\dot{V}_A \cdot - \dot{V}_{INF}) R \cdot F_{INS} + (\dot{V}_E - \dot{V}_A) F_{INS} + \dot{V}_{INF} \cdot F_{INF}$$

Rearranging, gives equation 5.

Note that 5 gives impossible answers when inflow exceeds alveolar ventilation because equation 1 no longer is correct.

Equation 5 says that the inspired concentration (F_{INS}) approaches the inflowing concentration (F_{INF}) (that is, F_{INS}/F_{INF} approaches 1) as the inflow rate ($\dot{V}_{INF}$) increases to the alveolar minute ventilation. R is the ratio of alveolar to inspired anesthetic concentrations and indicates the uptake of the anesthetic: a highly soluble agent has a small R. Notice that as R approaches zero, F_{INS}/F_{INF} approaches $\dot{V}_{INF}/\dot{V}_{A}$. That is, with highly soluble agents, the inspired concentration is nearly directly proportional to the inflow rate. The validity of equation 5 is suggested by the closeness of predicted values to those demonstrated by Eger and Ethans (9) in figures 12 and 13 of their work. Equation 5 also may be used to approximately predict F_{INS}/F_{INF} values for arrangements B, D and G in figure 13, 7. Actual values should be somewhat lower because these systems (particularly B) allow loss of fresh gas before all alveolar gas is discarded.

Equation 5 says that total minute ventilation has no effect on the inspired concentration (it doesn't even appear in the equation). The lack of an effect of total minute ventilation applies to all arrangements with overflow at the patient (B, D and G). This means that changes in dead-space ventilation do not alter the inspired concentration when overflow is at the patient. The reason for this is that regardless of dead-space increase the overflow valve opens when the same amount of alveolar gas remains to be expelled: thus the same amount of alveolar gas escapes through the overflow. This differs from the other arrangements of inflow and overflow (i.e., arrangement A, C, E or F in fig. 13, 7) where an increase in minute ventilation will decrease the inspired concentration.

The same constancy does not apply to changes in alveolar ventilation. Increases in alveolar ventilation lower the inspired concentration for all arrangements. The lower limit approached by the inspired concentration may be seen if we substitute for R (see equation 3) in equation 5 and rearrange:

$$\frac{F_{INS}}{F_{INF}} = \frac{F_{A}}{F_{INF}} + \frac{\dot{V}_{INF}}{\dot{V}_{A}} - \frac{F_{A} \cdot \dot{V}_{INF}}{F_{INF} \cdot \dot{V}_{A}} \qquad (6)$$

As alveolar ventilation ($\dot{V}_{A}$) becomes very large, the last two right-hand terms become small and may be discarded leaving F_{INS}/F_{INF} equal to F_{A}/F_{INF} which further reduces to F_{INS} equals F_{A}. This equality simply says that the inspired concentration (F_{INS}) approaches the alveolar concentration (F_{A}) when ventilation is very large—a result which is intuitively obvious.

Conservation of Fresh Gases: Arrangements C and F. A given inflow rate produces a lower inspired concentration when the overflow valve is moved from a position near the patient (arrangements B, D, G and H) to a position near the reservoir bag (arrangements A, D, E and F). The failure to conserve dead-space gas makes the arrangements with overflow near the reservoir less efficient than the arrangements placing the overflow near the patient.

Among the overflow arrangements positioned near the reservoir bag, C and F have the greatest efficiency with E less and A least. Arrangements C and F conserve fresh inflow gas and preferentially eject alveolar plus dead-space gas. Let us see how fresh inflow gas is conserved with arrangement C or F. During exhalation, dead-space plus alveolar gas move down the expiratory limb of the circle. By the time they reach the overflow valve, these gases are mixed. At midexpiration, the mixed exhaled gases move past the overflow valve towards the partially collapsed reservoir bag (fig. 13, 9*A*). The inflow gases concomitantly flow into the reservoir bag. When the bag is full, the overflow valve opens and allows the ejection of the mixed exhaled dead-space and alveolar gases through the remainder of expiration (fig. 13, 9*B*). At the same time, the inflow gases (which can no longer enter the filled reservoir bag) reverse

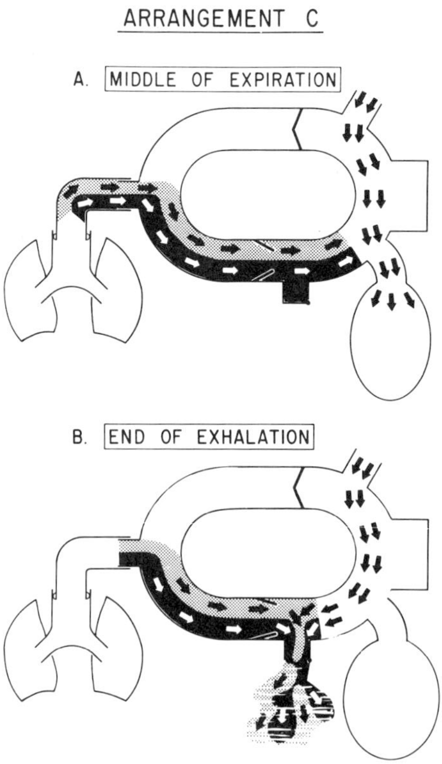

FIG. 13, 9. The symbols used for this demonstration of the function of arrangement C (or F) are identical to those in the previous figures. The pairing of the dead-space gas with alveolar gas is intended to show complete mixing of these volumes.

the flow of the mixed dead-space and alveolar gases which had reached the space between the overflow valve and reservoir bag. These gases are now driven backward and out the overflow valve. Note that only mixed alveolar and dead-space gases have exited through the overflow. No fresh gas can be lost until all the mixed alveolar and dead-space gases have been ejected.

The effect of this arrangement of the inspired concentration may be calculated* as:

$$\frac{F_{INS}}{F_{INF}} = \frac{\dot{V}_{INF} \cdot \dot{V}_E}{\dot{V}_E \cdot \dot{V}_A + \dot{V}_{INF} \cdot \dot{V}_D - R \cdot \dot{V}_A(\dot{V}_E - \dot{V}_{INF})} \tag{12}$$

where the symbols are those used in equation 5 with the addition of total minute ventilation ($\dot{V}_E$) and dead-space minute ventilation ($\dot{V}_D$). Equa-

---

* At equilibrium, the amount of anesthetic delivered to the system per minute in the inflow, $\dot{V}_{AINF}$, equals the amount taken up, $\dot{V}_U$, plus the amount lost through the overflow, $\dot{V}_O$:

$$\dot{V}_{AINF} = \dot{V}_U + \dot{V}_O \tag{7}$$

$\dot{V}_{AINF}$ also equals the inflow rate ($\dot{V}_{INF}$) times the inflow concentration (F_{INF})

$$\dot{V}_{AINF} = \dot{V}_{INF} \cdot F_{INF} \tag{8}$$

Uptake ($\dot{V}_U$) equals the inspired concentration (F_{INS}) times the alveolar minute ventilation ($\dot{V}_A$) minus the alveolar concentration (F_A) times the alveolar ventilation. The alveolar concentration is some fraction (R) of the inspired concentration. Then

$$\dot{V}_U = F_{INS} \cdot \dot{V}_A - R \cdot F_{INS} \cdot \dot{V}_A \tag{9}$$

The volume of anesthetic lost through the overflow ($\dot{V}_O$) equals the mixed expired concentration, F_{EX}, times the total volume of gas exiting. Assume that the flow rate of exiting gas equals the inflow rate ($\dot{V}_{INF}$), an assumption which ignores uptake of oxygen and anesthetic. Then

$$\dot{V}_O = \dot{V}_{INF} \cdot F_{EX} \tag{10}$$

The amount of anesthetic in the mixed expired gases equals that in the dead-space ventilation, $\dot{V}_D$, plus that in the alveolar ventilation. The concentration of anesthetic in the mixed expired gases (F_{EX}) equals the sum of anesthetic in dead-space and alveolar ventilation divided by the total volume in which they are contained ($\dot{V}_E$). Thus, we change 10 to

$$\dot{V}_O = \frac{\dot{V}_{INF}(\dot{V}_D \cdot F_{INS} + \dot{V}_A \cdot F_A)}{\dot{V}_E} = \frac{\dot{V}_{INF} \cdot F_{INS}(\dot{V}_D + R \cdot \dot{V}_A)}{\dot{V}_E} \tag{11}$$

Substituting 8, 9 and 11 into 7

$$\dot{V}_{INF} \cdot F_{INF} = F_{INS} \cdot \dot{V}_A - R \cdot F_{INS} \cdot \dot{V}_A + \frac{\dot{V}_{INF} \cdot F_{INS}}{\dot{V}_E} (\dot{V}_D + R \cdot \dot{V}_A)$$

Rearranging gives equation 12

P. Schreiber (10) has approached this problem from a slightly different viewpoint. The interested reader also may wish to review his approach.

tion 12 indicates that arrangements C and F are less efficient than H. Equation 12 suggests that no rebreathing occurs in arrangements C and F when the inflow rate ($\dot{V}_{INF}$) equals the *total* minute ventilation ($\dot{V}_E$). However, equation 5 suggests that no rebreathing occurs in arrangement H when inflow equals the *alveolar* minute ventilation.

Conservation of Fresh Gases: Arrangement A. Of all the arrangements in current use (and all the arrangements diagrammed in fig. 13, 7 are commercially available), A produces the lowest ratio of inspired/inflow concentrations at any given inflow rate. It is less efficient than F or C because it causes the ejection of fresh inflow gas as well as dead-space gas. We can see why this happens by examining the composition of the gases reaching the overflow valve. The expired mixture of dead-space and alveolar gases travels down the expiratory limb toward the partially collapsed reservoir bag (fig. 13, 10*A*). This does not differ from arrangements C or F. What does differ is that the introduction of the inflow past the inspiratory valve forces inflowing gas to accompany the exhaled mixture down the expiratory limb. The introduction of the

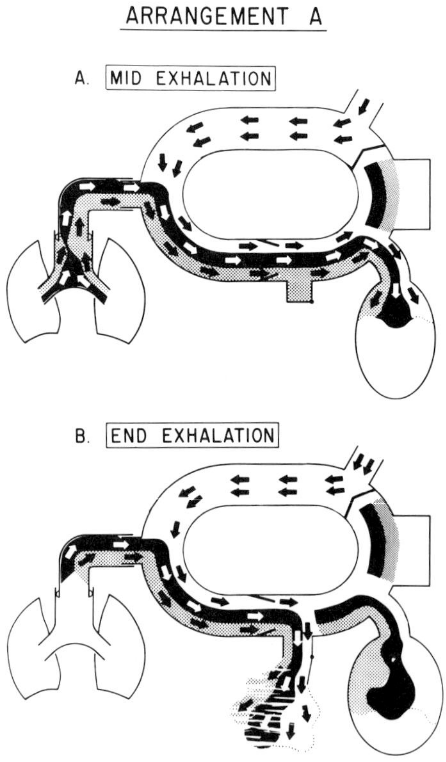

FIG. 13, 10. This figure illustrates the functioning of arrangement A. Again, the symbols representing alveolar, dead-space and inflow gases are those used previously.

inflow past the inspiratory valve prevents the inflowing gases from filling the bag by reverse flow. Thus, when the reservoir has filled and the overflow opens, the ejected gas is composed of fresh inflow gas as well as the dead-space and alveolar gases (fig. 13, 10*B*).

The mathematical description of the inspired concentration produced by arrangement A* is similar to but more cumbersome than the descriptions for arrangements C, F and H:

$$\frac{F_{INS}}{F_{INF}} = \frac{\dot{V}_{INF}(\dot{V}_E + R^1 \cdot \dot{V}_{INF})}{\dot{V}_{INF}[\dot{V}_D + R^1 \cdot \dot{V}_A + (1 - R^1)R \cdot \dot{V}_A + R^1 \cdot \dot{V}_{INF}] + \dot{V}_E \cdot \dot{V}_A(1 - R)} \quad (14)$$

where R^1 (the fraction of the respiratory cycle spent in exhalation) has been added to the symbols used previously.

With equations 5, 12 and 14 we can demonstrate the effect of different arrangements on the inspired anesthetic concentration. Figure 13, 11 illustrates such differences between arrangements and in addition, shows the importance of changes in 1) the ratio of alveolar to inspired concentration (R) and; 2) inflow rate. R is an inverse function of anesthetic uptake. An R of 0.2 (an alveolar concentration which is 20 percent of the concentration inspired) commonly is found with very soluble anesthetics such as methoxyflurane or ether. An R of 0.7 might be seen with halothane, fluroxene, enflurane or isoflurane but an R of 0.9 would occur only with poorly soluble agents such as cyclopropane or nitrous oxide.

A lower R results in a lower inspired concentration with all arrangements (fig. 13, 11). However, noticeable differences appear between

---

* As with systems C and F, the amount of anesthetic delivered to the system per minute in the inflow ($\dot{V}_{AINF}$) equals the amount taken up ($\dot{V}_U$) plus the amount lost through the overflow ($\dot{V}_O$) (equation 7). The amount delivered in the inflow is described by equation 8 and the amount taken up by equation 9. The amount lost through the overflow per minute is determined by the concentration reaching the overflow times the total volume ejected. As before, assume that the total volume ejected per minute equals the inflow rate ($\dot{V}_{INF}$). The concentration in the ejected gas is determined by the relative contributions of dead-space, alveolar and fresh anesthetic. The amount of anesthetic in the dead-space gas equals the dead-space ventilation ($\dot{V}_D$) times the concentration in the dead-space. The dead-space contains inspired gas and therefore has the inspired concentration (F_{INS}). The amount of anesthetic in alveolar gas equals the alveolar ventilation ($\dot{V}_A$) times the alveolar concentration (F_A or $R \cdot F_{INS}$). The contribution of the inflow is limited by the fraction of the respiratory cycle spent in exhalation (R^1). This fraction times the inflow rate ($\dot{V}_{INF}$) gives the total volume added by the inflow and this total volume times the inspired concentration (F_{INS}) equals the volume of anesthetic contributed by the inflow (this assumes that the inflow is well mixed with the inspired gases).

Now insert these equalities into equation 7:

$$F_{INF}\,\dot{V}_{INF} = \frac{F_{INS} \cdot \dot{V}_D + R \cdot F_{INS} \cdot \dot{V}_A + R^1 \cdot F_{INS} \cdot \dot{V}_{INF}}{\dot{V}_D + \dot{V}_A + R^1 \cdot \dot{V}_{INF}} \quad V_{INF} + F_{INS} \cdot V_A(1 - R) \quad (13)$$

Rearranging gives equation 14.

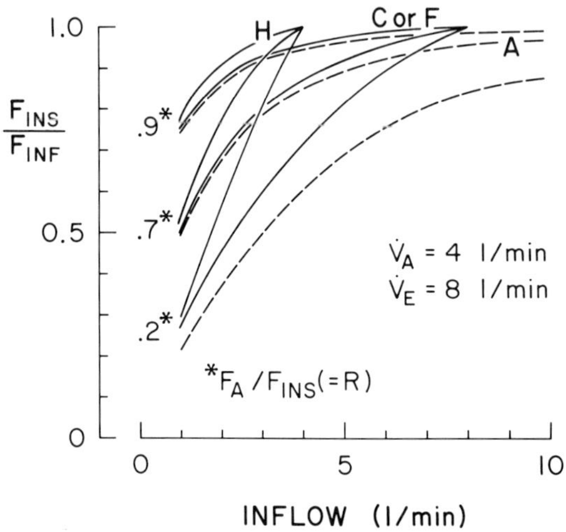

FIG. 13, 11. The inspired concentration of anesthetic (F_{INS}) is a fraction (F_{INS}/F_{INF}) of the concentration flowing into the anesthetic system (F_{INF}). Figure 13, 11 shows that the F_{INS}/F_{INF} ratio is a function of at least three factors: inflow rate, uptake (as reflected in the ratio, R, of alveolar to inspired (F_A/F_{INS}) anesthetic concentrations), and the arrangement of system components. Arrangement H is more efficient (higher inspired concentration for a given inflow rate and F_A/F_{INS} ratio) than arrangements C or F, which in turn are more efficient than arrangement A. Increasing either inflow or the F_A/F_{INS} ratio raises F_{INS}.

arrangements: at a given inflow rate, H (overflow at the patient) consistently produces a higher inspired concentration than C or F while C or F are always more efficient than A. For example, at a 4 liter/minute inflow rate and an R of 0.2, the inspired concentration with H is 1.67 times as great as with A and 1.41 times as great as with C or F. Thus, if 1 percent methoxyflurane were given with arrangement H, the alveolar concentration at a 4 liter/minute inflow might be 0.20 percent; with arrangement C it would be 0.14 percent and with arrangement A it would be 0.12 percent. Notice the difficulty this adds to the predictability of the effect of a given inflowing concentration. All arrangements are more efficient than an arrangement wherein the gases are continuously and completely mixed as described by equation 5 in Chapter 12 (but not shown in fig. 13, 11). Note that the simulation of the curves obtained in Chapter 12 assumed complete mixing of the circuit gases. This precludes any preferential conservation of fresh inflowing or dead-space gases and therefore gives the lowest possible inspired and alveolar rates of rise.

The differences in inspired concentrations between arrangements are small at very low inflows where rebreathing is nearly complete regardless of the position of inflow and overflow (fig. 13, 11). The differences are greatest in the 3 to 8 liter/minute range—the range most commonly used clinically. Above 8 to 10 liters/minute, the differences again decrease as inflow reduces or eliminates rebreathing in all systems. A nonrebreathing system is achieved with arrangement H when inflow equals the alveolar minute ventilation. Nonrebreathing occurs with C or F when the inflow equals the minute ventilation. Nonrebreathing occurs at very high inflow rates with system A and cannot be achieved when the circuit gases are mixed continuously (not shown).

Changes in dead-space ventilation (without change in alveolar ventilation) do not affect the inspired concentration with arrangement H. Similarly, the inspired concentration is not altered by dead-space changes when the circuit gases are completely mixed. These conclusions follow from equation 5 in this chapter or equation 5 in Chapter 12, neither of which contain a dead-space term. However, arrangements C, F and A all cause a decrease in inspired concentration when the dead-space is increased (fig. 13, 12). The effect is greatest at lower ratios of F_A to F_{INS}. The limit approached as dead-space enlarges is that found with complete mixing.

An increase in alveolar ventilation reduces the inspired concentration for all arrangements. However, the fall in the inspired concentration does not reduce the alveolar concentration. The rise in R (i.e., the rise in the alveolar/inspired concentration ratio) which accompanies hyperventilation more than compensates for the fall in inspired concentration and the alveolar concentration rise is therefore accelerated (see figs. 12, 9; 12, 10 and 12, 11).

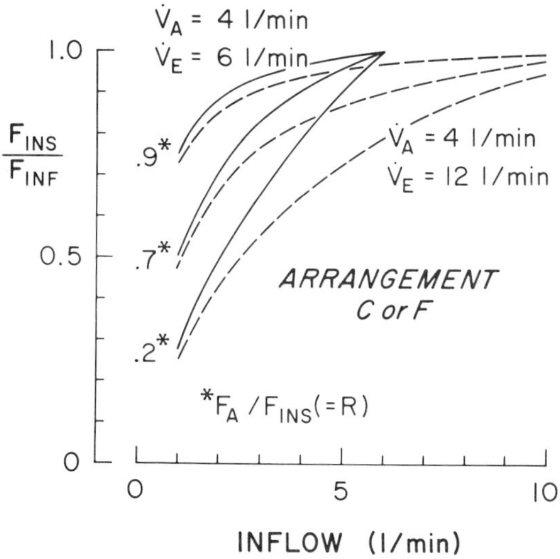

FIG. 13, 12. This figure differs from the previous one in that only the effects in one arrangement (C is functionally identical to F) is shown. It also differs in that the minute ventilation ($\dot{V}_E$) is 6 liters/minute (*continuous graphs*) or 12 liters/minute (*dashed graphs*). In both cases alveolar ventilation ($\dot{V}_A$) is 4 liters/minute. Note that the arrangement is less efficient at the higher ventilation.

Summary

Anesthetic systems range from simple open devices to complex absorption circuits. Each system serves three principal functions: 1) eliminate CO_2; 2) aid in monitoring and control of respiratory functions; and 3) sustain the inspired anesthetic concentration at predictable levels. Properly used, all systems prevent rebreathing of CO_2. However, the open systems fail to assist in monitoring and control of respiration nor do they cause predictable inspired anesthetic concentrations. The semiopen systems do provide these functions but at the cost of high inflow rates. The circle absorption systems may fulfill all three functions except that at low inflow rates the predictability of the inspired anesthetic concentration may be decreased or lost.

In a circle system, the inspired anesthetic concentration may be reduced from the inflowing concentration by rebreathing of anesthetic depleted gas. Two general arrangements of circle components aid in preserving the inspired anesthetic concentration by causing the preferential elimination of alveolar gas. Both those systems which place the overflow near the patient (at least during spontaneous respiration) and those systems which permit the flow of inflowing gas to move either toward the patient or the reservoir bag are more efficient in maintaining the inspired concentration.

QUESTIONS

1. Why is assisted respiration not possible with the Ayres T piece?
2. Explain how a ventilatory pattern of inspiration-expiration followed by a prolonged end-expiratory pause allows an inflow equal to the alveolar minute ventilation to prevent rebreathing with the Rees T.
3. If inflow to a Rees T piece, was twice the normal minute volume what would be the lowest $PaCO_2$ that could result from controlled ventilation if the dead-space normally was half the tidal volume and if the normal $PaCO_2$ was 40 torr? Why do lower inflow rates allow a better assessment of respiration?
4. The inflow required to prevent rebreathing with the Rees T is much increased by apneustic breathing. Why is the inflow not similarly affected with the Magill apparatus?
5. Explain how each of the systems in figure 13, 6 allows rebreathing of exhaled CO_2.
6. Using circle system H (fig. 13, 7) explain how alveolar gas is preferentially ejected when ventilation is controlled. Assume a spring-loaded overflow valve which opens as the pressure in the system is raised. Why doesn't fresh gas ejection preferentially occur during controlled ventilation as with the Magill attachment? Why does it occur with arrangement B, D or G?
7. With arrangement H, why does an increase in dead-space not alter the inspired concentration? (Why does the overflow valve always open when the same volume of gas remains to be expired?)

8. Why does a given inflow produce a lower inspired anesthetic concentration with arrangement A than arrangement C? Why should arrangement G be less efficient in sustaining an inspired concentration than arrangement H? Explain why arrangement E should be less efficient than arrangement C.
9. Using equation 12, show that when the inflow rate equals the total minute ventilation, arrangement C becomes a nonrebreathing system. Using equation 5 show that when the inflow rate equals the alveolar minute ventilation, arrangement H becomes a nonrebreathing system.
10. From figure 13, 11, calculate the inflowing concentration which will maintain MAC with halothane at a 4 liter/minute flow with arrangement H and with arrangement A.

REFERENCES

1. Moyers, J.: A nomenclature for methods of inhalation anesthesia. Anesthesiology 14: 609–611, 1953.
2. Arens, J. F.: A hazard in the use of an Ayre T-piece. Anesth. Analg. Curr. Res. 50: 943–946, 1971.
3. Munson, E. S., Farnham, M., and Hamilton, W. K.: Studies of respiratory gas flows. A comparison using different anesthetic agents. Anesthesiology 24: 61–67, 1963.
4. Rees, G. J.: Anaesthesia in the newborn. Brit. Med. J. 14: 1419–1422, 1950.
5. Mapleson, W. W.: The elimination of rebreathing in various semi-closed anaesthetic systems. Brit. J. Anaesth. 26: 323–332, 1954.
6. Woolmer, R., and Lind, B.: Rebreathing with a semi-closed system. Brit. J. Anaesth. 26: 316–322, 1954.
7. Kain, M. L., and Nunn, J. F.: Fresh gas flow and rebreathing in the Magill circuit with spontaneous respiration. Proc. Roy. Soc. Med. 60: 749–750, 1967.
8. Parmley, J. B., Tahir, A. H., and Adriani, J.: Disposable plastic breathing bags and tubes; hazards for inhalation therapy and anesthesia. J. A. M. A. 217: 1842–1844, 1971.
9. Eger, E. I., II, and Ethans, C. T.: The effects of inflow, overflow and valve placement on economy of the circle system. Anesthesiology 29: 93–100, 1968.
10. Schreiber, P.: Anaesthesia breathing systems. In *Anaesthesia Equipment Performance, Classification and Safety*, Ch. 8. Springer-Verlag, New York, 1972.

Chapter 14

Recovery from Anesthesia

Complete consciousness may return very slowly following general anesthesia. Although most patients appear to approach their preanesthetic state within minutes to hours, Davison *et al.* (1) found changes in cognitive functions and in symptoms for 2 to 4 days after halothane or isoflurane anesthesia in volunteers. Defining the exact point at which the full return of mental faculties occurs may be difficult or impossible. From the point of view of the anesthetist, a complete return of mental faculties is not immediately necessary. What is necessary is the restoration of those reflexes which protect against cardiorespiratory stresses. In particular, the patient should be able to overcome obstruction of the airway by tongue or foreign material. No studies have reported the anesthetic dose at which this may be expected, but our experiences suggest that it is close to "MAC awake." "MAC awake" is the alveolar concentration at which 50 percent of patients respond to a simple command such as "Open your eyes" (2). Patients at this dose maintain their airways without assistance. Studies of 4 anesthetics showed that the ratio of "MAC awake" to MAC was fairly constant and equalled 0.6. "MAC awake" also defines the brain anesthetic partial pressure at which "awakening" occurs. Thus, when the brain anesthetic partial pressure has fallen to half of MAC we may expect the patient to rouse in response to verbal stimulation and to maintain his airway.

This chapter will describe the factors which control the descent of the brain anesthetic partial pressure to this "safe" level of slightly below "MAC awake." Many of the factors which governed the rate at which induction was achieved also govern the rate of attainment of "MAC awake." However, these factors may take a different form or apply dissimilarly to recovery. Moreover, some new factors appear. Let us see how they influence recovery.

Factors Affecting Anesthetic Elimination from the Alveoli

Removal of the mask or endotracheal tube permits the patient to breathe room air. This corresponds to breathing from a nonrebreathing system containing an inspired anesthetic concentration of zero, and an inspired oxygen of 20 percent. If prolonged anesthesia has caused the equilibration of all tissues with the concentration inspired during anesthesia then the rate of fall of alveolar anesthetic concentration on breathing room air equals the rate of rise that occurred on induction (3, 4).

As discussed in Chapter 4, ventilation and uptake govern the rate of rise of anesthetic during induction. Ventilation causes the rise in alveolar concentration while uptake opposes that rise. Similarly, ventilation and anesthetic output govern the rate of fall of alveolar anesthetic on recovery. Normal ventilation clears the lung gases at a rapid rate (see fig. 4, 1). If unopposed, ventilation quickly would reduce the alveolar anesthetic concentration to zero. However, the effect of ventilation is opposed by the delivery of anesthetic to the lung from body tissues. The "output" of anesthetic into the lung is determined by the same three factors that determined uptake: solubility, cardiac output and the venous to alveolar anesthetic partial pressure difference. An increase in any of these three factors will increase output and oppose the tendency of ventilation to decrease the alveolar concentration.

Recovery is slow following anesthesia with a highly soluble agent such as methoxyflurane, but recovery is rapid following anesthesia with a poorly soluble agent such as nitrous oxide. This also is demonstrated by equation 12 in Chapter 4 which may be modified to apply to clearance of anesthetic from the blood passing through the lungs. If the venous anesthetic partial pressure is held constant at the partial pressure achieved during anesthesia, then:

$$(F_{AO} - F_A)/F_{AO} = \dot{V}_A/(\lambda \cdot \dot{Q} + \dot{V}_A) \qquad (1)$$

where the alveolar concentration which immediately preceded cessation of anesthetic administration (F_{AO}) minus the alveolar concentration (F_A) divided by F_{AO} equals the fraction of anesthetic cleared from the blood passing the lung. This in turn equals alveolar ventilation ($\dot{V}_A$) divided by the blood/gas partition coefficient (λ) times the cardiac output ($\dot{Q}$) plus V_A. Note that since the equation assumes that the tissues remain saturated with anesthetic, it therefore only applies to the first few minutes of recovery. The equation can be used to illustrate the differences between the clearance of various anesthetics. For example, at a ventilation of 4 liter/minute and a cardiac output of 6 liters/minute, the reduction in alveolar concentration would be 0.052 (5.2 percent) for ether, 0.222 for halothane, 0.322 for isoflurane and 0.587 for nitrous oxide. The importance of solubility is apparent.

The effect of cardiac output is intuitively obvious: an increase in cardiac output delivers more agent to the alveoli and therefore hinders the reduction in alveolar anesthetic by ventilation. The effect of cardiac output also may be seen from the above equation which predicts that an increase in $\dot{Q}$ reduces the clearance of anesthetic.

Initially (before any anesthetic is removed from the lungs) the venous and alveolar anesthetic partial pressures are identical. Lack of a venous to alveolar partial pressure difference prevents any anesthetic output. Similarly, a small venous to alveolar difference causes only small anesthetic output. This permits ventilation to induce a rapid reduction in alveolar concentration in the first minute of recovery (fig. 14, 1). The initial downsweep is soon halted by the development of a venous to alveolar anesthetic partial pressure difference which is large enough to cause an output which equals the removal of anesthetic by ventilation. The same output may be produced by different venous to alveolar

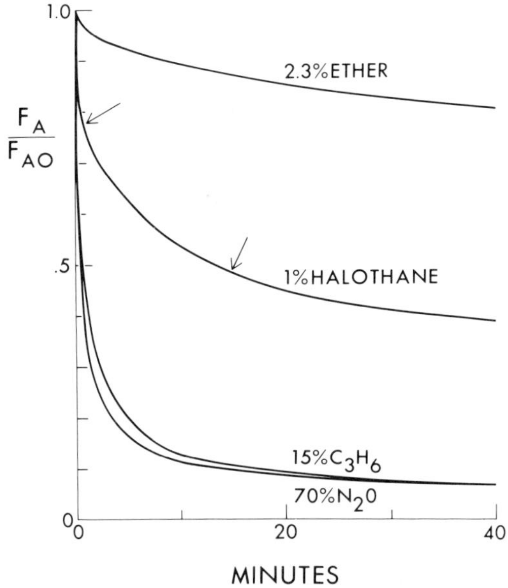

FIG. 14, 1. The downward path of the alveolar anesthetic concentration during the first 40 minutes of recovery has three parts. A rapid fall in the first minute results from ventilatory washout. The fall is slowed by output of anesthetic which balances the effect of ventilatory washout (for example, see the first *arrow* for halothane). The extent of the initial fall, and the subsequent level of each of the curves is inversely related to solubility: the greater the solubility, the smaller the fall. After the rapid initial fall, the downward path proceeds (at a less rapid rate) as a result of a decreasing output from the vessel rich group. Equilibration of the vessel rich group with the reduced arterial anesthetic pressure is nearly complete in 15 minutes (second *arrow*). The following slower decline in alveolar concentration is due to the progressive decrease in anesthetic output from muscle and fat as they too approach the arterial anesthetic partial pressure. F_A is the alveolar concentration. The alveolar concentration established during anesthesia is F_{AO} and is appended to the label of each curve.

differences: a high solubility allows a small difference to produce the same output as a large difference and a low solubility.

The initial balance between output and ventilatory removal is transitory. As the tissues give up their anesthetic stores the tissue partial pressure falls, thereby reducing the venous anesthetic partial pressure toward that in the coursing arterial blood. The rate of reduction in a particular tissue is a function of its time constant (see Chapter 4 and table 4, 3). The short time constant of the vessel rich group permits a rapid reduction in its anesthetic partial pressure, and a corresponding decrease in the venous to alveolar difference and anesthetic output. This results in a further fall in alveolar concentration from the concentration reached in the initial rapid decay. The effect exerted by the vessel rich group is large since it receives three-quarters of the cardiac output.

The longer time constants of muscle and fat delay the decay in their partial pressures and allow them a sustained effect on venous anesthetic pressure. After 10 to 15 minutes of recovery the decaying contribution of the vessel rich group becomes negligible and output results principally from the muscle and fat contributions. Subsequent reductions in alveolar concentration require the washout of muscle and fat—a slow process occupying hours to days.

The course of the alveolar curves is similar for all anesthetics: a rapid (1 to 2 minute) initial alveolar descent is followed by a slower (10 to 15 minute) but longer fall which is in turn followed by a still slower and more prolonged fall (fig. 14, 1). However, the position of the alveolar curves depends on solubility. Highly soluble agents have the slowest decay rates while poorly soluble agents have the fastest rates. The recovery from nitrous oxide or cyclopropane anesthesia is rapid but recovery from methoxyflurane and ether anesthesia is slow. In figure 14, 1 the anesthetizing concentrations were slightly more than MAC for ether, halothane and cyclopropane. If "MAC awake" is reached when F_A/F_{AO} equals 0.5, the differences between the recovery times become starkly obvious: recovery from a cyclopropane anesthesia requires a few minutes; from halothane perhaps 15; and from ether, several hours.

Differences between Induction and Recovery: The Concentration Effect

Recovery differs from induction by the absence of the concentration effect. Its disappearance stems from two factors. First, the uptake of nitrous oxide was drawn from an infinite inspired reservoir and anesthetic taken up was augmented by a further inspiration of gas. However, the output reservoir formed by the blood is finite, thereby limiting its possible contribution. Second, the blood volume is unaffected by the output of anesthetic whereas the alveolar gas volume was shrunk by uptake. The importance of this shrinking is obvious from figure 6, 1*D* where the reduction in gas volume is what prevents uptake of half the anesthetic from resulting in a 50 percent decrease in concentration.

The lack of an appreciable concentration effect during recovery is demonstrated in the boxes in figure 14, 2. In A the blood returning to the lungs contains 3 volumes percent. This blood is equilibrated with an equal volume of fresh gas. At a blood/gas partition coefficient of 0.5 the equilibration leaves 1 volume percent in blood (B). That is, the blood

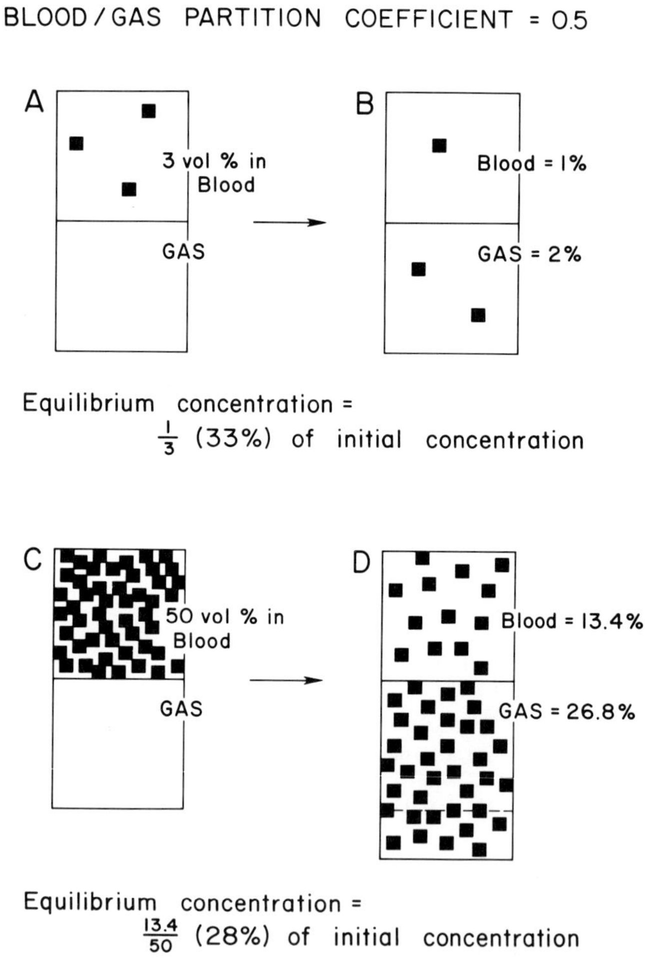

FIG. 14, 2. The initial blood concentration has only a small influence on the washout rate; the fraction removed from blood containing a low initial concentration (*A* to *B*, 67 percent removed) is only slightly less than the fraction removed from a high initial concentration (*C* to *D*, 72 percent removed). The blood/gas partition coefficient is 0.5. Note the expansion of the gas volume by the output of anesthetic in *D*.

anesthetic concentration falls to 33 percent of the original value. A far higher initial blood concentration of 50 percent (C) produces an equilibrium value of 13.4 percent in blood (D). (Note that it takes 100 volumes percent in the gas phase to produce 50 volumes percent in blood when the blood/gas partition coefficient is 0.5.) In this case the blood anesthetic partial pressure falls to 28 percent of the initial concentration, a decrease not greatly different from the 33 percent reduction obtained with the 3 percent initial concentration. Contrast this small difference with the large differences seen with the introduction of anesthetic during induction. Recall that uptake of anesthetic at a low alveolar concentration caused a proportional reduction of the alveolar concentration (see Chapter 6) while uptake from a lung containing 100 percent of an anesthetic did not affect the alveolar concentration.

Finally, note that the transfer of anesthetic from blood to gas has expanded the gas volume in figure 14, 2*D*. This must dilute other alveolar gases including CO_2. The reduction in CO_2 may depress ventilation (5). Such a result would further diminish the differences in washout rate between the low and high initial concentrations.

Diffusion Hypoxia

The dilution of alveolar gases by the outpouring of nitrous oxide may produce what Fink called "diffusion anoxia" (6). A reduction in arterial oxygen partial pressure (fig. 14, 3) or content results from the dilution of alveolar oxygen and from depression of respiration secondary to dilution of alveolar CO_2 (5–7). The time of maximum reduction in arterial oxygen is coincident with the time of maximum nitrous oxide output. Diffusion hypoxia is of no physiological significance if ventilation is normal and if no ventilation/perfusion abnormalities exist (8). However, if ventilation already is compromised or if ventilation/perfusion abnormalities are present, then the reduction in arterial oxygen may be of importance. In any case, hypoxia largely can be prevented by administration of oxygen during the time of greatest outpouring of nitrous oxide—that is during the first 3 to 5 minutes of recovery from anesthesia.

Influence of Ventilation on Rate of Recovery

As with induction an increase in ventilation hastens the alveolar rate of change during recovery (fig. 14, 4), and therefore accelerates recovery. The effect varies with the solubility of the anesthetic: with a very soluble agent (methoxyflurane), doubling ventilation nearly doubles the rate of change whereas there is no appreciable effect of increasing ventilation if the anesthetic is poorly soluble (nitrous oxide). However, the implications of these results differ from those on induction. On induction, doubling the rate of rise that might occur with methoxyflurane also

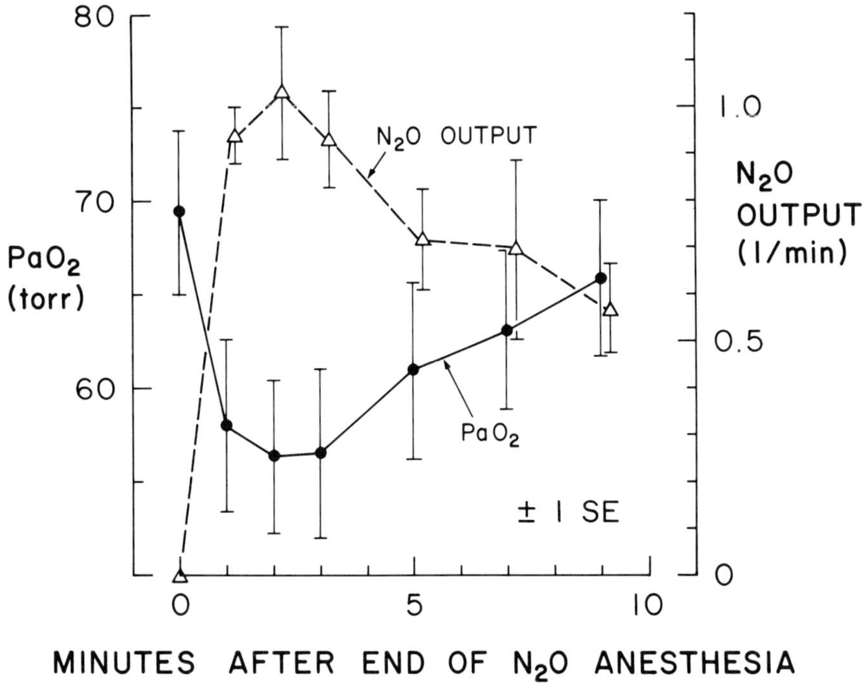

FIG. 14, 3. A change in the inspired gases from 21 percent oxygen/79 percent nitrous oxide to 21 percent oxygen/79 percent nitrogen causes a fall in arterial oxygen tension. The nadir of the fall is coincident with the period of greatest outpouring of nitrous oxide. As evidenced by direct measurement of exhaled volumes, the fall in PO_2 is not the result of a decrease in ventilation. (Adapted from Sheffer, L., Steffenson, J. L., and Birch, A. A.: Nitrous oxide-induced diffusion hypoxia in patients breathing spontaneously. Anesthesiology 37: 436–439, 1972.)

doubled the alveolar concentration and thereby doubled the anesthetic effect. In contrast, increasing the rate of fall does not produce a proportional decrease in the anesthetic concentration. For example, 20 minutes after recovery has begun, normal ventilation lowers the alveolar methoxyflurane to 82 percent of the concentration immediately preceding recovery (fig. 14, 4). Doubling ventilation does not halve this concentration but instead reduces the alveolar methoxyflurane to 70 percent (at 20 minutes). Thus, it has little effect on the anesthetic state. At the same time (20 minutes) doubling ventilation causes a fall from 46 to 30 percent of the prerecovery halothane concentration. Thus, recovery from halothane appears to be slightly more affected by an augmented ventilation than recovery from methoxyflurane. That is, the variation or "spread" in alveolar concentrations produced by different ventilations seems greatest with halothane, an agent of intermediate solubility.

Actually the differences between anesthetics in the effect of ventilation relate more to the duration of recovery than to solubility. The maximum separation of the curves for a 4 fold variation in ventilation is 30 to 40 percent for all agents. But with a poorly soluble anesthetic (nitrous oxide) this greatest "spread" occurs in the first few minutes of recovery. With a moderately soluble agent (halothane) the spread reaches a maximum between 10 and 30 minutes, while with a very soluble agent (methoxyflurane) the maximum spread is reached after several hours (not depicted in fig. 14, 4). The duration of maximum or near-maximum separation due to differences in ventilation also varies with solubility: it is brief with nitrous oxide; 2 to 3 hours with halothane; and several hours with methoxyflurane.

The clinical implication of these observations is that the greatest impact of augmenting ventilation on recovery is achieved with halothane: the effect of augmentation is too brief with a poorly soluble agent, too delayed with a very soluble agent, but "just right" with an agent of intermediate solubility. Note the contrast with induction of anesthesia: on induction an increase in ventilation has the greatest effect at all times on the most soluble agent.

These observations ignore the effect of CO_2 on cerebral blood flow: an increase in ventilation lowers cerebral blood flow by reducing $PaCO_2$. The effect on recovery from anesthesia is similar to that observed for induction (9) (see Chapter 7). The reduction in cerebral blood flow slows the clearance of anesthetic from the brain. Reduction may delay recovery

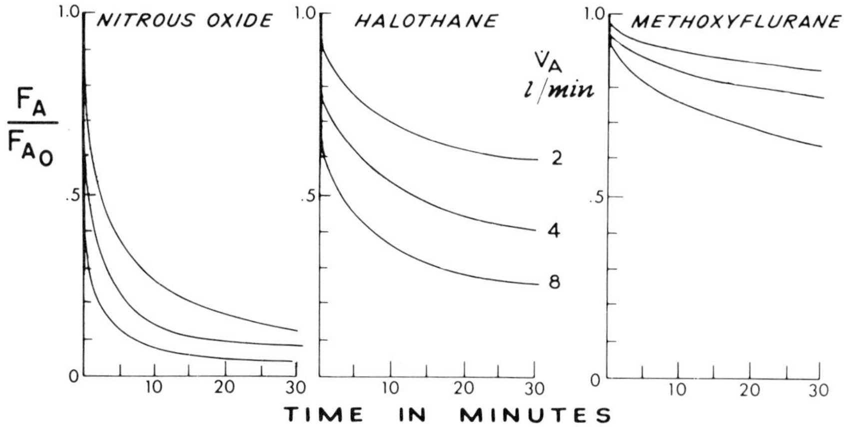

FIG. 14, 4. The rate of fall in alveolar concentration is accelerated by an increase in alveolar ventilation ($\dot{V}_A$). F_A/F_{AO} is the ratio of alveolar concentration during the course of recovery to the concentration immediately preceding recovery. (Reproduced with permission from Stoelting, R. K., and Eger, E. I., II: The effects of ventilation and anesthetic solubility on recovery from anesthesia: An in vivo and analog analysis before and after equilibration. Anesthesiology 30: 290–396, 1969.)

despite the augmented fall in alveolar anesthetic partial pressure achieved with hyperventilation. The delay is greatest with a poorly soluble anesthetic. The delay is reduced as solubility increases because of the compensatory acceleration of the alveolar decay curve.

The Influence of Cardiac Output on Recovery from Anesthesia

Changes in cardiac output alter the rate of recovery just as they alter induction (10). A reduction in cardiac output (ventilation constant) permits a more rapid decay of the alveolar concentration by reducing the anesthetic output. The opposing effect on tissue time constants concomitantly slows the initial fall in tissue anesthetic partial pressure (fig. 14, 5). If solubility is low (cyclopropane) the slightly accelerated alveolar rate of decay is unable to compensate for the effect on the brain time constant. The result is a delay in the recovery rate. If the solubility is high, the increased alveolar rate of fall balances the effect of the reduction in cerebral anesthetic clearance.

Note that this assumes a proportional reduction in both cardiac output and cerebral blood flow. If output is reduced but cerebral perfusion sustained at normal levels then recovery is accelerated for all anesthetics

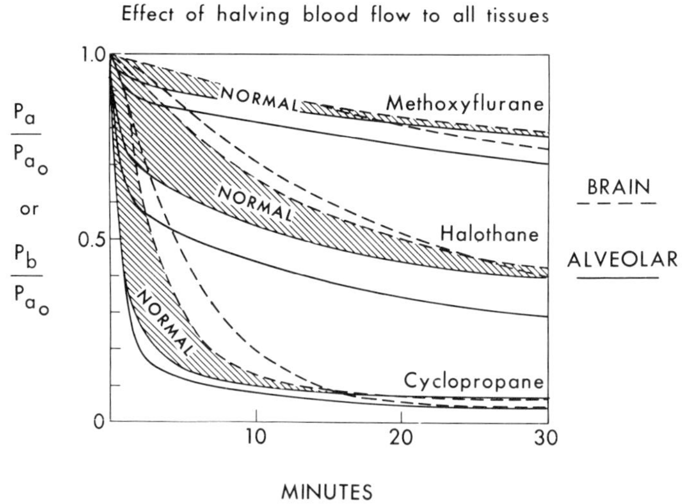

FIG. 14, 5. Halving blood flow to all tissues increases the anesthetic rate of fall in the alveoli but may retard the brain rate of fall by reducing cerebral blood flow. Alveolar anesthetic partial pressure (P_a) relative to the alveolar partial pressure prior to recovery (P_{aO}) is indicated by *continuous lines*. The brain partial pressure (P_b) is given as *dashed lines*. Alveolar and brain curves that result from a normal cardiac output are connected by the *shaded area*. (Adapted with permission from Munson, E. S., Eger, E. I., II, and Bowers, D. L.: The effects of changes in cardiac output and distribution on the rate of cerebral anesthetic equilibration: Calculations using a mathematical model. Anesthesiology 29: 533–537, 1968.)

(fig. 14, 6). Maintenance of normal brain blood flow may occur in shock. Similarly, halothane anesthesia may reduce cardiac output (11) but at the same time may increase cerebral blood flow (12).

Effect of Concomitant Increases in Cardiac Output and Ventilation

Conditions such as pain, shivering or delerium are likely to stimulate both ventilation and cardiac output. An increase in blood flow increases anesthetic output and thereby slows the fall in the alveolar anesthetic concentration. In contrast, an increase in ventilation accelerates the fall in the alveolar concentration by increasing the anesthetic removal from the lungs. It would appear that the effects of concomitant increases in ventilation and circulation should cancel each other. However, the combined effect ultimately is to accelerate the fall in alveolar anesthetic because the shorter tissue time constant conferred by an increase in blood flow results in the more rapid elimination of anesthetic from tissue stores.

As noted in Chapter 7, the immediate effect of increased ventilation and circulation depends on the distribution of the augmented cardiac output. If the increase in blood flow is proportionately distributed to all tissues (for example, as a result of hyperthermia) then the fall in alveolar

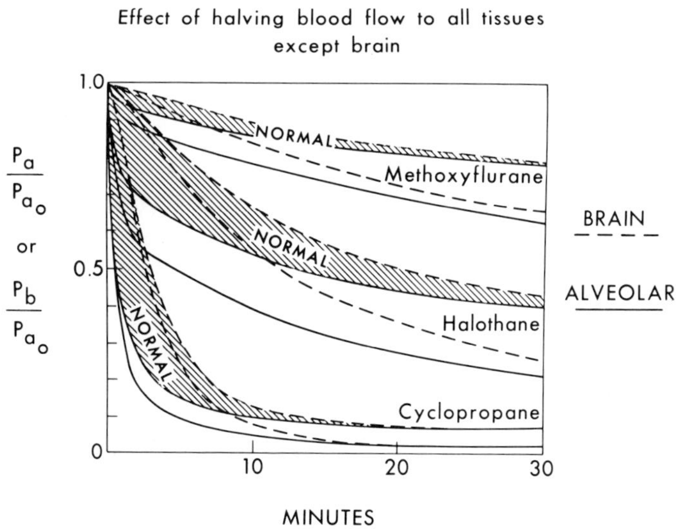

FIG. 14, 6. This graph is similar to figure 14, 5 except that cerebral blood flow is sustained at normal levels when flow to all other tissues is halved. (Adapted from Munson, E. S., Eger, E. I., II, and Bowers, D. L.: The effects of changes in cardiac output and distribution on the rate of cerebral anesthetic equilibration: Calculations using a mathematical model. Anesthesiology 29: 533–537, 1968.)

concentration will be more rapid than usual but the difference from normal will be relatively small. If the principle recipient of the increase in blood flow were a highly vascular tissue then the increase in flow and ventilation may considerably accelerate the fall in alveolar concentration. In practice, this might result from an increase in cerebral blood flow secondary to an elevated CO_2 or simply the presence of anesthetic (12). If the increase in blood flow mainly perfuses muscle or fat (for example, as a result of shivering or excitement) then the initial fall in alveolar concentration may be slowed although the ultimate result would be to accelerate recovery. Anesthesia itself may increase muscle blood flow. This occurs after long anesthesia with halothane, fluroxene, ether or cyclopropane (13). Isoflurane increases muscle blood flow acutely (14) and Cromwell *et al.* (15) have suggested that this increase in flow modifies recovery from isoflurane anesthesia. They demonstrated that the rate of fall of arterial isoflurane following isoflurane anesthesia in volunteers was slower than the rate of rise on breathing subanesthetic concentrations (fig. 14, 7). The measured muscle blood flow in the latter group was one-third of that in the former group.

Note that some of the conditions mentioned above (increased CO_2, hyperthermia, anesthesia) increase cerebral blood flow and therefore also may influence recovery by accelerating the approach of brain anesthetic partial pressure toward the falling arterial level.

The Effect of Ventilation/Perfusion Abnormalities on Recovery

Ventilation/perfusion abnormalities affect recovery just as they affect induction (see Chapter 8). Perfusion of unventilated alveoli delays the elimination of anesthetic from arterial blood. The effect is negligible for highly soluble agents and increases with decreasing solubility. Thus, recovery from cyclopropane or nitrous oxide may be less rapid than usual in the patient with pneumonia or atelectasis. Recovery from ether or methoxyflurane, while no more rapid than usual, would not be slowed.

Anesthesia may cause shunting of blood both through the lungs and through the body. As noted above, shunts through the lungs may slow recovery from anesthesia. On the other hand, concomitant body shunts or increases in flow to highly perfused organs (brain) will oppose the effect of the lung shunts (see Chapter 8).

Changes in Solubility

Two factors may alter solubility during the course of anesthesia. Replacement of blood lost with protein free solutions produces anemia and hypoproteinemia. The resulting decrease in blood solubility on the one hand will accelerate the fall in alveolar concentration but on the other hand, will lengthen the tissue time constant and hence delay the

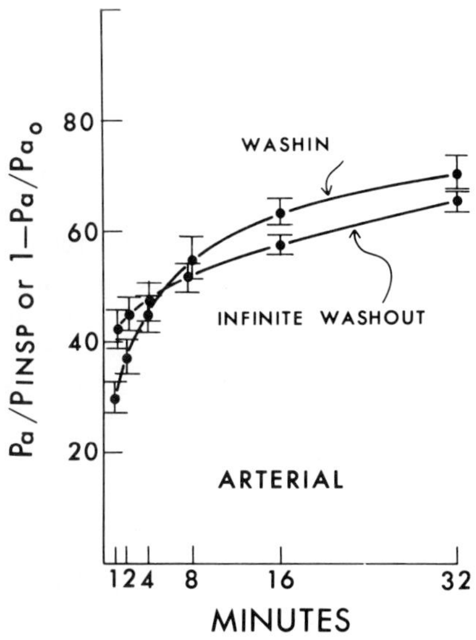

FIG. 14, 7. The arterial rate of rise of isoflurane (washin) is (after the first 4 minutes) more rapid than the rate of fall on recovery (infinite washout). Muscle blood flow during washout was 3 times the flow during washin and probably explains the difference between the curves. P_a is arterial insoflurane partial pressure; P_{INSP} is the inspired partial pressure; and P_{aO} is the arterial partial pressure immediately prior to discontinuance of isoflurane. (Reproduced with permission from Cromwell, T. H., Eger, E. I., II, Stevens, W. C., and Dolan, W. M.: Forane uptake excretion and blood solubility in man. Anesthesiology 35: 401–408, 1971.)

approach of tissue anesthetic partial pressures toward the falling arterial level. The initial balance between these opposing factors favors neither and the result is no alteration in the initial brain anesthetic decay (see Chapter 9). Of course, the lower alveolar concentration eventually leads to a lower brain anesthetic partial pressure.

Hypothermia frequently occurs during anesthesia. The increase in skin blood flow, a cold operating suite, and reduced metabolism all favor a heat loss which exceeds heat production. The result of hypothermia is an increase in both blood and tissue solubility. This increased solubility slows the fall of both the alveolar and the brain anesthetic partial pressures. Hypothermia also slows recovery by reducing ventilation and tissue blood flow.

During induction of anesthesia the effect of hypothermia on uptake was mitigated by its concomitant effect on MAC (see Chapter 9). Although the alveolar and tissue rates of rise were slower the levels to be reached were lower. However, on recovery, no such mitigation occurs: in fact, the decrease in anesthetic levels required to reach wakefullness during hypothermia may be lower than during normothermia.

The Effect of Metabolism on Recovery

Recall that the fraction of halothane (or fluroxene) removed from the hepatic blood flow of miniature swine is inversely related to the anesthetic partial pressure (16). The fraction extracted approaches zero at anesthetizing concentrations and conversely is nearly complete at 0.005 MAC. If these studies apply to man then anesthetic metabolism may play different roles during induction and recovery. During induction, the fraction of anesthetic removed by metabolism decreases and thus the fraction of anesthetic uptake due to metabolism becomes smaller as the anesthetic partial pressure rises. Although the initial rise in anesthetic partial pressure may be hindered by metabolism the later rise is little restrained. During recovery the hepatic anesthetic partial pressure initially is at a level which restricts metabolism. Only when the partial pressure has fallen can the metabolic contribution become a significant fraction of the output of agent from the body. Thus, the initial fall in alveolar anesthetic during recovery is not significantly affected by metabolism. However, the "tail" of anesthetic recovery may be greatly influenced. The influence is greatest with a very soluble agent such as methoxyflurane. For example, 5 percent of the methoxyflurane reaching the lungs may be cleared by ventilation (equation 1). The hepatic clearance may be much larger. The total hepatic blood flow is about 25 percent of the cardiac output. If all of the methoxyflurane in this blood is metabolized then the hepatic clearance of anesthetic is 5 times that at the lungs and obviously is the principal cause of the fall in methoxyflurane partial pressure!

The Effect of Incomplete Tissue Equilibration on Recovery

The above observations assumed that the anesthetic partial pressure in all tissues equals the arterial anesthetic partial pressure prior to the start of recovery. That is, they presumed a long period of anesthetic equilibration. However, most anesthesias are of short duration. Even our longer administrations do not usually saturate the fat group or even the muscle group. These tissues have attained only a fraction of the arterial anesthetic partial pressure when recovery begins. On recovery they therefore contribute less to, or may even continue to take up anesthetic and thereby reduce the returning venous anesthetic partial pressure. This permits a more rapid fall in alveolar anesthetic partial pressure. Thus, duration of anesthesia influences the rate at which recovery occurs: the longer the anesthetic the slower the recovery (4, 15).

The influence of anesthetic duration differs between anesthetics of different solubility. Recovery is rapid with nitrous oxide anesthesia regardless of duration. Although the alveolar rate of nitrous oxide fall is slowed by a prolonged compared to a brief anesthetic, the differences are small (fig. 14, 8). The differences increase with halothane, an agent of intermediate solubility. We found that human volunteers awaken slowly after 8 to 11 hours of halothane anesthesia, sometimes requiring 2 to 3 hours to reach "MAC awake." This is much longer than the time to recover from halothane in clinical practice where anesthesias are of far shorter duration. The greater variability related to duration of anesthesia results with an anesthetic of great solubility: here the difference in effect between a short 15 minute anesthesia and a 2 hour anesthesia may be enormous.

To demonstrate these differences between poorly soluble and highly soluble anesthetics, assume that "MAC awake" is reached when the alveolar concentration falls to 40 percent of the concentration immediately prior to the commencement of recovery. Then figure 14, 8 suggests that after either a 15 or 240 minute anesthesia with nitrous oxide "MAC awake" would be reached in a few minutes in the alveoli (and be reflected in the brain a few minutes later). After a 15 minute halothane anesthesia "MAC awake" would be reached in 3 to 4 minutes but would take 15 minutes after a 4 hour anesthesia. The time to "MAC awake" is increased to only 20 minutes after a 15 minute methoxyflurane anesthesia, but after 240 minutes of methoxyflurane anesthesia "MAC awake" is not reached for over 2 hours.

The above discussion presumes that the halothane and methoxyflurane anesthesias are not supplimented with nitrous oxide. Awaking will

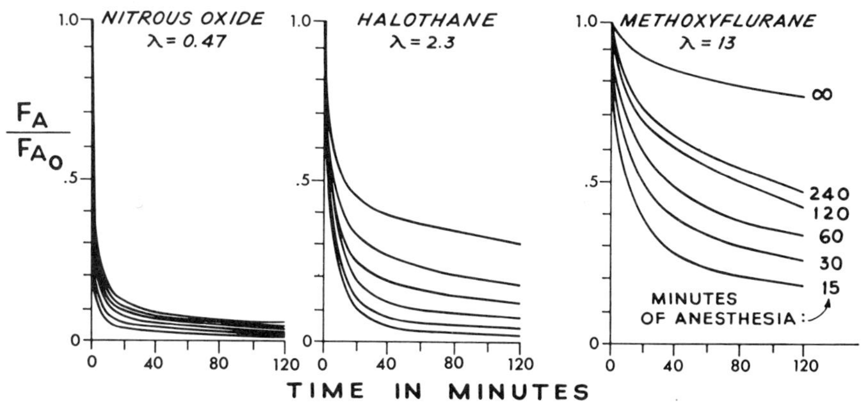

FIG. 14, 8. The fall in alveolar (F_A) anesthetic concentration from the concentration immediately preceding recovery (F_{AO}) is governed both by solubility and by duration of anesthesia. Increasing duration of anesthesia (15, 30, 60, 120, 240 or infinite minutes of anesthesia) prior to recovery delays the fall in alveolar concentration of all agents but is most evident with agents of high solubility. (Reproduced with permission from Stoelting, R. K., and Eger, E. I., II: The effects of ventilation and anesthetic solubility on recovery form anesthesia: An in vivo and analog analysis before and after equilibration. Anesthesiology 30: 290–296, 1969.)

occur more rapidly with supplementation since the added nitrous oxide permits a significant reduction in the highly soluble agent. Thus, on recovery, the rapid elimination of nitrous oxide leaves a subanesthetic residual of the more slowly declining effect of halothane or methoxyflurane.

Duration of anesthesia also influences the effect of changes in ventilation (fig. 14, 9) (4). A shorter anesthetic reduces the impact of changes in ventilation (i.e., the "spread" between the graphs for any one anesthetic) and the maximum separations of alveolar concentration occur sooner. The effect is similar to that which results from reducing solubility without reducing duration of anesthesia: note the similarity in position and "spread" for the halothane curves following 15 minutes of anesthesia and the nitrous oxide curves following 240 minutes of anesthesia. These curves imply that after an anesthetic of short duration (and negligible equilibration of muscle and fat depots), the rapid fall in alveolar concentration is little influenced by changes in ventilation. Only after a prolonged anesthetic with a moderately or highly soluble agent can an alteration of respiration significantly hasten or delay recovery.

The Effect of Changes in Ventilation during the Course of Recovery

In the above discussion we assumed that a given ventilation was constant throughout recovery. However, there are many causes for ventilation changes in the course of recovery. Hamilton and Devine (17)

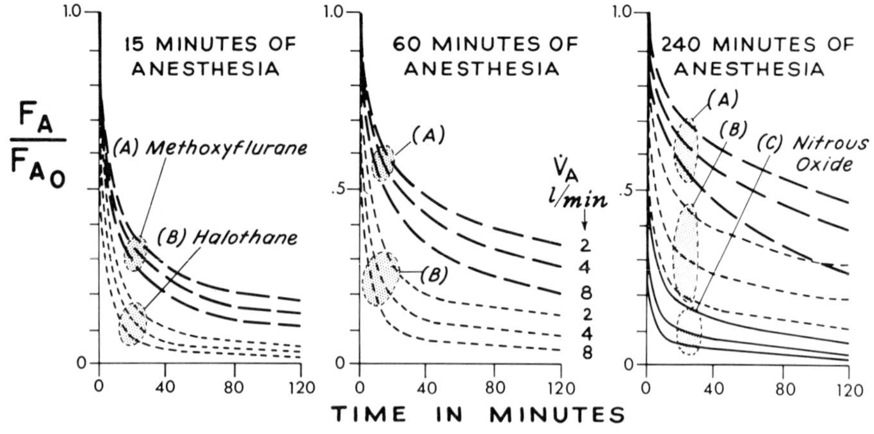

FIG. 14, 9. The coordinates are identical to those of figure 14, 8. The effect of different ventilations on alveolar anesthetic dose increase with increase in duration of anesthesia prior to recovery. (Reproduced with permission from Stoelting, R. K., and Eger, E. I., II: The effects of ventilation and anesthetic solubility on recovery from anesthesia: An in vivo and analog analysis before and after equilibration. Anesthesiology 30: 290–296, 1969.)

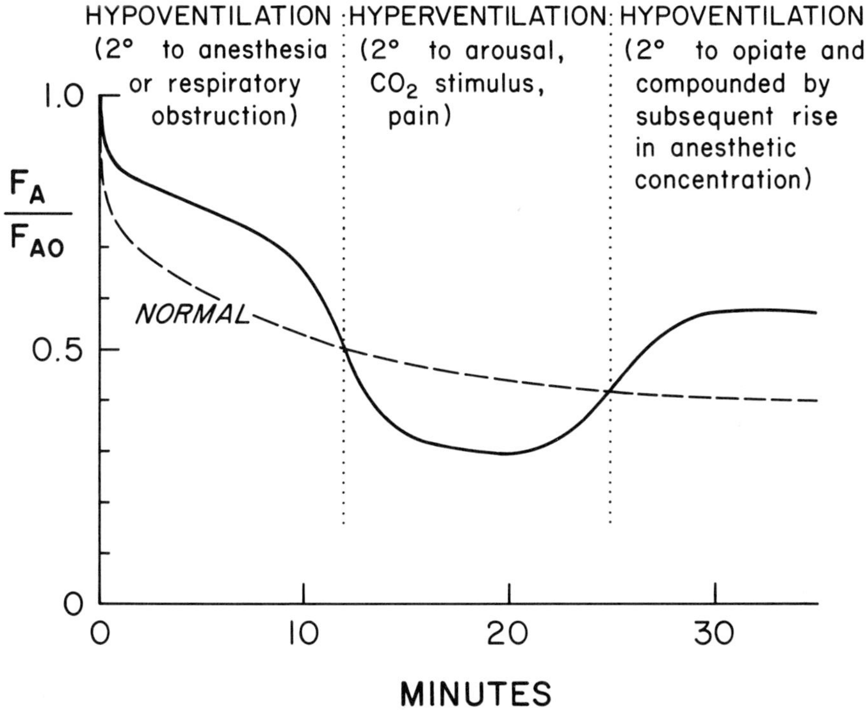

FIG. 14, 10. Ventilation may vary during the course of recovery. Such variations will cause deviations (*heavy continuous curve*) from a normal (*dashed line*) rate of alveolar fall of halothane. Hypoventilation during the first 12 minutes might be caused by anesthetic depression or obstruction or a "reset" of the CO_2 sensor and would produce a retarded rate of fall. In the next 12 minutes hyperventilation secondary to awakening, an increased perception of an elevated CO_2 and/or pain, might accelerate the rate of fall. After this, administration of a narcotic might relieve pain. Both relief of pain and a direct depressant effect might reduce ventilation and allow the alveolar anesthetic concentration to rise again.

found temporally related changes in $PaCO_2$ in the recovery room patient which may have related to factors such as residual anesthetic, initial CO_2 levels, the presence of pain, and respiratory obstruction. For example, the patient anesthetized with halothane (or isoflurane or enflurane or any anesthetic accompanied by a narcotic) may sustain considerable respiratory depression during anesthesia and as a consequence have sizeable increases in CO_2 stores (18–20). Because of the respiratory depression, the initial rate of recovery may be slower than usual (fig. 14, 10). As the anesthetic is eliminated, the brain increasingly appreciates the stimulus given by the elevated CO_2 and a progressive increase in ventilation follows. At its peak, the increased ventilation exceeds normal in order to eliminate both the normal contribution of metabolically produced CO_2 plus the excess in CO_2 retained during the period of hypoventilation. During this period the alveolar anesthetic concentration may fall below normal. This position may be sustained if hyperventilation is produced by the growing perception of pain. Conversely, two factors may oppose hyperventilation during recovery. The high CO_2 levels maintained during anesthesia may cause the central CO_2 chemoreceptor to be "reset" so that a higher $PaCO_2$ is accepted as normal (21, 22). If so, then hypoventilation, an elevated CO_2 and a slower fall in the alveolar anesthetic concentration result. However, Fourcade (unpublished data) found no elevation of arterial CO_2 following recovery from prolonged (greater than 5 hours) anesthesia in volunteers anesthetized with isoflurane. During anesthesia, the average $PaCO_2$ had exceeded 50 torr.

We also may decrease the respiratory response to a CO_2 stimulus when we relieve pain by the administration of a narcotic. This may eliminate the hyperventilation due to pain and add a depressant effect of its own. The result may be compounded by the effect on alveolar anesthetic

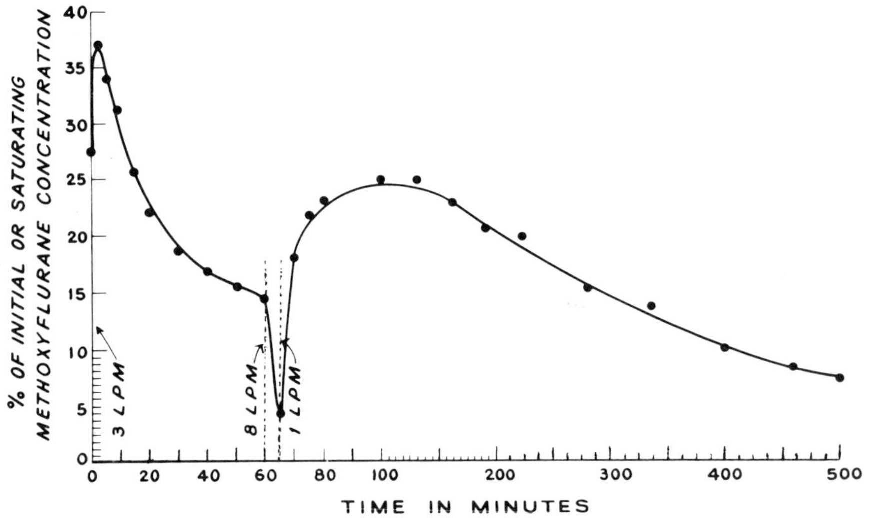

FIG. 14, 11. The rubber parts constituting a circle absorption system (5 liter rubber bag plus 2 corrugated hoses) were connected in a circle and the gases within the system maintained (continuously mixing) at 1.7 percent methoxyflurane (initial saturating concentration) for 17 hours. The system then was flushed with 8 liters/minute of pure oxygen for 3 minutes following which the oxygen inflow (no methoxyflurane) was reduced to 3 liters/minute . The concentration within the system fell over the course of an hour from a high of 37 percent of the initial saturating concentration to 15 percent. An 8 liter/minute inflow for 5 minutes reduced the concentration still further. Reversion to 1 liter/minute inflow allowed the concentration to rise to a quarter of the initial saturating concentration. (Reproduced with permission from Eger, E. I., II, and Brandstater, B: Solubility of methoxyflurane in rubber. Anesthesiology 24: 679–683, 1963.)

concentration (fig. 14, 10). The decrease in anesthetic elimination via respiration permits the alveolar concentration to rise and this rise itself may further depress respiration. These thoughts suggest caution in administration of narcotic during recovery from anesthesia. Note that the hazard applies mainly to more soluble anesthetics: respiratory depression cannot cause an appreciable alveolar rise of a poorly soluble anesthetic.

Effect of an Anesthetic Circuit

Following anesthesia we may require that the patient breathe oxygen from an anesthetic circuit in order to prevent hypoxia secondary to hyperventilation or to diffusion anoxia. The anesthetic circuit may alter recovery in several ways. Anesthetic which has been absorbed in rubber components may be released and limit the fall in inspired (and therefore alveolar) anesthetic concentration (fig. 14, 11) (23). This of course, only applies to highly rubber soluble anesthetics such as methoxyflurane and to a lesser extent, halothane.

A low inflow rate (1 to 3 liters/minute) causes a slow clearance of anesthetic from the gas contained in the circuit and in addition permits rebreathing of significant amounts of exhaled gas. High inflow rates (greater than 6 to 10 liters/minute) rapidly clear the circuit and prevent rebreathing. They also reduce or eliminate the contribution of anesthetic from rubber. Such inflow rates are necessary to assure a maximal rate of recovery from anesthesia.

Summary

Many of the factors governing recovery from anesthesia are identical to those which regulate induction. Ventilation rapidly lowers the alveolar anesthetic concentration at the end of anesthesia. Were the effect of ventilation unopposed, the alveolar anesthetic concentration would soon reach zero. But output of anesthetic from blood and tissues limits the fall in alveolar concentration. Output is a function of solubility, cardiac output and the venous to alveolar anesthetic partial pressure difference: an increase in any of these will increase output and thus oppose the effect of ventilation. Recovery differs from induction in that the concentration effect does not modify the ventilation-output relationship. However, there is a "concentration effect" on nonanesthetic gases: the outpouring of nitrous oxide at the end of anesthesia may dilute the alveolar oxygen and thereby produce "diffusion hypoxia."

A reduced cardiac output or increased ventilation permits a more rapid fall in the alveolar anesthetic concentration. These changes may accelerate recovery following anesthesia with more soluble agents but the concomitant increase in tissue washout time may delay recovery with poorly soluble agents. Concomitant increases in ventilation and circulation will accelerate recovery unless the increased perfusion is directed to tissues of normally low perfusion such as muscle or fat.

Recovery differs from induction in that the tissues are variably equilibrated with anesthetic at the end of anesthesia. Incomplete equilibration permits the alveolar anesthetic concentration to fall more rapidly on recovery than to rise on induction: a short anesthetic results in a very rapid fall, even with highly soluble agent. In addition, a short anesthetic reduces the impact of variations in ventilation or circulation on the rate of recovery. Finally, if the patient continues to breathe from the anesthetic circuit during recovery then recovery may be delayed both by re-entrance of anesthetic from rubber components and by rebreathing of previously exhaled agent.

QUESTIONS

1. In what ways may the alveolar curves obtained during recovery differ from those obtained during induction?
2. Using equation 1 what is the clearance of divinyl ether? of methoxyflurane?
3. Why is there no "concentration effect" on recovery?
4. Would diffusion anoxia occur if the blood solubility of nitrous oxide were 0.015 (i.e., the same as the solubility of nitrogen)? Why is ether unlikely to cause diffusion anoxia?
5. In what ways does an augmented ventilation alter recovery after anesthesia with a highly soluble agent differently from recovery after anesthesia with a moderately soluble agent?
6. How may an augmented ventilation accelerate the fall in alveolar anesthetic concentration yet delay recovery?
7. How may a reduction in cardiac output influence recovery?
8. Why does the alveolar concentration fall less rapidly when all blood flows are halved (fig. 14, 5) than when the brain is exempted from the reduction in flow (fig. 14, 6)?
9. Why do concomitant increases in cardiac output and ventilation usually tend to accelerate recovery? In what case may these increases delay recovery?
10. How may anesthesia influence its own elimination through the production of shunts?
11. What factors may alter anesthetic solubility during the course of anesthesia? How may these alterations affect recovery?
12. Is metabolism more likely to affect the early or the late part of recovery?
13. Why does a shorter anesthetic result in a more rapid recovery from anesthesia?
14. Why do differences in ventilation (or circulation) have less effect on recovery following a short anesthetic?
15. Why is the combination of nitrous oxide and methoxyflurane likely to result in a more rapid awakening than the use of methoxyflurane alone?

16. What factors may modify ventilation during the course of recovery?
17. In what ways may the continued use of the anesthetic circuit delay recovery?
18. Both halothane and cyclopropane may re-enter an anesthetic circuit from rubber components during recovery (i.e., while only oxygen is delivered to the circuit). Which is more likely to retard recovery?

REFERENCES

1. Davison, L. A., Steinhelber, J. C., Stevens, W. C., et al: The effects on anesthesia on mental functioning: illustration with halothane and Forane. To be published.
2. Stoelting, R. K., Longnecker, D. E., and Eger, E. I., II: Minimum alveolar concentrations in man on awakening from methoxyflurane, halothane, ether and fluroxene anesthesia: MAC awake. Anesthesiology 33: 5–9, 1970.
3. Mapleson, W. W.: Quantitative prediction of anesthetic concentrations. In *Uptake and Distribution of Anesthetic Agents*, edited by E. M. Papper, and R. J. Kitz, Ch. 9, pp. 104–119. McGraw-Hill, New York, 1963.
4. Stoelting, R. K., and Eger, E. I., II: The effects of ventilation and anesthetic solubility on recovery from anesthesia: An in vivo and analog analysis before and after equilibration. Anesthesiology 30: 290–296, 1969.
5. Rackow, H., Salanitre, E., and Frumin, M. H.: Dilution of alveolar gases during nitrous oxide excretion in man. J. Appl. Physiol. 16: 723–728, 1961.
6. Fink, B. R.: Diffusion anoxia. Anesthesiology 16: 511–519, 1955.
7. Sheffer, L., Steffenson, J. L., and Birch, A. A.: Nitrous oxide-induced diffusion hypoxia in patients breathing spontaneously. Anesthesiology 37: 436–439, 1972.
8. Frumin, M. J., and Edelist, G.: Diffusion anoxia: A critical reappraisal. Anesthesiology 31: 243–249, 1969.
9. Munson, E. S., and Bowers, D. L.: Effects of hyperventilation on the rate of cerebral anesthetic equilibration. Anesthesiology 28: 377–381, 1968.
10. Munson, E. S., Eger, E. I., II, and Bowers, D. L.: The effects of changes in cardiac output and distribution on the rate of cerebral anesthetic equilibration: Calculations using a mathematical model. Anesthesiology 29: 533–537, 1968.
11. Eger, E. I., II, Smith, N. T., Stoelting, R. K., Cullen, D. J., Kadis, L. B., and Whitcher, C. E.: Cardiovascular effects of halothane in man. Anesthesiology 32: 396–409, 1970.
12. Wollman, H., Alexander, S. C., Cohen, P. J., et al: Cerebral circulation of man during halothane anesthesia. Anesthesiology 25: 180–184, 1964.
13. Eger, E. I., II, Smith, N. T., Cullen, D. J., Cullen, B. F., and Gregory, G. A.: A comparison of the cardiovascular effects of halothane, fluroxene, ether and cyclopropane in man: A resume. Anesthesiology 34: 25–41, 1971.
14. Stevens, W. C., Cromwell, T. H., Halsey, M. J., Eger, E. I., II, Shakespeare, T. F., and Bahlman, S. H.: The cardiovascular effects of a new inhalation anesthetic, Forane, in human volunteers at constant arterial carbon dioxide tension. Anesthesiology 35: 8, 1971.
15. Cromwell, T H., Eger, E. I., II, Stevens, W. C., and Dolan, W. M.: Forane uptake excretion and blood solubility in man. Anesthesiology 35: 401–408, 1971.
16. Sawyer, D. C., Eger, E. I., II, Bahlman, S. H., et al: Concentration dependence of hepatic halothane metabolism. Anesthesiology 34: 230–235, 1971.
17. Hamilton, W. K., and Divine, J. C.: The evaluation of respiratory adequacy in immediate post operative period. Surg. Gynec. Obstet. 105: 229–232, 1957.
18. Munson, E. S., Larson, C. P., Jr., Babad, A. A., Regan, M. J., Buechel, D. R., and Eger, E. I., II: The effects of halothane, fluroxene and cyclopropane on ventilation: a comparative study in man. Anesthesiology 27: 716–728, 1966.
19. Fourcade, H. E., Stevens, W. C., Larson, C. P., Jr., Cromwell, T. H., Bahlman, S. H.,

Hickey, R. F., Halsey, M. J., and Eger, E. I., II: Ventilatory effects of Forane—a new inhaled anesthetic. Anesthesiology 35: 26–31, 1971.

20. Linde, H. W., Lamb, V. E., Quimby, C. W., et al: The search for better anesthetic agents: clinical investigation or Ethrane. Anesthesiology 32: 555–559, 1970.
21. Eger, E. I., II, Kellogg, R. H., Mines, A. H., Lima-Ostos, M., Morrill, C. G., and Kent, D. W.: Influence of CO_2 on ventilatory acclimatization to altitude. J. Appl. Physiol. 24: 607–615, 1968.
22. Edelist, G., and Osorio, A.: Postanesthetic initiation of spontaneous ventilation after passive hyperventilation. Anesthesiology 31: 222–227, 1969.
23. Eger, E. I., II, and Brandstater, B.: Solubility of methoxyflurane in rubber. Anesthesiology 24: 679–683, 1963.

Chapter 15

Diffusion May Limit or May Increase Anesthetic Uptake

Gases brought to the alveoli by inspiration must diffuse to the alveolar walls before they may be taken up. Similarly, uptake by the tissues requires diffusion of anesthetic from tissue capillaries.

We have assumed that diffusion presents no barrier to the attainment of equilibrium at either the lungs or tissues. Like many of our assumptions, this one is mostly (or usually) true, but deviates sufficiently from reality to merit further study. Paradoxically, incomplete diffusion equilibrium may both limit and accelerate the rise of alveolar uptake of anesthetic. Let use see where each may occur.

Diffusion Barriers at the Lung

Until recently, we believed that diffusion rapidly and completely mixed the gases within an alveolus. Mixing was thought to occur so quickly that no significant intra-alveolar gas concentration differences could exist. However, several experiments have demonstrated that a gas entering an alveolus does not instantly equilibrate with all of the alveolar gas. The most convincing evidence pointing to this conclusion comes from Georg *et al.* (1) and Cumming *et al.* (2). In their experiment a mixture of helium or neon and sulfur hexafluoride (1) was inspired and immediately exhaled. The relative concentrations of these gases in the expired mixture were found to be related to the volume exhaled. Both investigators found that the ratio of the heavier gas (SF_6) to the lighter gas (He or Ne) progressively decreased as the expired volume increased (fig. 15, 1). Although the decline in the ratio was exaggerated in emphysemous subjects, it cannot be explained by regional differences in ventilation. Such differences might cause variations in the concentrations of both gases, but the ratio of these concentrations would be unaffected. Nor can differences in solubility explain these results: He, Ne and SF_6 all are almost completely insoluble.

Presumption of a diffusion limitation offers a satisfactory explanation to the inverse relationship of the SF_6/He ratio to the tidal volume size

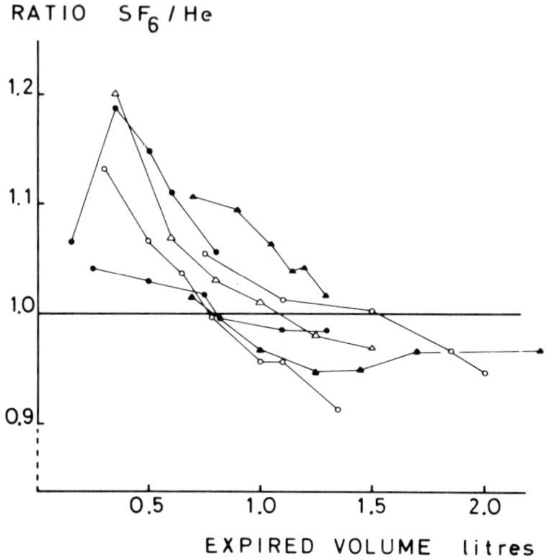

FIG. 15, 1. If a gas mixture containing equal parts of SF_6 and He is inspired, then the ratio of SF_6/He in the exhaled gas depends on the volume expired; it tends to be greater than 1 for volumes below 1 liter and less than 1 for volumes above 1 liter. (Reproduced with permission from Georg, J., Lassen, N. A., Millmgaard, K., and Vinther, A.: Diffusion in the gas phase of the lungs in normal and emphysemous subjects. Clin. Sci. 29: 525–532, 1965.)

(fig. 15, 2). Inspiration delivers the SF_6 and He (or Ne) to the alveolar ducts. From there they must diffuse into the alveolus (A). The He diffuses 6 times more rapidly (diffusion is inversely related to the square root of the density of the gas) than SF_6. This more rapid diffusion moves He into the alveolus ahead of the SF_6 (B and C). The result is a relative increase in the concentration of He in the alveoli and distal portion of the alveolar duct and a relative decrease in He concentration in the proximal portion of the alveolar duct. Thus, since the first part of exhalation comes from the proximal gas, it carries a higher SF_6/He ratio than the latter part which comes from the distal portion of the alveolar duct.

Further evidence that the change in SF_6/He ratio (fig. 15, 1) is due to different diffusion rates comes from breath holding experiments. When a breath of SF_6 and He (or Ne) mixture was inspired and held for 30 seconds rather than immediately expired, the SF_6/He ratios from the exhalate were identical regardless of the volume expired. In 30 seconds the slower diffusing SF_6 was able to equilibrate with the alveolar gas just as the He had in a far shorter span of time.

Halothane, methoxyflurane, isoflurane and enflurane are more dense than SF_6 while fluroxene is only slightly less so. A diffusion limitation must apply to these gases and probably also to a lesser extent to the less dense nitrous oxide, cyclopropane, and ether. This limitation should result in a gradient between end-expired and arterial anesthetic partial pressures. Such indeed, is normally the case (see fig. 8, 1) and the previous explanation of these gradients as due to ventilation/perfusion abnormalities must be amended to include diffusion. Both a diffusion barrier and ventilation/perfusion abnormalities may impede changes in anesthetic partial pressure in blood and tissues and thus hinder the development or elimination of the anesthetic state. The hindrance likely is exaggerated in emphysematous patients because the enlarged alveoli or ducts increase the distance over which the anesthetic molecules must diffuse.

Nitrous oxide administration may alter the hindrance that diffusion imposes on a concomitantly administered anesthetic such as halothane or isoflurane. Uptake of nitrous oxide may not only increase the "inspired ventilation" (as described under the second gas effect in Chapter 6) but also may increase the bulk flow into the alveolar sac. That is, the void left by uptake of nitrous oxide from the alveolar sac would draw in gas from the distal portion of the alveolar duct. The anesthetic molecules in this indrawn gas would have a shorter diffusion path, and hence diffusion would present less of a barrier to equilibration with pulmonary capillary blood.

Diffusion Limitations at the Tissues

It appears that there is little or no diffusion limitation to the movement of anesthetic from arterial blood to highly perfused tissues

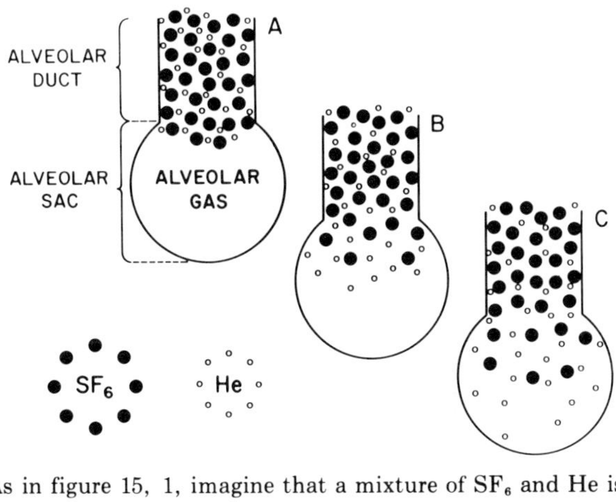

FIG. 15, 2. As in figure 15, 1, imagine that a mixture of SF_6 and He is inspired. Bulk flow carries this mixture to the termination of the alveolar duct (*A*). To reach the alveolar sac wall, the molecules must diffuse through the alveolar gas (*B* and *C*). The smaller He molecules move with 6 times the velocity of the larger SF_6 molecules and their spread into the alveolar gas is more rapid. Thus, when exhalation occurs (*C*), the first gas exhaled (that in the upper part of the alveolar duct) has relatively less He while the last gas exhaled (that in the lower duct and alveolus) has relatively more.

(VRG). The small diffusing distances apparently do not impose a significant barrier. This may not be the case in muscle and fat where diffusion distances are larger. However, with muscle the barrier to diffusion cannot be a major one since determination of muscle blood flow by gas washout (xenon 133) agrees with flow measurements made with other techniques, including direct measurement (3, 4). The flow measurements would likely not correlate well if diffusion imposed any significant barrier to the transfer of gas between tissue and blood. Inert gas uptake (5) or clearance (6) techniques also have been used to determine fat blood flow. The values obtained reasonably suggest that diffusion also is not a gross barrier to equilibration in fat.

For the purpose of describing the rate of rise of anesthetic in arterial blood, complete equilibration in fat or muscle is not important. The capacity of fat or muscle for most agents is so large that clearance would be essentially complete even in the presence of a considerable gradient between blood and tissue. For example, presume that with complete equilibration, fat removed 99 percent of the anesthetic from the blood perfusing that tissue. Even if the amount that the fat failed to remove were increased 10 fold, the clearance still would be 90 percent. The difference between this and 99 percent would only slightly increase the arterial anesthetic rate of rise.

Other Diffusion Limitations: Percutaneous Loss of Anesthetic

Where then may diffusion limit the rise of tissue anesthetic partial pressure? We shall examine three possibilities: one in which the diffusion barrier is too great and two in which the diffusion barrier is not great enough.

The skin presents a significant barrier to equilibration. The 1 mm thickness of epidermis plus dermis prevents the percutaneous loss of most of the anesthetic delivered to the dermis (7). The greatest percutaneous loss occurs with nitrous oxide and represents less than 10 percent of the nitrous oxide delivered to the skin. Percutaneous loss of ether or halothane is less than 1 percent of the amount delivered. These *in vivo* studies have been confimed *in vitro* and extended to amniotic membrane which shows similar properties (8). We may conclude that a 1 mm layer of lean tissue represents a very large barrier to diffusion.

Intertissue Diffusion

Diffusion of anesthetic from one tissue to an adjacent tissue will occur when a partial pressure difference exists between the two tissues. The difference may result because one tissue is perfused and the other is not or because one tissue has a far greater capacity to hold anesthetic. Cartilage, ligaments, tendons and bone are essentially avascular and the rise of the anesthetic partial pressure in these tissues depends on diffusion of anesthetic from adjacent, better perfused tissues such as muscle. In contrast, fat is not avascular but the anesthetic partial pressure in fat remains low because of the large anesthetic capacity conferred by solubility. As adjacent tissues attain higher anesthetic partial pressures (by virtue of higher perfusion and/or lower solubility) transfer of anesthetic to fat must occur. Such adjacent tissues might be muscle or dermis (next to subcutaneous fat); intestine (next to omentum); or kidney (next to perirenal fat). The transfer of anesthetic from one tissue to another in effect increases the capacity of the first tissue to hold anesthetic. In this way, intertissue diffusion may significantly increase total anesthetic uptake (9). For example, adding the capacity of the omental fat to the capacity of the intestine might increase halothane uptake by 25 to 50 percent over the course of a 2 or 3 hour anesthetic. Cohen *et al.* (10) have reported an experiment which probably directly demonstrated the existence of intertissue diffusion (11). The brains of monkeys given an intravenous dose of radioactive halothane were examined by radioautography. As would be expected from its greater perfusion, grey matter received the preponderance of radioactivity immediately after injection (left side of fig. 15, 3). The greater partial pressure of halothane in grey matter caused the movement of halothane into the adjacent white matter. Subsequently, the high perfusion of the grey matter removed the halothane from that tissue, leaving a band of halothane in the less well perfused adjacent white matter (right side of fig. 15, 3).

Unfortunately we do not know the overall extent of intertissue diffusion or its impact on total uptake. An elegant experiment by Rackow, Perl and associates (12, 13) suggested a large effect, but recent evidence undermined their conclusions by demonstrating that one of their assumptions was untrue. Rackow *et al.* (12) measured the alveolar rates of rise of tracer concentrations of nitrous oxide and cyclopropane when administered concomitantly. If these gases were identically soluble in all tissues except fat, then their alveolar rates of rise should have been close if no intertissue diffusion to fat occurred. In fact, however, they found a much slower rise in alveolar cyclopropane, suggesting intertissue diffusion. We have duplicated their experiment (unpublished data) and although we found less of a difference between the nitrous oxide and cyclopropane curves, our results in general confirm their findings. Unfortunately, the assumption that cyclopropane and nitrous oxide are identically soluble in all tissues except fat is untenable. As noted in Chapter 9, at low concentrations cyclopropane is significantly more soluble in blood than nitrous oxide. A greater solubility also may apply to tissues such as muscle. The higher cyclopropane solubility by itself can explain the slower rise in the alveolar concentration.

Thus, the question of the importance of intertissue diffusion is

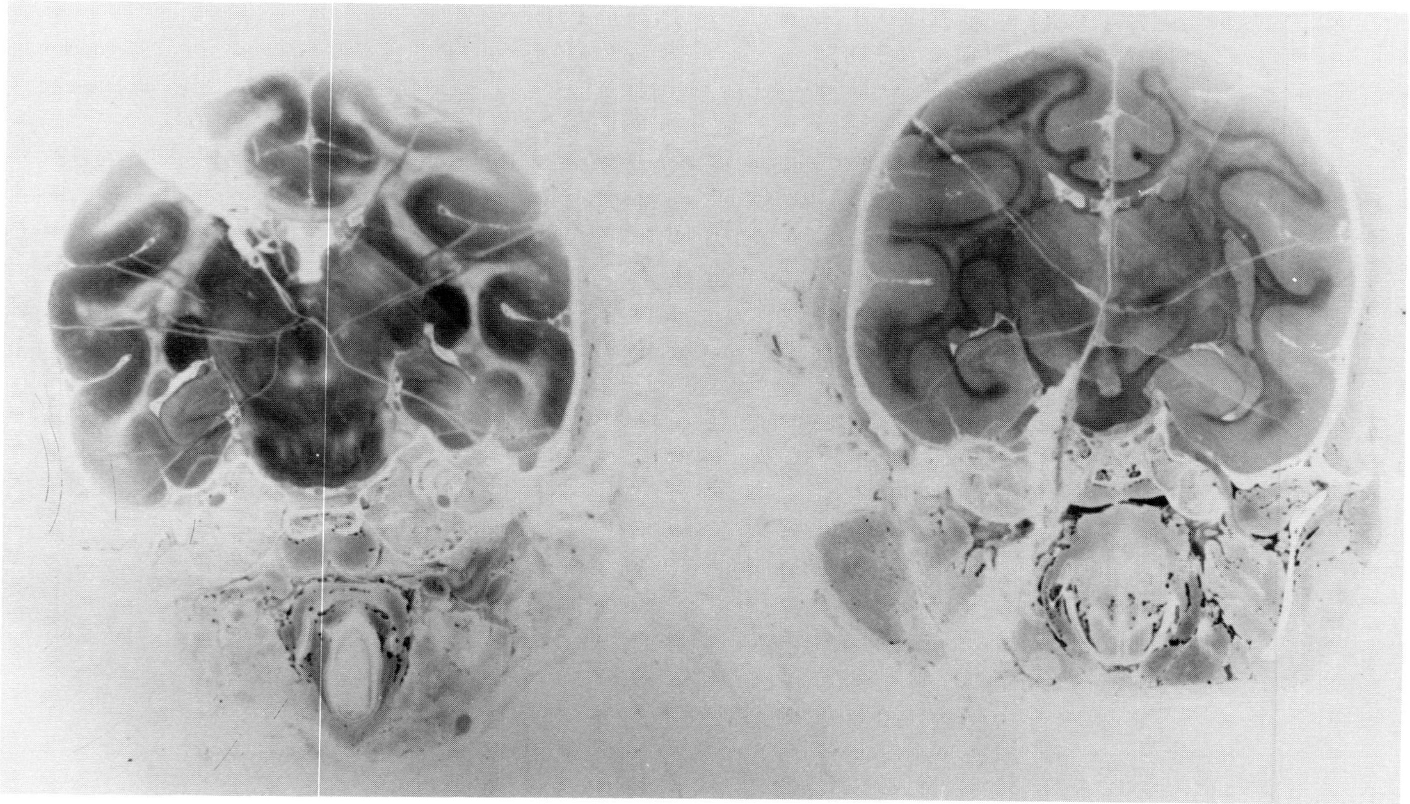

FIG. 15, 3. Two minutes after the intravenous injection of radioactive halothane into a monkey, most of the halothane is in the grey matter as indicated by the dark cortical band in the left hand radioautograph (10). Three minutes later, the darkest band (greatest radioactivity) lies at the interface of white and grey matter, with the preponderance probably in white matter. The band of white matter radioactivity can be explained by the transfer of halothane from adjacent grey matter (intertissue diffusion). The transferred halothane persists (and so is apparent in the radioautograph) in the white matter because of the lower perfusion of white matter, and the greater solubility of halothane in white matter (11). (Reproduced with permission from Cohen, E. N., Chow, K. L., and Mathers, L.: Autoradiographic distribution of volatile anesthetics within the brain. Anesthesiology 37: 324–331, 1972.)

unresolved. We know that such diffusion must occur, but have not yet measured its extent. However, we may predict one limitation to intertissue diffusion from the studies of percutaneous diffusion (see above): if intertissue diffusion is to be significant, anesthetic must pass through a lean tissue slab of less than 1 mm thickness.

Intervascular Diffusion

Except for the pulmonary circulation, veins, and arteries run in parallel and contiguous courses. The propinquity of vessels makes possible the direct transfer of anesthetic from arterial to venous blood on induction and from venous to arterial blood on recovery (intravascular diffusion; 4, 14, 15). This reduces the effective tissue perfusion. A decreased uptake of anesthetic must occur on induction and a decreased clearance on recovery.

Although the evidence is limited, it appears that intervascular diffusion is small and has little influence on tissue anesthetic rate of change. For highly soluble agents, the effect on the rate of change in tissues must be negligible, because of the opposing change that results in arterial blood. That is, suppose on induction a shunt existed at the tissues so that the effective tissue flow were halved. As noted in Chapter 7, this would halve uptake at the lungs and permit a considerable elevation of the arterial anesthetic partial pressure. This elevation would increase uptake and thereby compensate for the reduction in effective tissue flow. No such compensation is possible with poorly soluble agents, since the alveolar (arterial) concentration is little influenced by changes in uptake.

Summary

Diffusion limitations may hinder the rate at which anesthetics equilibrate with some tissues. These limitations may cause alveolar to arterial or venous to tissue anesthetic partial pressure difference. On the other hand, diffusion of anesthetic from a more richly perfused tissue to a less well perfused tissue (intertissue diffusion) may accelerate the rate of rise of anesthetic in the less well perfused tissue. This would increase total anesthetic uptake per unit time. Finally, anesthetic molecules may move from artery to vein and hence never reach the tissue perfused by the blood in which they are carried. Although each of the above undoubtedly affects anesthetic uptake and distribution, their total impact remains unknown.

QUESTIONS

1. When breathed for the first time, which of these gas pairs should produce the greatest end-tidal to arterial partial pressure ratio (assume all these gases are nearly insoluble): a) H_2 and N_2; b) Ne and N_2; c) SF_6 and CF_4?

2. Give three reasons why concomitant nitrous oxide and halothane administration should produce a more rapid rate of rise of arterial halothane partial pressure.
3. An anesthetic has a fat/blood partition coefficient of 10. Blood flow to fat is 2 ml/100 ml of fat/minute. At the start of the anesthesia, what fraction of the anesthetic in blood will be removed as the blood passes through the fat if there is no diffusion limitation? What is the fraction removed if there is a diffusion limitation such that the anesthetic only equilibrates with 10 percent of the fat? Notice that removal by fat is nearly complete even with the smaller volume of equilibration.
4. Babies may have smaller alveoli and breathe more rapidly than adults. How would these differences influence transfer of anesthetic from the alveolar duct to pulmonary capillary? Many anesthetics cause tachypnea: how might this affect the rate of rise of anesthetic in arterial blood?
5. The arteries that pass to the dermis must traverse subcutaneous fat: how might this affect uptake of anesthetic?
6. Why would intertissue diffusion to fat be of greater importance than intertissue diffusion to ligaments, tendons or cartilage?
7. Why would intervascular diffusion affect brain anesthetic rate of rise less than the rate of rise in muscle or fat.?

REFERENCES

1. Georg, J., Lassen, N. A., Mellemgaard, K., and Vinther, A.: Diffusion in the gas phase of the lungs in normal and emphysemous subjects. Clin. Sci. 29: 525–532, 1965.
2. Cumming, G., Horsfield, K., Jones, J. G., and Muir, D. C. F.: The influence of gaseous diffusion on the alveolar plateau at different lung volumes. Res. Physiol. 2: 386–398, 1967.
3. Lassen, N. A., Lindbjerg, I. F., and Dahn, I.: Validity of the ^{133}Xenon method for measurement of muscle blood flow evaluated by simultaneous venous occlusion plethysmography. Circ. Res. 16: 287–293, 1965.
4. Sejrsen, P., and Tønnesen, K. H.: Inert gas diffusion method for measurement of blood flow using saturation techniques. Comparison with directly measured blood flow in isolated gastrocnemius muscle of the cat. Circ. Res. 22: 679–693, 1968.
5. Lesser, G. T., and Deutsch, S.: Measurement of adipose tissue blood flow and perfusion in man by uptake of ^{85}Kr. J. Appl. Physiol. 23: 621–630, 1967.
6. Larsen, O. A., Lassen, N. A., and Quaade, F.: Blood flow through human adipose tissue determined with radioactive xenon. Acta Physiol. Scand. 66: 337–345, 1966.
7. Stoelting, R. K., and Eger, E. I., II: Percutaneous loss of nitrous oxide, cyclopropane, ether and halothane in man. Anesthesiology 30: 278–283, 1969.
8. Cullen, B. F., and Eger, E. I., II: Diffusion of nitrous oxide, cyclopropane, and halothane through human skin and amniotic membrane. Anesthesiology 36: 168–173, 1972.
9. Perl, W.: Large-scale diffusion between body compartments. In *Uptake and Distribution of Anesthetic Agents*, edited by E. M. Papper and R. J. Kitz, Ch. 18, pp. 224–227. McGraw-Hill, New York, 1963.
10. Cohen, E. N., Chow, K. L., and Mathers, L.: Autoradiographic distribution of volatile anesthetics within the brain. Anesthesiology 37: 324–331, 1972.
11. Eger, E. I., II: Intertissue diffusion of anesthetics. Anesthesiology 38: 201, 1973.

12. Rackow, H., Salanitre, E., Epstein, R. M., et al.: Simultaneous uptake of N_2O and cyclopropane in man as a test of compartmental model. J. Appl. Physiol. 20: 611–620, 1965.
13. Perl, W., Rackow, H., Salanitre, E., et al.: Intertissue diffusion effect for inert fat-soluble gases. J. Appl. Physiol. 20: 621–627, 1965.
14. Calusen, J. P., and Lassen, N. A.: Muscle blood flow during exercise in normal man studied by the ^{133}Xenon method. Cardiov. Res. 5: 245–254, 1971.
15. Stosseck, K.: Hydrogen exchange through the pial vessel wall and its meaning for the determination of the local cerebral blood flow. Pflueger Arch. 320: 111–119, 1970.

Chapter 16

Mechanisms of Barbiturate Action

L. J. SAIDMAN

Barbiturates can impede impulse transmission through all parts of the nervous system. Although the critical concentration causing blockade at one site may be higher than at another, blockade eventually is achieved at all sites at a sufficiently high concentration. As with the inhaled anesthetics, barbiturates can block peripheral nerve conduction (1–3) and they can impair synaptic transmission through neuromuscular junctions (4–6), autonomic ganglia, the spinal cord (7–10) and the brain (11, 12). The specific principle gross site of barbiturate action is unknown, and, in fact, there may be no single site.

Effect on Axonal Transmission

While several gross anatomic areas of the central nervous system seem to be equally eligible as the primary site of barbiturate action, at a microscopic level there are only two sites which can explain the observed effects—the axon and the synapse. Like general and local anesthetics, barbiturates can inhibit axonal impulse transmission by reducing sodium conduction without altering transmembrane potential (1). The uncharged molecule is likely the active species (2, 3). Evidence for this comes from studies of the effect of pH changes on potency. A decrease in pH increases the ionized form (see section on pH effect in next chapter) and decreases potency (2).

The similarity between the effect of barbiturates and local and inhaled anesthetics on axonal conduction suggests a common mode of action. Thus, we may speculate that barbiturates reduce sodium conductance perhaps by direct obstruction of the sodium pore or perhaps indirectly by increasing the surface pressure of the excitable membrane. Unfortunately, the concentrations required to inhibit axonal transmissions are far in excess of those required to produce sedation and anesthesia. Thus, these speculations as to cause are of no importance unless they also describe a mechanism of action at a more susceptible site.

Action of Barbiturates at the Synapse

Barbiturates depress many levels of synaptic transmission at concentrations far less than those required for axonal block. It would appear that this site of action accounts for the major anesthetic effects of barbiturates. The most vulnerable portion of the synapse and the particular synapses which invariably must be affected to produce anesthesia are unknown. Studies of the impairment of transmission at several sites will be described in the succeeding sections. Some of these sites obviously are not the site of action (for example, the neuromuscular junction) but a mechanism discovered at this site may apply equally at the true site.

Neuromuscular Junction

Barbiturates can depress both presynaptic and postsynaptic transmission at the myoneural junction. In the presence of barbiturates, the postsynaptic membrane of amphibia is insensitive to acetylcholine (postsynaptic effect) (4). Pentobarbital depresses repetitive antidromic firing in motor nerves (presynaptic effect) (5). Concentrations of pentobarbital that depress strength of contraction 20 to 80 percent also prolong the absolute refractory period and decrease the resting end-plate potential, but do not affect miniature end-plate potential amplitude (6). This suggests that although pre- and postsynaptic effects are present, the primary action of pentobarbital is on motor nerve terminals (presynaptic).

Autonomic Ganglia

Both thiopental (13) and pentobarbital (14) depress transmission through sympathetic ganglia. Pentobarbital, 0.25 mM, blocks synaptic conduction, whereas 10 times that dose is required for block of axonal conduction (14). It appears that the effect either is on the presynaptic terminal or the ganglion cell itself. This ganglionic block in part might account for the fall in blood pressure following barbiturate administration.

Spinal Cord

Intracellular electrode studies in spinal motor neurons show that barbiturates depress the excitatory postsynaptic potential without affecting electrical properties of the postsynaptic membrane. A concomitant reduction in spike amplitude in the nerve terminal indicates a presynaptic effect (7). Input resistance of the motor neuron is not affected by thiopental (no postjunctional effect) and 10 mg/kg of thiopental to cats decreases the quantal content of neurotransmitter (presynaptic effect) (8). A 25 percent decrease in transmitter release theoretically might decrease monosynaptic reflex transmission by 50 to 80 percent (15), a figure close to the 40 to 60 percent decrease seen by Weakley (8). Somjen (9), on the other hand, while not ruling out decreased transmitter release, suggested that stabilization of the postsynaptic membrane was the most likely explanation for decreased synaptic transmission.

Other CNS Sites

Pentobarbital impairs transmission through the cuneate nucleus (11). The subsynaptic membrane appears to be affected to a greater degree than the presynaptic nerve terminal although at higher doses, a presynaptic effect can be demonstrated.

In a number of CNS networks, small doses of barbiturate have little effect on the transmission of the first of a train of pulses, but do impair transmission of succeeding pulses (16). This effect on repetitive activity likely would impair wakefulness and thus may be important to the hypnotic effect of barbiturates.

Some Theories of Barbiturate Action

A Physical Effect on the Neural Membrane

The above sections point to a synaptic site of action for barbiturates. Evidence exists for both pre- and postsynaptic effects with a suggestion that the presynaptic locus is most important. None of these studies describe how barbiturates act at these sites but all imply an effect on the cell membrane.

The mechanisms of barbiturate action may be identical to those proposed for the inhaled anesthetics. The nerve action potential at the nerve terminal may be reduced—with a consequent reduction in transmitter release—by a decreased sodium conductance. As noted in the above section on axonal transmission, barbiturates may obstruct sodium pores directly by their presence in the pore or indirectly by their presence in the cell membrane. The latter effect may be achieved through an increase in the lateral membrane pressure. Such a hypothesis also would explain a decrease in subsynaptic sensitivity through similar effect on the ionic channels opened by transmitter.

The evidence suggesting membrane expansion as the mechanism of barbiturate action comes from the same sources as those which supported a similar mechanism for the inhaled anesthetics. If barbiturates act by expanding the membrane, then this action should be opposed by any force which compresses the membrane. Consonant with this argument, pentobarbital anesthesia in tadpoles and mice can be reversed by high hydrostatic pressure (100 to 200 atmospheres) (17).

The protection against hypotonic hemolysis of red blood cells afforded by inhaled anesthetics or pentobarbital also suggests the importance of membrane expansion by these agents (18). Anesthetizing concentrations of these agents all cause similar expansion of the erythrocyte membrane and a similar degree of protection against hemolysis. This study also suggests an alternative hypothesis: perhaps barbiturates impair the disruption of the synaptic vesicles just as they impair the disruption of erythrocytes. Such an impairment would reduce transmitter release. How barbiturates would act to strengthen the membrane is uncertain.

Another similar theory proposed for the inhaled anesthetics also might apply to barbiturates. Inhaled anesthetics expand olive oil roughly in proportion to their potency (19). Perhaps barbiturates interact with membrane lipids to expand or distort the membrane. It is known that spacing of phospholipid molecules affects the interaction of calcium with phospholipids (20), and such an interaction may be of considerable importance to membrane excitability. For example, the calcium-phospholipid link may form a portion of the "latch" to the sodium pore gate (see Chapter 2). Along these lines, Johnson and Bangham (21) suggest that the reversible anesthetic block of the axonal action potential is due to foreign molecules which sterically impede rearrangement of the membrane lipid groups responsible for sodium conduction during depolarization. Although these authors studied other agents, their conclusions also may apply to barbiturates. Finally, the importance of lipid solubility is suggested by the direct relationship between the octanol/water partition coefficient of barbiturates and their potency as anticonvulsants (22).

An Effect on Oxidative Metabolism

Barbiturates decrease oxidative metabolism. However, the decreased metabolism may be only a secondary result of decreased activity rather than the result of some primary effect. Even if the decrease is a manifestation of a primary effect, it still is just a manifestation and only indicates a direction for investigation. Certainly a decrease in metabolism per se does not produce anesthesia. Hypothermia or hypothyroidism can reduce metabolism more then barbiturates without producing anesthesia. Perhaps barbiturates impair the production of high energy phosphate bonds (23, 24), but there is little evidence for this being a consistent effect for all barbiturates. Even if it were consistent, it is unclear how this would induce the almost instantaneous anesthesia produced by the ultrashort acting barbiturates.

Summary

Barbiturates can depress all macroscopic levels of central nervous system conduction, but no one level seems particularly sensitive. On a microscopic level, synaptic transmission is blocked by far lower doses of barbiturate than axonal transmission and the synapse thus must be the principle site of action. Presynaptic nerve terminal function seems to be more readily depressed by barbiturates than subsynaptic membrane function.

The precise molecular mechanism by which barbiturates act remains speculative. The fact that potency appears related to lipid solubility, that the active form appears to be the undissociated molecule, that membranes are expanded by barbiturate anesthesia and that hydrostatic pressure reverses the anesthetic effect, all suggest a hydrophobic site of action and mechanisms similar to those proposed in the chapter on theories of narcosis for inhalation agents (Chapter 3). For example, the physical pressure of the drug in the cell membrane may alter surface activity and thereby decrease sodium conductance. Alternatively, transmitter release may be hindered by the effect of barbiturate on the synpatic vesicle membrane.

Finally, although barbiturates depress oxidative metabolism as well as neural transmission, the question as to which is cause and which effect is uncertain. It appears unlikely that depression of oxidative metabolism is the specific mechanism by which barbiturates act.

QUESTIONS

1. Compare the relative sensitivity of the axon and the synapse to the effects of barbiturates.
2. What is the evidence that a physical effect on neural membranes might be the same for both barbiturates and inhaled anesthetics?
3. How is lipid solubility of barbiturates related to anesthetic potency?
4. Why aren't barbiturates used as local anesthetics?
5. What does the extremely rapid onset of action of ultrashort acting barbiturates imply about their mechanism of action?
6. Some barbiturates (not used clinically) are convulsants. Suggest a mechanism by which they might act which also would be consistent with the mechanism producing barbiturate anesthesia.

REFERENCES

1. Schoepfle, G. M.: Pentothal block of single nerve fibers and subsequent revival by means of anodal polarization. Fed. Proc. 16: 114, 1957.
2. Krupp, P., Bianchi, C. P., and Suarez-Kurtz, A.: On the local anaesthetic effect of barbiturates. J. Pharm. Pharmacol. 21: 763–768, 1969.
3. Narahashi, T., Frazier, T., Deguch, T., Cleaves, C. A., and Ernau, M. C.: The active form of pentobarbital in squid giant axons. J. Pharmacol. Exp. Ther. 177: 25–33, 1971.
4. Thesleff, S.: The effect of anesthetic agents on skeletal muscle membrane. Acta Physiol. Scand. 37: 335–349, 1956.
5. Riker, W. F., Jr., Werder, G., Roberts, J., and Kuperman, A.: Pharmacologic evidence

of the existence of a presynaptic event in neuro-muscular transmission. J. Pharmacol. Exp. Ther. 125: 150–158, 1959.
6. Galindo, A.: Procaine, pentobarbital and halothane: effects on the mammalian myoneural junction. J. Pharmacol. Exp. Ther. 177: 360–368, 1971.
7. Loyning, T., Oshima, T., and Yokota, T.: Site of action of thioamylol sodium on the monosynaptic spinal reflex pathway in cats. J. Neurophysiol. 27: 408–428, 1964.
8. Weakly, J. N.: Effect of barbiturates on "quantal" synaptic transmission in spinal motoneurons. J. Physiol. (London) 204: 63–77, 1969.
9. Somjen, G. G.: Effects of ether and thiopental on spinal presynaptic terminals. J. Pharmacol. Exp. Ther. 140: 396–402, 1963.
10. Banna, N. R.: Antagonism of barbiturate depression of spinal transmission by catechol. Experientia 26: 1330–1331, 1970.
11. Galindo, A.: Effects of procaine, pentobarbital, and halothane on synaptic transmission in the central nervous system. J. Pharmacol. Exp. Ther. 169: 185–195, 1969.
12. Clark, D. L., and Rosner, B.: Neurophysiological effects of general anesthesia. Anesthesiology 38: 564–582, 1973.
13. Larrabee, M. G., and Holaday, D. A.: Depression of transmission through sympathetic ganglia during general anesthesia. J. Pharmacol. Exp. Ther. 105: 400–408, 1952.
14. Larrabee, M. G., and Posternark, J. M.: Selective action of anesthetics on synapses and axons in mammalian sympathetic ganglia. J. Neurophysiol. 15: 91–114, 1952.
15. Rall, W.: Experimental monosynaptic input-output relations in the mammalian spinal cord. J. Cell. Comp. Physiol. 46: 413–437, 1955.
16. Sharpless, K.: Hypnotics and sedatives I. The barbiturates. In *The Pharmacological Basis of Therapeutics*, edited by L. S. Coodman, and A. Gilman. Macmillan Co., New York, 1970.
17. Lever, M. J., Miller, K. W., Paton, W. D. M., and Smith, E. B.: Pressure reversal of anaesthesia. Nature 231: 368–371, 1971.
18. Roth, S., and Seeman, P.: Anesthetics expand erythrocyte membranes without causing loss of K^+. Biochim. Biophys. Acta 255: 171–177, 1972.
19. Sears, D. F., and Fuller, E. L.: Volume changes of polar and nonpolar liquid hydrocarbon exposed to pressures of gases. Res. Physiol. 5: 175–186, 1968.
20. Shah, D. O., and Schulman, J. H.: Binding of metal ions to monolayers of lecethins, plasmalogens, cardiolipids, and diacetyl phosphate. J. Lipid Res. 6: 341–349, 1965.
21. Johnson, S. M., and Bangham, A. D.: The action of anesthetics on phospholipid membrane. Biochim. Biophys. Acta 193: 92–104, 1969.
22. Lien, E. J.: Structure-activity correlations for anticonvulsant drugs. J. Med. Chem. 13: 1189–1191, 1970.
23. Eiler, J. J., and McEwen, W. K.: The effect of pentobarbital on aerobic phosphorylation in brain homogenates. Arch. Biochem. 20: 163–165, 1949.
24. Kozawa, S., Fujita, N., Yoshie, S., and Ozawa, Y.: Effect of narcotic and convulsant on lactic acid, phosphate esters, and acetylcholine content of the brain. Jap. J. Pharmacol. 3: 50–61, 1953.

Chapter 17

Uptake, Distribution and Elimination of Barbiturates

L. J. SAIDMAN

Although barbiturates and inhaled gases are administered in different ways, both consist of highly lipid soluble, freely diffusable molecules distributed to tissues in proportion to each tissue's blood flow. Thus, uptake and distribution of barbiturates follow many of the principles described in earlier chapters. Just as an understanding of uptake and distribution of inhaled agents makes their administration safer, so too should this knowledge help prevent untoward responses in patients receiving barbiturates. The purpose of this chapter then is to outline principles of barbiturate uptake and distribution, including a discussion of factors that alter the normal response to these drugs. Thiopental will serve as our model, both because of its popularity and because more is known about this agent than any other.

Solubility, Blood Flow and "Partial Pressure" as Applied to Barbiturates

Tissue/Blood Partition Coefficient

As with inhaled anesthetics, the factors governing the distribution of barbiturates are tissue/blood partition coefficient, tissue blood flow and the barbiturate "partial pressure" difference between blood and tissues. Tissue/blood partition coefficient defines the ratio of drug in tissue to that in blood when equilibrium has been achieved, i.e., no further net movement of drug between blood and tissue. This definition is identical to that for the tissue solubility of inhaled agents. Table 17, 1 lists tissue/blood partition coefficients for some barbiturates.

Tissue Blood Flow

Again, as with inhaled agents, we can describe the distribution of barbiturates with a multicompartment model in which each tissue (or group of tissues having similar blood flow per unit volume of tissue and

TABLE 17, 1

Tissue/blood partition coefficients for various barbiturates

Drug	Species	Tissue	Tissue/Blood Partition Coefficient
Thiopental	Human (1)	Brain	1.4
		Heart	1.2
		Liver	1.9
		Kidney	2.0
		Muscle	1.5
		Fat	11.0
	Rabbit (2)	Muscle	0.83
		Brain	0.97
		Lung	1.20
		Kidney	3.73
		Heart	1.23
		Liver	2.96
	Dog (3)	Brain*	1.03
Pentobarbital	Rabbit (2)	Muscle	1.0
		Brain	1.4
		Lung	1.6
		Kidney	2.0
		Heart	1.6
		Liver	2.7
	Dog (3)	Brain*	1.3
Phenobarbital	Rabbit (2)	Muscle	0.70
		Brain	0.67
		Lung	0.72
		Kidney	0.9
		Heart	0.85
		Liver	1.15
	Dog (3)	Brain*	1.1

* Tissue/plasma partition coefficients. However, data from Reference 2 indicate close agreement between plasma and blood barbiturate concentrations.

similar tissue/blood partition coefficients) receives drug in proportion to its blood flow. The rate at which each tissue equilibrates with barbiturates (i.e., the time constant) is determined by the capacity of the tissue (volume times the tissue/blood partition coefficient) relative to its perfusion. The vessel rich group tissues come into equilibrium with blood before the less well perfused tissues of the body. In the same vein, muscle equilibrates more rapidly than fat because its capacity for anesthetic is less than fat.

Partial Pressure

Partial pressure (or "activity") is an easily understood concept for inhaled anesthetics but perhaps is somewhat confusing when applied to barbiturates. Partial pressure in either case is the net force that influences movement of anesthetic molecules from one phase to another. Recall that a tissue/blood partition coefficient defines the relative concentrations in two phases when equilibrium has been established between the phases. At equilibrium no net transfer of anesthetic occurs (i.e., the concentrations remain constant) because the net forces—that is, the partial pressures—in both phases are equal. For example, the thiopental fat/blood partition coefficient is 11 and thiopental molecules will move from blood to fat as long as the concentration in fat is less than 11 times that in blood. In other words, until the partial pressure concentration in fat is 11 times that in blood, thiopental partial pressure is higher in blood and drug will move from blood to fat. As with inhaled drugs, partial pressure does NOT refer to concentration or amount.

Factors Influencing Onset of Action and Duration of Narcosis

Since all barbiturates given intravenously reach the cerebral circulation at the same speed, the onset of narcosis from various barbiturates is related to their rates of penetration into the central nervous system. Molecular size, ionization, protein binding and lipid solubility each influence the rate of penetration.

Molecular Size

The speed of diffusion across a membrane is inversely related to molecular size, but since the barbiturates come in relatively similar sizes, this factor does not account for differences in onset or the duration of narcosis.

Ionization

Barbiturates are weak acids which normally are prepared as the salt of a strong base (e.g., sodium thiopental). Once inside the body, the ionized base can combine with hydrogen ions to form the nonionized acid:

$$NaP \rightleftharpoons Na^+ + P^- \tag{1}$$

and

$$H^+ + P^- \overset{Ka}{\rightleftharpoons} HP \tag{2}$$

where P^- represents the barbiturate radical (i.e., the thiopental of sodium thiopental) and Ka is the dissociation constant. The formation of the nonionized HP is of great importance since only the nonionized molecule can readily cross biological membranes. The law of mass action allows us to rewrite equation 2 as

$$Ka = [H^+][P^-]/[HP] \tag{3}$$

or

$$[HP]/[P^-] = [H^+]/Ka \tag{4}$$

Equation 4 illustrates that the fraction of nonionized barbiturate varies directly with the concentration of the hydrogen ion. Since the Ka for barbiturates and physiological concentrations of $[H^+]$ are close to each other, an appreciable fraction of barbiturate exists in the nonionized form and therefore is available for penetration of biological membranes.

Equation 3 usually is written in the familar Henderson/Hasselbach form:

$$pKa - pH = \log [HP]/[P^-] \tag{5}$$

As noted in table 17, 2, pKa for most barbiturates is slightly greater than a physiological pH of 7.4 and therefore over half of *in vivo* barbiturate would exist as nondissociated molecules.

Although they do not limit the passage of barbiturates across membranes, ionization and pH may considerably influence the distribution of a barbiturate within the body. At equilibrium the concentration of the nonionized form is the same between blood, extracellular fluid and the hydrophilic portion of the cell. However, because pH affects the fraction of ionized barbiturate and because intracellular pH differs from extracellular pH, the fraction of ionized barbiturate may differ between the inside and outside of the cell. Accordingly, there may be a concentration difference of total barbiturate (ionized and nonionized) across the cell membrane. The relationship between the extracellular and intracellular concentrations are described by:

$$H_o^+ + P_o^- \rightleftharpoons HP_o = HP_i \rightleftharpoons H_i^+ + P_i^- \tag{6}$$

where the subscripts "o" and "i" refer to species, respectively, outside and inside of a cell. The ratio (R) of barbiturate concentration inside as

TABLE 17, 2 (4)

	Thiopental	Pentobarbital	Barbital
pKa	7.6	8.1	7.5
Fraction bound to protein at pH 7.4	0.75	0.40	<0.02
Fraction nonionized at pH 7.4	0.61	0.83	0.557
n-Heptane/water partition coefficient for nonionized species	3.3	0.05	0.002
"Effective partition coefficient" *	2.0	0.042	0.001
Penetration rate constant (min^{-1})†	0.50	0.17	0.026

* Calculated by multiplying fraction ionized times n-heptane water partition coefficient.
† Determined from rate of appearance of drug in CSF after intravenous injection.

opposed to outside the cell may be expressed as:

$$R = \frac{1 + 10^{pHi - pKa}}{1 + 10^{pHo - pKa}} \quad (7)*$$

Changes in either extra or intracellular pH therefore alter the distribution of drug between the two phases. An increase in extracellular pH without any alteration in intracellular pH draws barbiturate out of the cell. Table 17, 3 shows the progressive fall in the ratio (R) of intracellular to extracellular barbiturate concentrations that attends an extracellular alkalosis. These calculated values are supported by *in vivo* data. Plasma phenobarbital concentrations are increased by metabolic alkalosis in dogs (5). Similarly, the median anesthetic dose of phenobarbital in mice is raised 20 percent by bicarbonate treatment (6). Note that these changes in distribution may not apply when *both* intracellular and extracellular pH concomitantly change in the same direction. Thus, a respiratory alkalosis or acidosis has much less influence on the distribution of barbiturate.

TABLE 17, 3

pH_i (plasma pH)	pH_o (intracellular pH)	R*
7.0	7.0	1.0
7.4	7.0	.77
7.8	7.0	.48

* R is the ratio of intracellular to extracellular barbiturate concentrations The pKa is assumed to equal that of thiopental (7.6).

---

* By definition

$$R = \frac{[HP_i] + [P_i^-]}{[HP_o] + [P_o^-]} \quad (8)$$

From equation 3,

$$[P_i] = [HP_i]Ka/[H_i^+] \text{ and } [P_o] = [HP_o]Ka/[H_o^+]$$

Substituting into 8,

$$R = \frac{[HP_i] + [HP_i]Ka/[H_i^+]}{[HP_o] + [HP_o]Ka/[H_o^+]} \quad (9)$$

But $[HP_i]$ equals $[HP_o]$. Therefore,

$$R = \frac{1 + Ka/[H_i^+]}{1 + Ka/[H_o^+]} \quad (10)$$

which also may be written as equation 7.

Protein Binding

Protein binding is a reversible combination of a small molecule (e.g., barbiturates) and a protein. A greater binding indicates a greater attractiveness of the protein binding sites for barbiturate. Binding and solubility may be thought of as being synonymous. Thiobarbiturates are bound to a greater extent than their oxygen analogs. For example, roughly twice as much thiopental is bound to protein than pentobarbital (figs. 17, 1; 17, 2). The difference probably relates to the effect of the sulfur substitution on the affinity for a hydrophobic portion of the protein. As indicated in table 17, 2 the fraction bound decreases with a decrease in the N-heptane/water partition coefficient—i.e., with a decrease in lipid solubility. First, the fraction increases with pH to a maximum at a pH of about 8.0 (2) (fig. 17, 1). Second, the fraction decreases with the saturation of binding sites that occurs at higher drug concentrations (fig. 17, 2). Third, as a corollary to the second factor, an increase in protein concentration increases the fraction (and amount) of drug bound at a given barbiturate concentration (2). Fourth, there may be competition for the barbiturate binding site by other drugs which may be given concomitantly (2, 5).

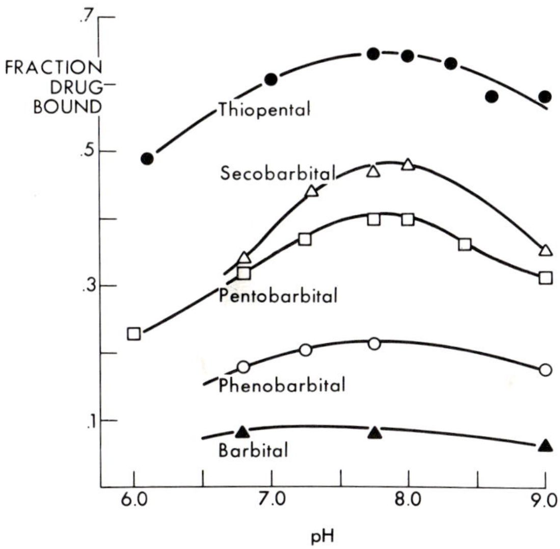

FIG. 17, 1. Binding of 0.001 M substituted barbituric acids by 1 percent bovine serum albumin reaches a peak in the physiological pH range. (Adapted with permission from Goldbaum, L. R., and Smith, P. K.: The interaction of barbiturates with serum albumin and its possible relation to their disposition and pharmacological actions. J. Pharmacol. Exp. Ther. 111: 197, 1954.)

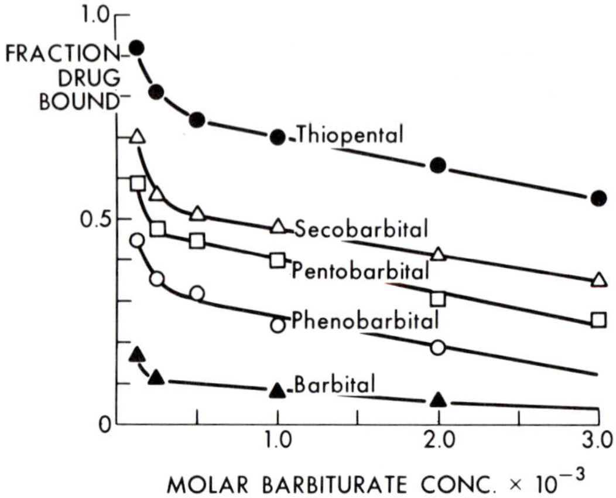

FIG. 17, 2. An increase in barbiturate concentration reduces the fraction bound by one percent bovine serum albumin, presumably by saturation of binding sites. (Adapted with permission from Goldbaum, L. R., and Smith, P. K.: The interaction of barbiturates with serum albumin and its possible relation to their disposition and pharmacological actions. J. Pharmacol. Exp. Ther. 111: 197, 1954.)

As noted above, an increase in binding to blood proteins is synonymous to an increase in blood solubility or to a decrease in the tissue/blood partition coefficient. An increase in binding thus lowers partial pressure or activity. Binding therefore can slow the rate of disappearance of barbiturate from blood. This presumes that any change in blood protein binding is not accompanied by an identical change in tissue binding. Concomitant identical changes will produce counterbalancing effects on distribution which tend to cancel each other.

The tissue/blood partition coefficient is of great importance to the rate of loss from the body by excretion or metabolism. An increase in the partition coefficient slows the elimination process by limiting the delivery of barbiturate to the organ(s) of metabolism or excretion. This may be readily seen at the extreme represented by a tissue/blood partition coefficient of infinity: no drug then is carried by blood and hence none can be eliminated. This concept is of importance to an understanding of how other nondepressant drugs can alter the effect of barbiturates by altering protein binding. The capacity of blood protein to bind barbiturate may be reduced by prior or concomitant administration of drugs which compete for the same site. As a result, barbiturate will be displaced from blood to tissues thereby intensifying the anesthetic effect. Furthermore, the clearance rate of barbiturate from tissues will be decreased and the delivery of barbiturate to the liver will be reduced by the reduction in blood solubility. As a result, the effect of the barbiturate will be prolonged. *In vivo* studies support this hypothesis. For example, pretreatment of rats with sodium acetrizoate, a contrast material highly bound to plasma protein, results in a 70 percent increase in duration of narcosis from pentobarbital (5). Similarly, hypoproteinemia may reduce blood barbiturate concentration and prolong narcosis.

Lipid Solubility

The lipid solubility of a barbiturate is determined almost entirely by the solubility of the nonionized molecule: the ionized molecule is poorly soluble in lipid. The factors determining solubility of the nonionized molecule are unclear although it is known that the thiobarbiturates are more lipid soluble than their oxygen analogs (table 17, 2) (3).

In general, the greater the lipid solubility of the nonionized molecule, the faster the rate of penetration into the central nervous system and hence the more rapid the onset of action. The relative importance of lipid solubility, protein binding and ionization to penetration into the brain has been studied by measuring rates of entry of three barbiturates into cerebrospinal fluid (2). As noted above, protein binding is related to lipid solubility and it would appear that this latter factor also is crucial to the rate of penetration (table 17, 2).

Duration of narcosis is a function of the rate at which the blood level falls, which in turn is a function of redistribution to muscle and fat and of metabolism (see discussion on influence of metabolism). An additional factor to consider is that of acute tolerance. Patients receiving higher initial doses of thiobarbiturates recover consciousness at higher blood thiopental levels than those receiving small initial doses (7). The reason for this is not understood.

A General Description of Thiopental Uptake and Distribution

The initial distribution of an intravenous injection of thiopental is to the central blood volume of the body. Dilution by blood establishes a certain initial concentration which then is further decreased by distribution of thiopental to tissues. The amount going to any one tissue is proportional to tissue blood flow. The amount of barbiturate taken up by that tissue is determined by the same three factors which determined the tissue uptake of an inhaled anesthetic. These are: 1) tissue solubility; 2) blood flow per unit volume of tissue; and 3) the blood to tissue barbiturate partial pressure difference. An increase in any of these factors will increase uptake and a decrease will decrease uptake. Because of its high blood flow, the VRG initially receives the majority of the drug, and narcosis (or cardiovascular depression) rapidly ensues. In contrast to the constantly rising blood level seen on induction with inhalation agents, the blood level with barbiturates rapidly falls, and within 1 minute, thiopental partial pressure in the VRG exceeds that in blood coming to it (i.e., concentration ratio of VRG to blood is greater than the VRG/blood partition coefficient). Drug now re-enters blood (fig. 17, 3). At the same time, fat and muscle accumulate drug at a rate dependent on solubility, tissue volume and blood flow. As for the inhaled anesthetics, these factors determine the time constants for equilibration. The lower blood flow relative to capacity (capacity is tissue volume times the tissue/blood partition coefficient) of muscle and fat causes their approach to equilibrium to be far slower than the approach of the VRG and the drug that has re-entered blood from VRG is redistributed to muscle, fat and the VPG. Muscle equilibrates in about 20 minutes after which it too loses drug to blood. Fat, because of its huge capacity for thiopental, is the last tissue to equilibrate with the falling blood level.

Alterations in blood volume or in the distribution of blood flow to tissues may alter the distribution of thiopental. For example, hypovolemia may decrease blood flow to muscle and fat but allow maintenance of flow to brain and heart. The initial blood thiopental concentration

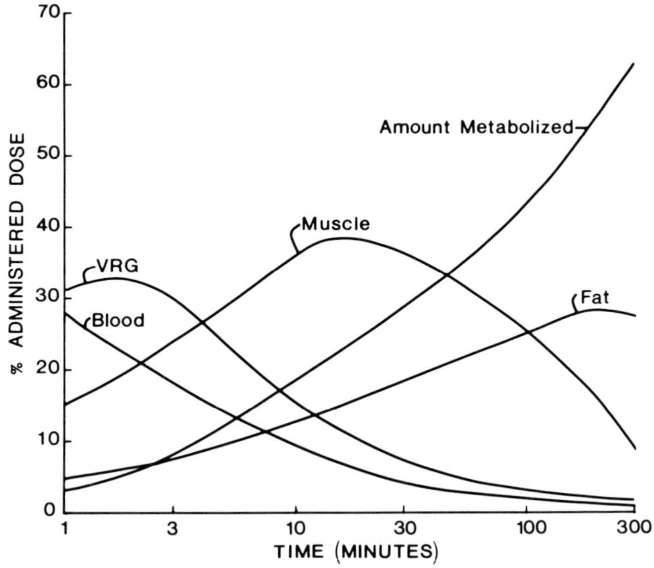

FIG. 17, 3. Following an intravenous bolus, the percent of thiopental remaining in blood rapidly decreases as drug moves from blood to body tissues. Time to attainment of peak tissue levels is a direct function of tissue capacity for barbiturate relative to blood flow. Thus, a larger capacity or smaller blood flow is related to a longer time to a peak tissue level. Initially, most thiopental is taken up by the VRG because of its high blood flow. Subsequently, drug is redistributed to muscle and to a lesser extent to fat. Throughout this period, small but substantial amounts of thiopental are removed by the liver and metabolized. Unlike removal by the tissues, this removal is cumulative. Note that the rate of metabolism equals the early rate of removal by fat. The sum of this early removal by fat and metabolism is the same as the removal by muscle.

must be higher than normal due to less dilution in the central blood volume. Higher brain and heart concentrations would result and the rate of loss to muscle and fat would be decreased. Hypovolemia thus may increase drug depression, extend the duration of depression and increase adverse hemodynamic effects. On the other hand, apprehension may increase muscle blood flow without altering cerebral perfusion. The more rapid redistribution to muscle should accelerate the decrease in brain concentration and thereby shorten the period of narcosis.

Little change in onset or depth of narcosis should be seen in obese patients when a "normal" dose of thiopental is given. This is because fat normally receives relatively little blood flow, and obesity is not accompanied by a proportional increase in perfusion. Thus, the immediate amount of thiopental diverted from brain to fat is normally small and is not greatly increased by obesity. Of course, fat has an enormous capacity to hold thiopental and obesity might prolong anesthesia after a very large dose which is given over a long time (8).

As with the inhaled anesthetics, we may speculate on how the barbiturates may influence their own uptake by altering circulation. Increases in cutaneous blood flow that attend anesthetic induction may lead to a more rapid reduction in the blood level through a greater initial distribution to skin. Conversely, a dose of barbiturate which causes a decrease in cardiac output may produce a prolonged effect because of the delay in redistribution to muscle and fat.

Metabolism and Excretion

Barbiturates ultimately are eliminated by hepatic metabolism and (to a far smaller extent) by renal excretion. We will not discuss the specific metabolic pathways involved in biodegradation of barbiturates but will describe the effect of elimination on duration of action as reflected by plasma and tissue drug levels.

Originally, the ultrashort action of thiopental was attributed to rapid metabolism (9–11). This hypothesis soon was discarded and for several years it was acceped that the evanescent effect of thiopental was primarily due to redistribution to muscle and, to a lesser extent, to fat (1). The evidence against metabolism as a factor was the finding that several hours following injection, the decay in plasma barbiturate levels was only 10 to 15 percent/hour (12). The observation that plasma decay rates determined several hours after injection may not reflect the metabolic rate immediately following injection resurrected metabolism as an important codeterminant of early awakening (8). Let us examine the arguments for the importance of metabolism to the ultrashort action of thiopental and other barbiturates.

Evidence for an Effect of Metabolism

Removal of 85 percent of the liver in rats significantly increases the duration of action of intravenously injected thiopental (13). Similarly, inclusion of the liver in a heart-lung dog preparation accelerates the rate of decline of plasma thiopental concentration (14). Awakening from thiopental is prolonged indefinitely after production of an Eck fistula (15). Normal humans given 4 mg/kg of thiopental intravenously can stand without support after 163 seconds, whereas humans with liver dysfunction require 488 seconds (16).

Late versus Early Plasma Decay Rates

How can we reconcile these data with the finding that 4 or 5 hours following injection, plasma thiopental concentrations decay at a rate of only 10 to 15 percent/hour? The difficulty lies in the interpretation of the plasma decay rates. Although they indeed are dependent on metabolism, they also are determined by the distribution of the drug to be metabolized. For example, suppose that an intravenously administered drug were confined to the intravascular space and suppose that the liver destroyed all of the drugs brought to it. It is easy to see that the blood levels of this drug would rapidly decrease. If we assume a blood volume of 4.5 liters and a liver blood flow of 1.5 liters/minute, we can calculate a time constant of 3 minutes for the decay rate (i.e., 63 percent destroyed in 3 minutes). A different hepatic metabolism would result in a different time constant. If the liver destroyed only half of the drug brought to it, then the effective liver blood flow (as far as biodegradation of the drug is concerned) would be reduced by half. The time constant in this case would be 6 minutes or twice the time constant obtained when all the drug was destroyed.

But the metabolic rate (fraction of drug removed from the hepatic blood flow) is not the only factor which influences the time constant. Equally important is the volume of distribution of the drug. If we doubled the blood volume, this too would double the time constant. Similarly, if the drug were not confined to blood, then its volume of distribution and hence its time constant would be increased. The volume of distribution may vary with time. Immediately following an intravenous injection, all of the drug is contained in blood and the time constant is short. But as the drug is distributed and redistributed, the volume in which it is contained increases and thereby increases the time constant. Thus, a plasma decay rate of 10 to 15 percent obtained several hours after injection does not indicate the percent metabolized on induction.

Another way of viewing this is to consider that the liver receives only a fraction of the total drug contained within the body. If it receives a large fraction then it may destroy a large fraction and thereby cause a rapid fall in the total body stores of drug. However, if most of the drug is sequestered in tissues such as muscle and fat, then the liver receives only a small fraction of the body stores and no matter how efficiently it attacks the drug, the fall in total body stores must be slow. Thiopental destruction fits both descriptions. Immediately following injection, the liver receives a large fraction of the total dose contained within the body. In the first circulation, the liver receives 25 percent of the drug since that is the liver's share of the cardiac output. If hepatic destruction of thiopental were complete, then 25 percent of the injected dose would be destroyed in less than 1 minute. After several hours, most of the thiopental body stores lie in fat and the fraction of drug delivered to the liver is far less than in the first minute.

Hepatic Extraction of Thiopental; Impact on Blood Levels

Let us return to the fraction of thiopental removed from hepatic blood flow. Studies in humans suggest that the extraction is variable. In a group of patients afflicted with liver disease the fraction removed ranged from zero up to 49 percent (17). One patient with no liver dysfunction removed 35 percent. These values were obtained minutes to hours following injection of thiopental. The reader may question the validity of applying such values to earlier times when higher concentrations may have produced enzyme saturation and hence a lower fraction of removal. However, rat liver slices metabolize a constant fraction of thiopental (first order kinetics) at concentrations in excess of those used clinically (18) suggesting that enzyme saturation probably does not occur.

If we assume various values for the fraction of hepatic blood flow which is cleared of thiopental, then we can estimate the effect of metabolism on the plasma decay rate and therefore on awakening time (fig. 17, 4) (8). As expected, increasing metabolism decreases the arterial (presumably tissue) thiopental concentration. For example, 20 minutes after injection, the blood concentration is 3.5 percent of the initial arterial concentration when the metabolic rate is 30 percent (i.e., when 30 percent of the hepatic blood flow is cleared of thiopental). Without metabolism, this level is not reached until 100 minutes. Since, in a given individual, there is probably some correlation between drug level and awakening, it follows that alterations in metabolism will alter the duration of narcosis. This model also may be used to show the large differences in the fraction of the total body stores which are metabolized at different times following injection. For example, with a metabolic rate of 30 percent, only 5.3 percent of the remaining drug is metabolized in the sixth hour after injection. In the first hour, 30.8 percent is metabolized.

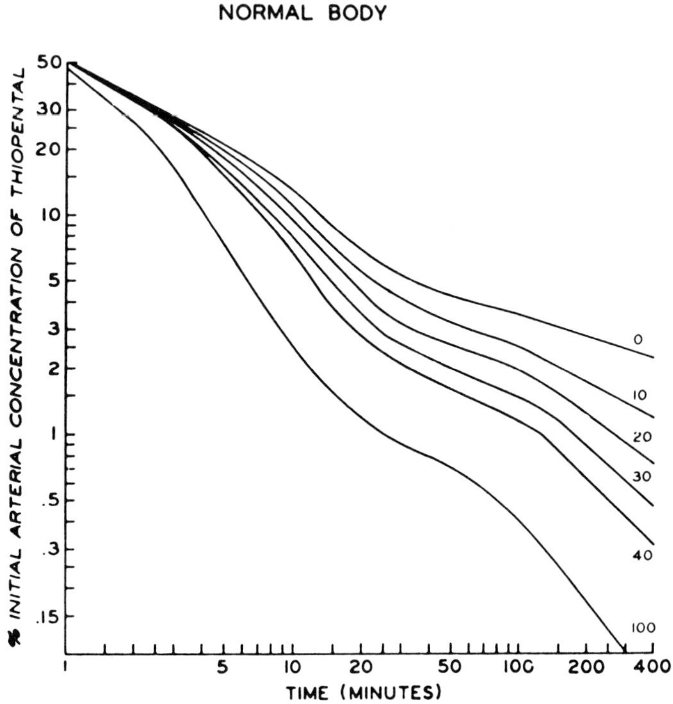

FIG. 17, 4. The numbers above each curve indicate the fraction of thiopental which is extracted from (and metabolised in) the liver blood flow. An increase in this fraction accelerates the rate of fall or arterial thiopental and thereby hastens recovery. (Reproduced with permission from Saidman, L. J., and Eger, E. I., II: The effect of thiopental metabolism on duration of anesthesia. Anesthesiology 27: 118–126, 1966.)

Factors Altering Hepatic Metabolism

Metabolism either may be increased or decreased in any one individual. Such changes should be anticipated since they can lead to unexpected responses. Prior exposure to barbiturates or other drugs can increase metabolism by induction of the enzymes responsible for metabolism. For example, pentobarbital hydroxylase activity in man and rats is increased by prior ethanol administration (19). Similarly, administration of one dose of alcohol to rats is followed within 17 hours by an increase in the *in vivo* and *in vitro* hepatic metabolism of hexabarbital (20). Perhaps this explains the apparent tolerance to barbiturates seen in chronic alcoholics. Chronic administration of phenobarbital, pentobarbital or hexabarbital increases their own metabolism—resulting in decreased blood levels and drug effect after a given dose (21). Finally, and perhaps most importantly, an increased requirement for thiopental has been found in those patients chronically exposed to urban atmosphere pollution (Montreal) as compared to patients from areas with little pollution (London, Ontario) (fig. 17, 5) (22).

Inhibition of microsomal enzyme activity should prolong the effect of metabolized barbiturates and indeed such is the case. Diphenyldipropylacetamide (SKF 525A) administration to rats more than doubles the duration of action and the half-life of hexabarbital (23). Other drugs also may inhibit metabolism and may thereby affect barbiturate narcosis. In contrast to chronic alcohol administration, acute intoxication inhibits barbiturate metabolism (19). Is the "drunk" patient more readily anesthetized and will his recovery be slower? The widely used stimulant methylphenidate retards metabolism of phenobarbital and other drugs in man (24). Will the patient treated with methylphenidate be anesthetized with an unexpectedly small dose of barbiturate?

The significance of altered metabolism (either increased or decreased) lies in the decreased predictability of response to a dose of drug. An individual may require far greater or lesser amounts of drug than "usual" to reach a given end-point. Obviously, prior and concomitant drug therapy and the effects of such therapy upon drug metabolism must be

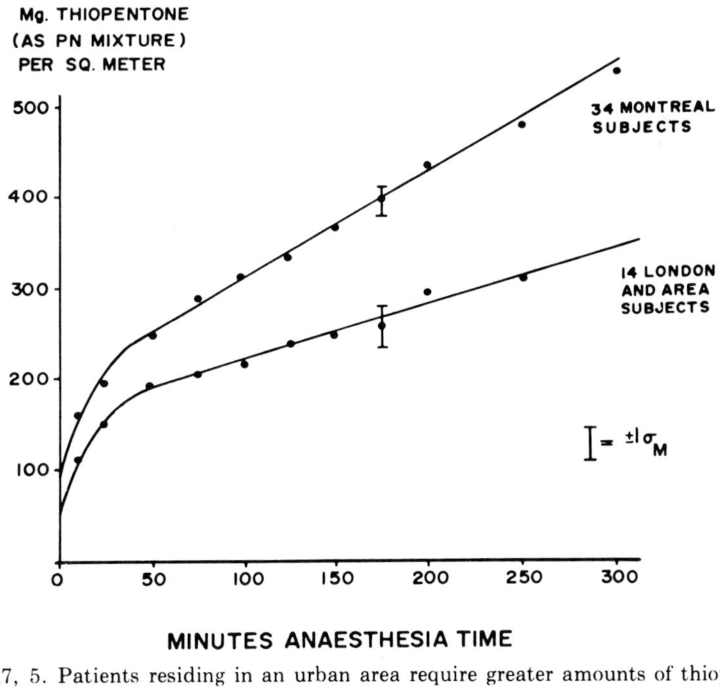

FIG. 17, 5. Patients residing in an urban area require greater amounts of thiopental-oxymorphone (PN) to induce and maintain anesthesia than patients residing in a rural area (London, Ontario). (From unpublished data kindly given the author by Dr. M. Kerri-Szanto.)

known if we are to properly gauge our administration of barbiturates.

Site of Administration and Metabolism

The position of the injection site relative to the liver will influence the effect of metabolism on blood and tissue levels of drug. Thiopental metabolism should be increased if blood leaving the injected area must pass through the liver before reaching the general circulation (25). For example, if 30 percent of thiopental is cleared from the blood passing through the liver and if all thiopental passes through the liver (oral administration) then 30 percent never reaches the general circulation. With intramuscular, intravenous or subcutaneous doses, all of the drug reaches the circulation before hepatic extraction can occur. When liver extraction equals 30 percent, the brain concentration after oral administration is only 50 percent of what it is after an identical intramuscular dose (figs. 17, 6 and 17, 7). These observations also suggest that altered hepatic function (increased or decreased) will alter the ultimate amount of thiopental available for pharmacological action more after oral or rectal administration than after intramuscular or intravenous administration.

Extravascular Administration of Barbiturates

Barbiturates are given by many routes. Sedation may be achieved with oral or intramuscular barbiturates. Anticonvulsive therapy similarly may require oral or intramuscular administration and rectal thiopental may be used for induction of basal narcosis in children. In addition to the factors thus far discussed (alteration in hydrogen ion concentration, protein binding and metabolism), special features of each injection site may affect blood and tissue barbiturate levels. These features include the injection site blood flow, the barbiturate solubility in the injected area and the presence of foreign diluting material (food or feces).

Intramuscular and Subcutaneous Injection

Absorption of barbiturates from subcutaneous or intramuscular sites depends on ease of penetration of the capillary wall and the injection site blood flow. With lipid soluble drugs such as barbiturates, the capillary wall presents a negligible barrier to diffusion. Thus, local blood flow relative to tissue capacity appears to be the major factor determining uptake. Uptake will be enhanced by increased blood flow (hyperthermia, excitement) and diminished by decreased blood flow (hypothermia, shock). Local hyperemia also may result from the trauma of injection. A more rapid uptake produces an earlier and high peak drug level (fig. 17, 8) (25). The effects of increased muscle blood flow and local uptake may be countered by a more rapid distribution to the hyperperfused muscle

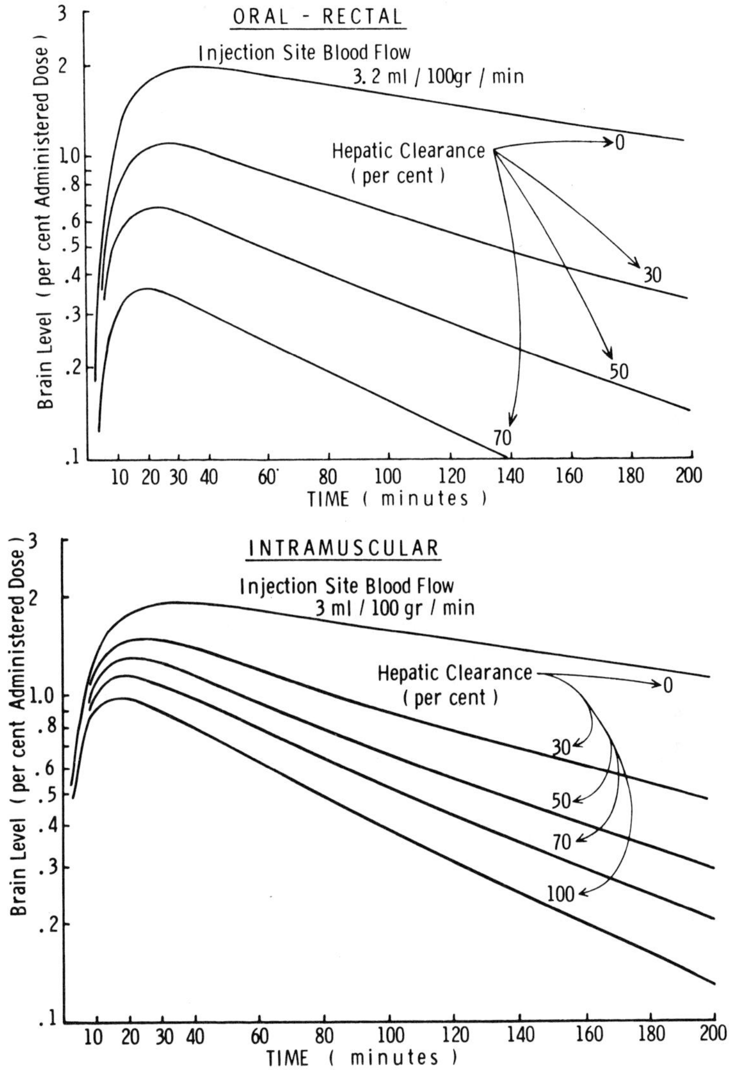

FIGS. 17, 6 and 17, 7. Oral administration of thiopental produces the same peak brain level of thiopental as an intramuscular injection of the same dose if no hepatic metabolism occurs. In the presence of metabolism the peak brain level is lower following oral administration. For both an oral and intramuscular administration, a higher rate of metabolism results in a lower peak level. (Reproduced with permission from Saidman, L. J., and Eger, E. I., II: Uptake and distribution of thiopental after oral, rectal or intramuscular administration. Clin. Pharmacol. Ther. 14: 12–20, 1973 (25).)

group (unless, of course, the only area with enhanced flow is the injected area itself). For a highly fat soluble barbiturate, injection into subcutaneous fat may produce a slower onset and lower peak effect than an

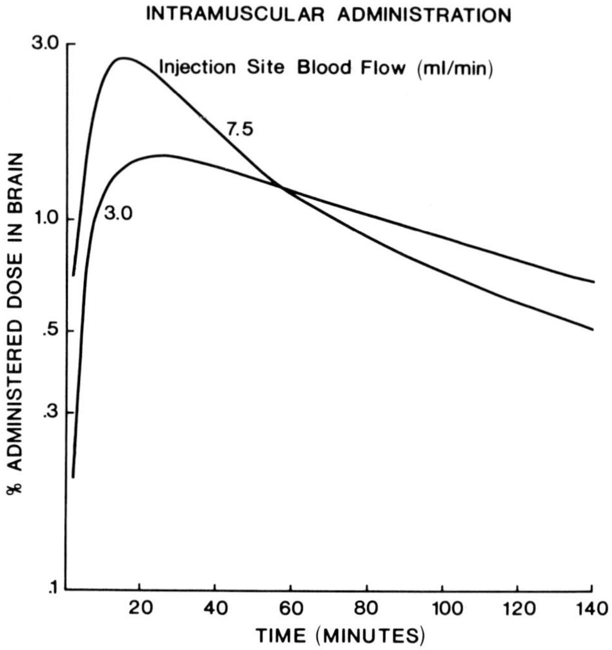

FIG. 17, 8. An increase in blood flow at the site of an intramuscular injection of thiopental produces an earlier and higher peak brain level of thiopental. (Reproduced with permission from Saidman, L. J., and Eger, E. I. II: Uptake and distribution of thiopental after oral, rectal or intramuscular administration. Clin. Pharmacol. Therap. 14: 12–20, 1973 (25).)

intramuscular injection. This results partly from a lower fat blood flow but more from the increased time constant for absorption imposed by the high fat capacity.

Oral Administration

Gastric pH, blood flow, drug solubility in gastric juice and the presence of food are important to the absorption of orally administered barbiturates. Since gastric epithelium is permeable to uncharged drug, barbiturates may be rapidly absorbed from the stomach (26). On the other hand, the decreased solubility of barbiturates in acid may cause precipitation which would diminish the rate of gastric absorption. The volume of gastric contents may reduce the absorption rate by diluting the administered dose. Since the rate of absorption is related to concentration, absorption will be inversely proportional to the volume of gastric contents (26). Blood flow for normal stomach has been estimated at 20 to 50 ml/100 ml/minute (27). If gastric absorption like muscle were flow rate limited, absorption would be much faster than actually observed. In fact, actual uptake of thiopental from human stomach corresponds to what uptake would be if flow rate were 3.2 ml/100 ml/minute (25). In other words, a number of factors (solubility, intragastric volume, hydrogen ion concentration and gastric blood flow) act simultaneously to produce an effective blood flow for drug uptake which is far less than actual blood flow.

Rectal Administration

Similarly, drug absorption after rectal administration is altered by several factors. Fecal material will dilute the drug and slow absorption, whereas the less acidic pH is less likely to precipitate drug and therefore may enhance absorption. Finally, the amount of drug which reaches the general circulation depends in part on how high into the rectum the drug is injected. Drug injected into the proximal rectum is absorbed into the superior hemorrhoidal veins and thence transported via the portal system to the liver where it is exposed to metabolism before entering the systemic circulation (28). On the other hand, drug absorbed from a low rectal injection reaches the general circulation without first passing the liver. These factors in a large part explain the unpredictable response which follows rectal (or oral) thiopental.

Summary

The factors which govern the uptake and distribution of inhaled agents apply with equal force to the barbiturates. These include solubility, tissue blood flow and the partial pressure (activity) difference between blood and tissues. The distribution of blood flow causes a rapid equilibration with the VRG, and a slower subsequent equilibration with muscle and fat. The barbiturates differ from the inhaled anesthetics in that they are normally given in an intravenous bolus and therefore the blood levels start at their highest and progressively fall. As the blood partial pressure falls below that in various tissues, the tissues cease taking up anesthetic and instead return agent to blood. Metabolism of barbiturate will accelerate the rate of fall and (unlike the inhaled anesthetics) will have its greatest influence immediately following the injection of agent. A decreased binding of barbiturate to blood proteins is analogous to a decrease in blood solubility. A reduction in solubility will accelerate the initial shift of barbiturate into tissues and hasten and augment the narcotic effect. It will also prolong that effect by hindering the delivery of barbiturate to the organ(s) of metabolism. The binding capacity of blood proteins may be reduced by hypoproteinemia or the administration of drugs which compete for protein binding sites.

Alterations in blood volume or the distribution of tissue blood flow will alter the distribution of thiopental. Hypovolemia concentrates the initial dose and its effect, and through a reduction in muscle and fat blood flow delays the redistribution of agent. Excitement may do the opposite.

Onset of barbiturate induced narcosis is slightly slowed by ionization. Penetrance of a barbiturate into the brain is most affected by its lipid solubility: increased solubility accelerates entrance into the brain. Through its effect on ionization, pH may significantly alter the distribution of barbiturate. If the intracellular pH is constant, the extracellular barbiturate concentration is increased by an increase in extracellular pH.

The site of barbiturate administration influences the onset, peak effect and duration of narcosis by influencing the rate of absorption. A low blood flow relative to the capacity of the injection site will slow absorption. In addition, injection into a site (stomach or rectum) whose blood flow must pass through the liver prior to entering the general circulation will produce a lesser effect because of a greater initial metabolism.

Both the prevention of excessive cardiorespiratory depression as well as the achievement of anesthesia are the major goals of barbiturate administration. In the past, untoward reactions or failure to induce anesthesia with "normal" doses of agent has been ascribed to "idiosyncracy"'(cardiovascular depression) or to "high tolerance" (inadequate anesthesia). Many of the factors presented in this chapter would explain these "mysterious" reactions and therefore would allow their prediction and prevention.

QUESTIONS

1. How may a fever influence the effect of a "standard" dose of thiopental?
2. Why may administration of a given dose of thiopental have a more profound effect in someone moderately anesthetized with halothane than in the unanesthetized patient?
3. At one time, thiopental was used as the sole anesthetic to induce and maintain anesthesia. Why might a patient anesthetized by this technique awaken quickly after a short procedure, but sleep for a long time after a long procedure?
4. What factors may influence the binding of thiopental to blood proteins? How does an increased binding to blood proteins influence the onset, duration and intensity of narcosis produced by a given dose of barbiturate?
5. How may a change in extracellular pH influence the distribution of thiopental if the intracellular pH remains constant?
6. Why might a plasma barbiturate decay of only 10 to 15 percent between the fifth and sixth hour of anesthesia not indicate that metabolism has little influence on the plasma decay rate during the first hour of anesthesia?
7. Laboratory animals often are anesthetized with intraperitoneal doses of barbiturate. Why is this route of administration likely to produce a lower peak brain concentration than the same dose given intravenously? Why is an

intragastric injection of the same dose likely to produce a lower brain peak than the intraperitoneal dose?

8. Assume a subcutaneous blood flow of 2 ml/100 ml of tissue/minute. If a barbiturate with a subcutaneous/blood partition coefficient of 5 were injected into this tissue, how long would it be until 95 percent of the drug was taken up? How long would it be if the injection were into muscle with a flow of 3 ml/100 ml/minute and a partition coefficient of 1? Why is the absorption of pentobarbitol not affected by subcutaneous versus intramuscular injection as much as thiopental?
9. How might acute alcohol intoxication alter the response to thiopental? Chronic alcoholism?
10. How might hypoproteinemia, hypovolemia, metabolic acidosis and liver dysfunction interact to alter the response to thiopental?

REFERENCES

1. Price, H. L., Kornat, P. J., Safar, J. N., Connor, E. H., and Price, M. L.: The uptake of thiopental by body tissues and its relation to the duration of narcosis. Clin. Pharmacol. Ther. 1: 16–22, 1960.
2. Goldbaum, L. R., and Smith, P. K.: The interaction of barbiturates with serum albumin and its possible relation to their disposition and pharmacological actions. J. Pharmacol. Exp. Ther. 111: 197–209, 1954.
3. Mark, L. C., Burns, J. J., Brand, L., Campomanes, C. I., Trousof, N., Papper, E. M., and Brodie, B. B.: The passage of thiobarbiturates and their oxygen analogs into brain. J. Pharmacol. Exp. Ther. 123: 70–73, 1958.
4. Goldstein, A., Aronaow, L., and Kalman, S. M.: *Principles of Drug Action*, p. 172. Harper and Row, New York, 1969.
5. Waddell, W. J., and Butler, T. C.: The distribution and excretion of phenobarbital. J. Clin. Invest. 36: 1217–1226, 1957.
6. Lasser, E. C., Elizondo-Martel, G., and Granke, R. C.: Potentiation of pentobarbital anesthesia by competitive protein binding. Anesthesiology 24: 665–671, 1963.
7. Dundee, J. W., Price, H. L., and Dripps, R. D.: Acute tolerance to thiopental in man. Brit. J. Anaesth. 28: 344–352, 1956.
8. Saidman, L. J., and Eger, E. I., II: The effect of thiopental metabolism on duration of anesthesia. Anesthesiology 27: 118–126, 1966.
9. Delmonico, E. J.: Tests for derivatives of barbituric acid. Proc. Mayo Clin. 14: 109–112, 1939.
10. Goodman, L. S., and Gilman, A.: *The Pharmacological Basis of Therapeutics*. MacMillan, New York, 1941.
11. Jarler, J. W., and Goldbaum, L. R.: Studies on the plasma concentration and tissue distribution of sodium pentothal (sodium ethyl (1-methylbutyl) thiobarbiturate). J. Lab. Clin. Med. 31: 1344–1349, 1946.
12. Brodie, B. B., Mark, L. C., Papper, E. M., Lief, P. A., Bernstein, E., and Rovenstein, E. A.: The fate of thiopental in man and a method for its estimation in biological material. J. Pharmacol. Exp. Ther. 98: 85–96, 1950.
13. Shideman, F. E., Kelly, A. R., and Adams, B. J.: The role of the liver in the detoxification of thiopental (pentothal) and two other barbiturates. J. Pharmacol. Exp. Ther. 91: 331–339, 1947.
14. Kelly, A. R., and Shideman, F. E.: Liver as major organ involved in detoxification of thiopental by dog. Fed. Proc. 8: 306, 1949.

15. Meyers, F. H., and Peoples, D.: The positive role of the liver in the rapid metabolism of thiopental. Anesthesiology 15: 146–149, 1954.
16. Shideman, F. E., Kelly, A. R., Lee, L. E., Lowell, V. F., and Adams, B. J.: The role of the liver in the detoxification of thiopental (pentothal) by man. Anesthesiology 10: 421–428, 1949.
17. Mark, L. C., Brand, L., Kamvyssi, S., Britton, R. C., Perel, J. M., Landran, M. A., and Dayton, P. G.: Thiopental metabolism by human liver *in vivo* and *in vitro*. Nature 206: 1117–1119, 1965.
18. Gould, T. C., and Shideman, F. E.: The *in vitro* metabolism of thiopental by a fortified cell-free preparation of the rat. J. Pharmacol. Exp. Ther. 104: 427, 1952.
19. Rubin, E., and Lieber, C. L.: Hepatic microsomal enzymes in man and rats: induction and inhibition by ethanol. Science 162: 690–691, 1968.
20. Mallov, S., and Baesl, T. J.: Effect of ethanol on rates of elimination and metabolism of zoxazolamine, hexabarbitol, and warfarin sodium in the rat. Biochem. Pharmacol. 21: 1667–1678, 1972.
21. Conney, A. H.: Pharmacological implications of microsomal enzyme induction. Pharmacol. Rev. 19: 317–366, 1967.
22. Keeri-Szanto, M., and Pomeroy, J. A.: Atmospheric pollution, enzyme induction and intravenous anesthetic requirements: a causal correlation? Abstracts of Scientific Papers, Annual Meeting of American Society of Anesthesiologists, pp. 139–140, 1970.
23. Axelrod, J., Reichenthal, J., and Brodie, B. B.: Mechanisms of the potentiating action of B-diethylaminoethyl diphenylpropylacetate. J. Pharmacol. Exp. Ther. 112: 49–54, 1954.
24. Garrettson, L. K., Perel, J. M., and Dayton, P. G.: Methylphenidate interaction with both anticonvulsants and ethyl biscournacetate. J. A. M. A. 207: 2053–2056, 1969.
25. Saidman, L. J., and Eger, E. I., II: Uptake and distribution of thiopental after oral, rectal, or intramuscular administration. Clin. Pharmacol. Ther. 14: 12–20, 1973.
26. Hogben, C. A. M., Schanker, L. S., Tocco, D. J., and Brodie, B. B.: Absorption of drugs from the stomach. II: The human. J. Pharmacol. Exp. Ther. 120: 540–545, 1957.
27. Wade, O. L., and Bishop, J. M.: *Cardiac Output and Regional Blood Flow*. Blackwell Scientific Publications, Oxford, 1962.
28. Woodburne, R. T.: *Essentials of Human Anatomy*, p. 149. Oxford University Press, New York, 1957.

Chapter 18

Mode of Action of Muscle Relaxants

R. A. EPSTEIN

An understanding of the action of muscle relaxants presupposes an understanding of the physiology of excitable membranes in general and of neuromuscular junction in particular. The physiology of excitable membranes was discussed in Chapter 2 and will be briefly reviewed here.

Physiology of the Myoneural Junction

The nerve action potential (NAP) passes from the motor neuron located in the spinal cord to the nerve terminal at the myoneural junction. The NAP causes the release of quanta of acetylcholine from the synaptic vesicles in the nerve terminal adjacent to the synaptic cleft. The number of quanta (the quantal content) is only a small fraction ("readily releaseable fraction") of the total quanta present. The quantal content is increased by an increase in calcium or a decrease in magnesium. It also is augmented by an increase in the amplitude of the NAP at the nerve terminal. Thus, the hyperpolarization that follows an impulse may predispose to a greater release of acetylcholine during the subsequent impulse. However, frequently repeated impulses also have another effect: they partially exhaust the acetylcholine available in the readily releaseable fraction. This exhaustion is primarily responsible for the "fade" seen with tetanic stimulation during curarization. The major portion of quanta exists in a form which is unavailable for immediate release (the "depot" stores). The depot stores replace the quanta in the readily releaseable stores which have been lost by release. The transfer rate to the readily releaseable fraction is increased (after a time lag) by increased demands as, for example, during and immediately following tetanic stimulation. The facilitation of neuromuscular transmission occurring after tetanic stimulation (post-tetanic potentiation) is caused by such increased mobilization.

In less than a millisecond the released acetylcholine crosses the synaptic cleft and acts on the closely opposed subsynaptic membrane (muscle end-plate). Acetylcholine interacts with the end-plate receptors to increase permeability to *both* sodium and potassium. As a result, the end-plate potential rises towards −15 mV, a point midway between the potential due to permeability to potassium alone (−90 mV) and to sodium alone (+60 mV). The magnitude of the potential change produced by acetylcholine is a function of the amount of acetylcholine released. Single quanta of spontaneously released acetylcholine cause brief increases of less than 1 mV. These potentials aptly are called miniature end-plate potentials (mepp). In contrast to the single quanta released spontaneously, the NAP releases a large number of quanta with a correspondingly larger increase in end-plate potential (epp). The epp is short-lived because acetylcholine rapidly diffuses away from the end-plate receptors or is quickly hydrolyzed by cholinesterase.

Acetylcholine affects only the end-plate permeability; the rest of the muscle membrane responds to changes in potential but not to acetylcholine. The epp changes the potential of (i.e., depolarizes) the muscle membrane adjacent to the end-plate. This depolarization produces a regenerative impulse based on the same factors which govern the propagation of the NAP. The regenerative impulse in turn results in muscle contraction.

Some Limitations to Studies of Neuromuscular Impulse Transmission

The act of contraction makes studies of neuromuscular transmission more difficult than studies of conduction at other synapses. Only the initial portion of the epp can be recorded during a normal muscle contraction; the larger muscle action potential masks the remainder of the epp. In addition the resulting muscle contraction usually dislodges the fragile glass pipette electrode used for recording. For these reasons most work comes from preparations which diminish the epp or in some way prevent the generation of the action potential normally caused by the epp. Such preparations may be abnormal ionic environments which lower quantal output, partial curarization which competes with released acetylcholine or the cutting of the muscle fibers which partially "short circuits" the membrane. Another preparation uses a hypertonic sucrose environment which prevents contraction without abolishing the action potential. Observations of epps during contraction have been made by prestretching the muscle which tends to hold the electrode in place. The most elegant, recent work involves "voltage clamping." In voltage clamping the membrane potential is artificially maintained constant preventing a propagated action potential. Changes in permeability may be measured as changes in current required to keep the membrane potential constant. The amount of end-plate current required to maintain the potential constant is analagous to the epp. All of these techniques except perhaps voltage clamping may themselves cause abnormal physiological changes. Extrapolation of results from these studies to *in vivo* effects must be done with restraint.

Margin of Safety of Neuromuscular Transmission

The normal myoneural junction differs from other synapses in that the arrival of a NAP at the junction almost invariably causes a regenerative impulse in the muscle membrane. A considerable reserve protects this system against failure. Each nerve impulse releases at least 5 times the acetylcholine required to produce an epp which can reach threshold levels. This "margin of safety" (1) of neuromuscular transmission has manifold pharmacological and clinical implications. Normal muscle contraction may persist despite a decrease in the release of acetylcholine, the occupancy of receptor sites by a competing drug or a decreased sensitivity of the receptors. Further addition of a subparalytic dose of another drug or any other factor which impairs transmission might then produce paresis even if the factor had a different site of action. Thus, a normally subparalytic dose of curare may cause paralysis in the presence of halothane (2) which decreases the sensitivity of the postjunctional membrane to acetylcholine (3). A subparalytic dose of curare may cause paralysis in the presence of large doses of local anesthetics or quinidine, either of which depress sodium conductance, reduce the NAP and thereby decrease quantal release. Tetanic stimulation which depletes stored acetylcholine or administration of hemicholinium which inhibits acetylcholine synthesis and decreases quantal size (4) would predispose to paralysis. Similarly, halothane fails to cause paresis in normal man, but may block neuromuscular transmission in a myasthenic individual (5). Tetanic stimulation also causes fade in the unanesthetized myasthenic. This fade differs from fade during tetanus in a normal curarized individual in that it is prolonged and far outlasts the period of tetanic stimulation (6). The fatigue which accompanies a continuous effort in an awake partially curarized or myasthenic patient is analogous to tetanic fade.

In clinical practice it is important to understand that normal contractile strength (twitch) in response to nerve stimulation does not require a normal neuromuscular junction. For example, subsequent doses of nondepolarizing muscle relaxants have a greater blocking effect per milligram than the original dose, despite a return of the evoked twitch tension to normal between doses (7). This presumably results from residual receptor occupancy which is not sufficient to impair transmission of a single impulse. A patient with a normal evoked twitch or even tetanic response still may be unequal to the stress of a required sustained muscular effort.

Pharmacology of Neuromuscular Transmission

Muscle activity depends upon a sequence of events starting at the central nervous system and ending with muscle contraction. Drugs acting anywhere along this chain can modify muscle activity. Inhibition may result from an action on the central or peripheral nervous system, the neuromuscular junction or the muscle.

Central Nervous System Effects

Although muscle relaxant drugs depress cortical activity when directly applied to the exposed brain, the blood-brain barrier normally blocks their passage into brain tissue (and probably into peripheral nerves as well). Thus, systematic administration of relaxants is unlikely to produce central effects. However, the central effects of other more penetrant drugs may contribute to the paralytic effect of muscle relaxants. Certain drugs used to release spastic states, such as diazepam (Valium) act on the brain stem reticular system to inhibit spinal reflexes and thereby produce muscle relaxation. The relaxation produced by general anesthetics when used in the absence of muscle relaxants likewise appears to be due to central effects. Several experimental methods may be used to distinguish between central and peripheral effects. Peripheral effects may be quantified as the muscle tension or electromyogram which results from electrically stimulating a motor nerve. Similarly, the central effect may be judged by the reflex muscle contraction which results from stimulating the cut central end of a sensory nerve. In the decerebrate cat inhaled anesthetics depress such reflex muscle contractions at concentrations which do not affect the contraction evoked by motor nerve stimulation (8). An elegant application of an analogous method in man has been the study of the "H"-reflex (9). Electrical stimulation of a mixed peripheral nerve produces central and peripheral impulses in *both* motor and sensory fibers. Two compound action potentials may be seen on the electromyogram:* an initial "M" wave which results from motor nerve stimulation followed by a reflex "H" wave. The "H" wave results from the monosynaptic depolarization of spinal motor neurons by the centrally directed sensory impulse. These sensory fibers come from stretch receptors. Clinical concentrations of halothane depress the (reflex) "H" wave but not the "M" wave.

Central and peripheral effects of inhaled anesthetics also may be distinguished in man by comparing the effects of anesthesia on spontaneous muscle activity (using electromyography) and on the muscle

* The electromyogram measures the change in potential of a large number of muscle fibers. An extracellular electrode is used which may be placed intramuscularly or simply on the surface of the skin.

contraction produced by motor nerve stimulation. In one such study ether and halothane depressed only spontaneous activity thereby implying a central action (10, 11). These results must be interpreted with caution since an accessory respiratory muscle (abdominal) was used to measure spontaneous activity and the depression observed may have represented a depression of central respiratory drive rather than a generalized central relaxant action. However, taken together these studies provide strong evidence for a central "relaxant" action of anesthetics. However, they do not exclude a significant peripheral effect appearing only as a decreased margin of safety of neuromuscular transmission. In addition, the reflexes studied are not necessarily typical of the reflexes that produce the muscle tension which interferes with surgery.

Peripheral Effects

Despite the general agreement on much of the basic physiology of neuromuscular transmission, the site and mode of drug action at the neuromuscular junction is subject to much controversy. The reasons for controversy are due in part to the diverse methods used to investigate neuromuscular activity. Most investigators believe that anesthetics and relaxants act mainly at the postjunctional (muscle end-plate) membrane. However, a sizeable minority hold that the presynaptic (nerve terminal) membrane is the most important site of action. The former suggest that acetylcholine and curare compete for postjunctional receptor sites which control permeability to sodium and potassium ions, and believe that other drugs change the "sensitivity" of such receptors to acetylcholine. The latter suggest that curare, succinylcholine and anesthetics depress the release of acetylcholine from nerve terminals. These two groups do not confront each other with conflicting data generated by similar methods. Rather, their methods vary widely and do not always permit us to discriminate between the relative importance of each site of relaxant action. The excessive release of acetylcholine (margin of safety) during normal transmission compounds the methodological problems. Thus, the demonstration of a pre- or postsynaptic action during paresis may not exclude a more subtle effect at a different site from lower nonparalytic concentrations of drug.

Postjunctional Effects

The classic studies of Dale (12) support a postjunctional site of relaxant drug action. Using perfused eserinized muscle Dale demonstrated that: 1) muscle contraction induced by motor nerve stimulation was accompanied by the release of acetylcholine; but 2) contraction of chronically denervated muscle induced by direct electrical stimulation of the muscle did not release acetylcholine; and 3) muscle paralyzed with curare released the usual amount of acetylcholine when the motor nerve was stimulated despite lack of muscle contraction. This work established acetylcholine as the chemical transmitter at the neuromuscular junction and also indicated that curare blocked the action of acetylcholine rather than its release. Numerous subsequent studies have confirmed that curare blocks the action of acetylcholine (13). Curare blocks the muscle contraction produced by acetylcholine applied exogenously in a muscle bath, administered by intra-arterial injection or applied directly to the end-plate through a micropipette. Curare decreases the magnitude and duration of the epp resulting from nerve stimulation or from direct iontophoretic application of acetylcholine to the end-plate. A sufficient concentration of curare reduces the epp below the threshold required to produce an action potential. Curare does not change the threshold that must be attained to depolarize the end-plate nor does it alter the electrical excitability of the muscle membrane. Contraction of the curarized muscle can be restored by the administration of sufficient acetylcholine or by administration of a cholinesterase inhibitor such as neostigmine which prevents the hydrolysis of endogenous acetylcholine. Carbachol, a drug which acts like acetylcholine but is not hydrolized by cholinesterase, also completely restores the contractile response.

Relaxant drugs can be divided into two classes based on whether they compete or do not compete with acetylcholine. A determination of the presence or absence of competition first requires measurement of the relationship between the dose of acetylcholine and the degree of muscle activation. The acetylcholine may be applied to the medium of a muscle bath, by intra-arterial injection, or by iontophoretic application via pipettes to the end-plate region. The degree of muscle activation may be judged by tension output, electromyography, or the size of the epp. Although administration of curare increases the amount of acetylcholine required to achieve a given degree of muscle activation, full activation can be achieved with a sufficiently high dose of acetylcholine. That is, curare acts as though it were competing with acetylcholine for end-plate receptors. In general, all nondepolarizing relaxants (e.g., gallamine, pancuronium) act competively. In contrast, addition of acetylcholine will not completely reverse the action of succinylcholine and decamethonium. At best, blockade may be partially reversed, but it actually may be increased. These drugs produce a noncompetitive block. Depolarizing relaxant drugs generally fall into this category.

The competitive and noncompetitive nature of relaxant drugs suggests at least two different sites of action. Waser's (14, 15) studies of binding sites for acetylcholine and for blocking drugs by autoradiographic techniques also suggest such a difference. Radioactive drugs are injected intravenously, the animal sacrificed and a muscle specimen (diaphragm) apposed to x-ray film. Alternately, an isolated muscle is bathed with labelled drug and then apposed to x-ray film after the degree of neuromuscular block is determined. The locus of the radioactive drug drug-receptor complex as well as the number of drug molecules in any end-plate region is determined from the location and intensity of the image formed on the film. Unfortunately acetylcholine is destroyed too rapidly by cholinesterase to be studied directly. The location and binding properties of the (cholinergic) receptors concerned with depolarization are determined with more stable depolarizing drugs such as decamethonium or carbachol. These radioautographic studies demonstrate a considerable difference between decamethonium and curare. Curare is clearly localized to the end-plate. As expected from the margin of safety of neuromuscular transmission, curare can occupy a considerable portion of the receptors without producing blockade. Unlike curare, depolarizing drugs such as decamethonium bind to a broad diffuse area around the end-plate. This area, but not the remaining muscle surface, is sensitive to directly applied acetylcholine. Muscle denervation increases both the area of decamethonium binding and the area sensitive to direct stimulation with acetylcholine. However, no curare binds to these "new" cholinergic receptors. Another difference exists between curare and depolarizing drugs in their interaction with receptors. Disregarding cholinergic receptors located outside the end-plate area, decamethonium must occupy many more binding sites than must curare to produce the same degree of paresis. Because of the many differences in the way curare and cholinergic drugs bind to muscle, Waser (14, 15) postulated that the curare receptors and cholinergic receptors were distinct. A third receptor, cholinesterase, was also postulated.

Thus, although curare and acetylcholine act competitively they probably do not compete for the same receptor site. From these data, Waser hypothesized that the large curare molecules occupy and thereby obstruct the pores in the membrane which allow flux of potassium and sodium ions during depolarization. The more numerous molecules of acetylcholine act on nearby sites to open the pores and thereby permit the ionic flux required for depolarization (fig. 18, 1).

The nature of the block produced by noncompetitive agents is more complicated (16). While curare opposes the action of acetylcholine and thereby decreases the epp, cholinergic agents initially mimic acetylcholine. Succinylcholine may cause depolarization sufficient to produce a muscle contraction (fasciculation). Blockade with decamethonium does not require depolarization to threshold and clinically used doses of decamethonium produce only a small depolarization generally without consequent contraction. If the membrane potential is held at approxi-

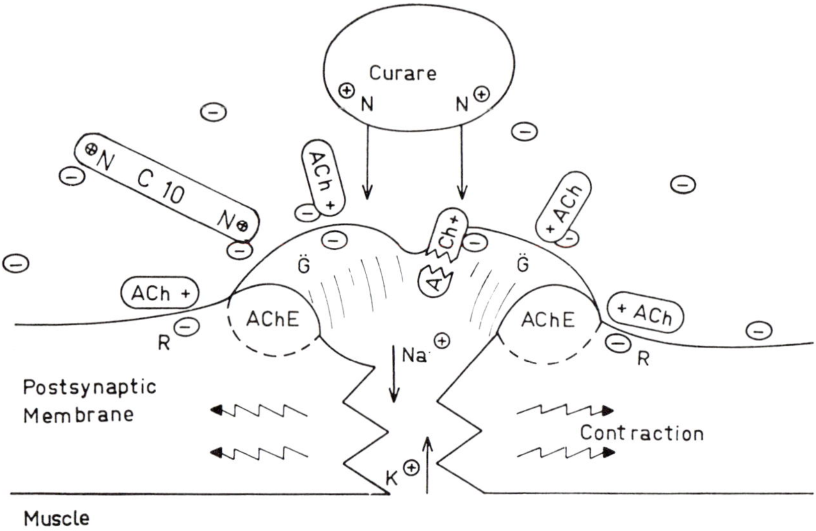

FIG. 18, 1. This schematic cross-section of the receptor area of the end-plate illustrates the sodium-potassium pore and the surrounding receptor area. Acetylcholine (ACh) interacts with cholinergic receptors (minus sign points) to open the pore to sodium and potassium ions. Many molecules of acetylcholine are required to open one pore. Decamethonium (C 10) molecules also attach to the cholinergic receptors. One molecule of curare is sufficient to block the pore. The opening to the pore is enclosed by two molecules of acetylcholinesterase (AChE). (Reproduced with permission from Waser, P. G.: On receptors in the postsynaptic membrane of the motor end plate. In *Ciba Foundation Symposium on Molecular Properties of Drug Receptors*, edited by R. Porter, and M. O'Connor, pp. 59–70. J. & A. Churchill, London, 1970.)

mately −55 mV by application of currents through intracellular electrodes or by the use of depolarizing drugs such as succinylcholine or decamethonium, the muscle fiber becomes inexcitable (17). Partial depolarization thus renders the end-plate insensitive to an increase in acetylcholine applied either by electrophoretic injection or by nerve stimulation. In addition, despite continued cholinergic stimulation the membrane potential returns toward normal. The muscle remains paralyzed and is then said to be desensitized to acetylcholine. Thus, with cholinergic drugs neuromuscular blockade is first accompanied by depolarization but later by a normal or near normal membrane potential. The depolarization block also is termed a phase I block, while the desensitization block is termed a phase II block. The end-plate potential is normal or near normal in both the curarized and desensitized block. But acetylcholine administration competitively antagonizes the first and causes the second. Likewise, cholinergic stimulation from succinylcholine, decamethonium, carbachol or the anticholinesterases neostigmine and edrophonium can partially antagonize a curare block. During a desensitization block the end-plate may still respond *briefly* to application of high acetylcholine concentrations. Thus, neostigmine first may antagonize a desensitization block after which it prolongs the block. Since both the antagonistic and synergistic effects are unpredictable the use of neostigmine to reverse a desensitization block clinically is discouraged.

There has been relatively little success in explaining the phenomenon of desensitization. Prolonged exposure to a depolarizing drug may change the conformation of the receptor to a form insensitive to acetylcholine (18) or depolarizing drugs. Alternatively, the open pore configuration may be unstable and may revert to the closed position despite the continued occupancy and action of cholinergic drugs at the acetylcholine receptor site. Supporting this notion is the persistant presence of decamethonium at the acetylcholine receptor sites during the desensitization period (14). Recent work demonstrates that calcium ions are required for the receptor inactivation. This work suggests that a prolonged cholinergic block allows intracellular Ca^{++} to combine with anionic membrane sites which normally act as carrier molecules for Na^{+} and K^{+} (19). This implies that carrier molecules are essential to the Na^{+} and K^{+} transfer occurring during depolarization. Such a concept is in conflict with the pore theory.

The epp decreases during repetitive stimulation. The decrease is greater with higher rates of stimulation, but may be demonstrated at stimulus rates as low as 1/second. The rate of decrease also is greater with higher rates of stimulation. This depression is due to decreased quantal output of acetylcholine per nerve stimulus. In uncurarized muscle there is a sufficient margin of safety of neuromuscular transmission so that despite this depression during tetanus the epp reaches threshold and depolarization occurs. Thus, tetanus normally is well maintained; that is, depolarization and sustained contraction occur thoughout tetanus despite the decrease in quantal output of acetylcholine. However, in the presence of a drug such as curare which competes with acetylcholine or in the presence of a drug such as decamethonium which decreases receptor sensitivity, the progressive depression of epp amplitude during tetanus may be sufficient to prevent some or all muscle fibers from reaching threshold and depolarizing. The decreased number of fibers responding to a stimulus during the latter part of tetanus (fade) can be measured clinically as a decreasing electromyographic compound action potential or as a decreasing muscle contraction (fig. 18, 2). Such studies also suggest that despite a continuing tetanic stimulation, the fade does not always persist at the level attained initially. In some cases both the electromyogram and contractile strength recover considerably—sometimes even to above control levels. Such recovery may be

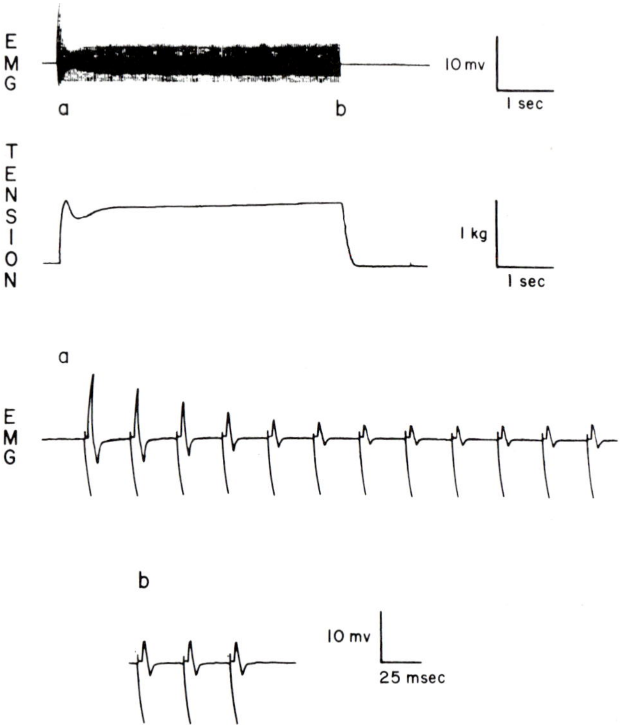

FIG. 18, 2. Tetanic fade can be demonstrated in a patient anesthetized with halothane in nitrous oxide 15 minutes after the intravenous administration of 0.1 mg/kg curare. The upper traces show the electromyogram (EMG) and tension of the adductor pollicis during tetanic stimulation (30 Hz). There is an initial fade of both EMG and tension followed by recovery. This recovery during tetanus seen in some subjects masks the fade on tension records. Recovery may be due to an increase in readily releaseable fraction or to a displacement of the curare by the released acetylcholine (20). The lower traces show the individual compound action potentials of the EMG at the start (*a*) and end (*b*) of tetanus. (Reproduced with permission from Epstein, R. A., and Epstein, R. M.: The electromyogram and mechanical response of indirectly stimulated muscle in anesthetized man following curarization. Anesthesiology 38: 212–223, 1973. The figure has been retouched to improve clarity.)

explained either by an increase in the readily releaseable fraction of acetylcholine at the nerve terminal, or by a displacement of curare from the postjunctional receptors (20).

A depolarizing block may be distinguished from either a desensitizing or competitive block by the absence of fade. If a partially paralytic dose of succinylcholine or decamethonium is administered, initially some fibers are depolarized (and completely inexcitable) while others are normal. Although the reduction in the number of normal fibers must decrease the electromyographic or contractile response to nerve stimulation, those fibers which do respond are normal and therefore do not fade during tetanus.

Depletion of transmitter during tetanus increases its synthesis and mobilization. This process continues for a period after tetanus and leads to an increased availability of transmitter in the post-tetanic period. The post-tetanic quantal content therefore is increased and the post-tetanic epp is greater than the pretetanic epp. If the pretetanic epps already caused depolarization of all muscle fibers, an increase in the epp could not cause any further increase in depolarization. On the other hand, in the curarized muscle, the additional acetylcholine released may partially or completely overcome the competitive block and thereby depolarize more muscle fibers. This post-tetanic potentiation (PTP) is a useful sign of curarization (fig. 18, 3). As noted above, the additional acetylcholine released by tetanic stimulation may displace curare from the receptor site (20). The reduced occupancy of these sites may contribute to PTP. PTP also may be seen with a desensitization block but is absent with a depolarization block. Clinical use of motor nerve stimulation to distinguish between a desensitization and depolarization block is at best difficult since desensitization is a gradually developing process which begins as soon as depolarization occurs (23).

Tetanic fade is a more reliable indicator of residual curare block than twitch depression or PTP. Even with a partial receptor block the epp may be large enough to cause depolarization because of the margin of safety of neuromuscular transmission. Twitch or PTP both would be normal. However, reduction of the epp by tetanus still might cause fade. An increase in the tetanic frequency increases transmitter depletion and further augments the fade (fig. 18, 4) (22).

Administration of a competitive blocker also may differentiate a depolarization block. Curare antagonizes a depolarizing block (although the dose is too critical to be of practical use) while it augments the effect of a desensitization block. Relaxant interactions may be too complex to predict in practice. First, the same muscle may contain fibers with different types of block. Second, a drug may possess mixed blocking characteristics. For example, gallamine, a competitive blocker, has limited depolarizing properties and neostigmine, a cholinesterase inhibitor, has some blocking properties. Third, changes in the margin of safety (as may occur with inhaled anesthetics) modify the effects of blocking drugs and of tetanic stimulation. Finally, effects at sites other than the postsynaptic junction (for example the nerve terminal or the muscle membrane) may alter drug interactions.

Postjunctional Effects of Anesthetics

Inhalational anesthetics long have been known to intensify the blocking action of curare. Early investigators believed that ether pos-

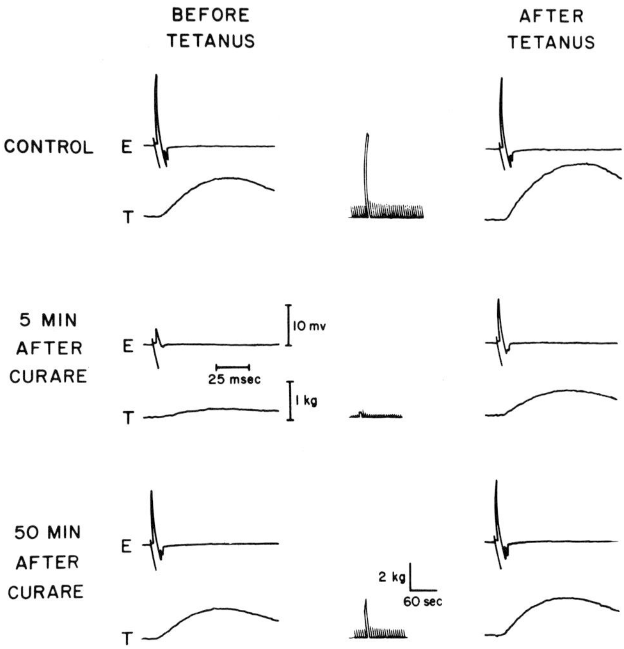

FIG. 18, 3. Post-tetanic potentiation (PTP) in the electromyogram (E) and evoked tension (T) are demonstrated in a patient anesthetized with halothane in nitrous oxide before (control) and after the intravenous administration of 0.1 mg/kg curare. Before curare *all* the muscle fibers were depolarized and therefore the increased epp after tetanus could cause no increase in the electromyogram. Five and 50 minutes after curare there was blockade and the increase in acetylcholine release after tetanus did cause PTP increase in the electromyogram (PTP). The same general result is seen on tension recordings. The situation is, however, less clear because there is also "PTP" in the control state caused by a phenomenon involving muscle contractility but not neuromuscular transmission. Tension recordings are therefore of less use in detecting curarization. (Reproduced with permission from Epstein, R. A., and Epstein, R. M.: The electromyogram and mechanical response of indirectly stimulated muscle in anesthetized man following curarization. Anesthesiology 38: 212–223, 1973. The figure has been retouched for clarity.)

sessed a "curare-like" action. Like curare, anesthetics decrease the ability of carbachol and acetylcholine to depolarize the postjunctional membrane. However, moderate ether or halothane concentrations prolong the time course of the mepps and epps *in vitro*, while curare decreases the size of the epp without altering the time course. Unlike curare, edrophonium or succinylcholine does not antagonize the neuromuscular block produced *in vitro* by anesthetics. Simultaneous recordings of electrical activity from the nerve terminal and the postjunctional membrane suggest that there is normal presynaptic depolarization in the presence of a depressed epp. The anesthetics thus desensitize the postjunctional membrane. This "desensitization", however, may be unrelated to the "desensitization" produced by depolarizing blockers. In any case, anesthetics decrease the margin of safety of neuromuscular transmission and thereby potentiate the blocking effect of curare and enhance tetanic fade (10, 11, 24, 25).

Prejunctional Effects of Relaxants and Other Drugs

The methodology of those advocating postjunctional mechanisms is not impervious to criticism. The application of depolarizing agents such as acetylcholine or carbachol to test for the presence of a postsynaptic block cannot be limited to a postjunctional site. The demonstration of presynaptic cholinergic receptors raises the possibility that the exogenously applied acetylcholine also acts at this locus (26, 27). However, this

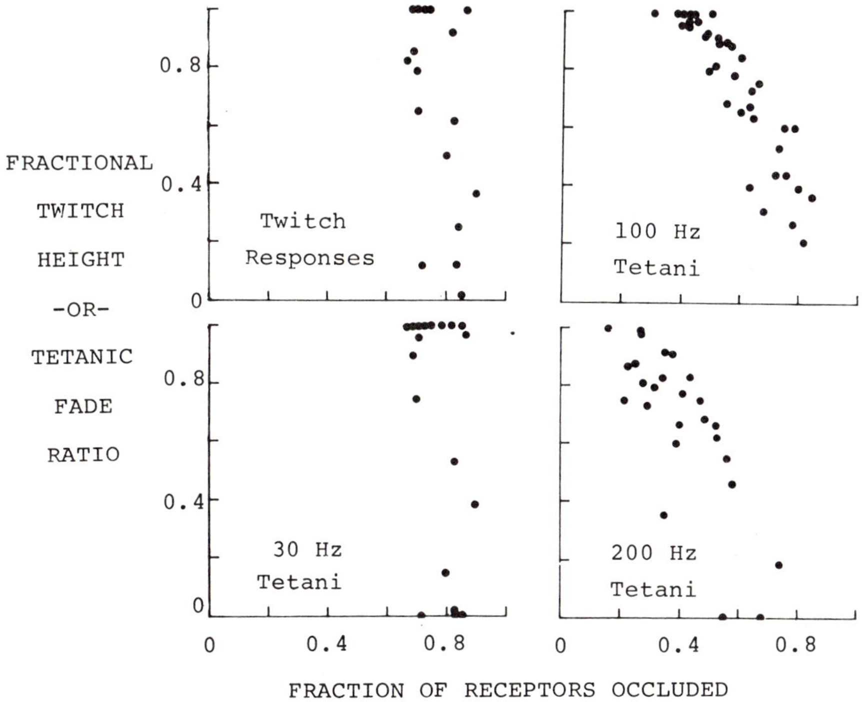

FIG. 18, 4. *Top left*, the evoked twitch tension in a cat was not depressed until about 80 percent of the receptors were occluded by curare. *Bottom left*, fade during tetanus at 30 Hz did not occur until about the same degree of receptor occlusion. *Top and bottom right*, with tetanus at higher frequencies (100 and 200 Hz) fade is seen with less receptor occlusion because of the rapid depletion of acetylcholine. (Reproduced with permission from Waud, B. E., and Waud, D. R.: The relation between tetanic fade and receptor occlusion in the presence of competitive neuromuscular block. Anesthesiology 35: 456–464, 1971.)

presynaptic cholinergic receptor cannot be demonstrated in all species. Other evidence supports the importance of presynaptic loci. Certain drugs have undisputed effects at the nerve terminal. Thus, hemicholinium blocks acetylcholine synthesis by nerve terminals, and botulinus toxin, calcium deficiency and high magnesium inhibit acetylcholine release. Finally the defect in myasthenia gravis is thought to be presynaptic.

There is no doubt that neuromuscular blocking drugs have presynaptic actions, but the importance of such actions remains in dispute. Two lines of evidence suggest a prejunctional site. First, following a period of high frequency tetanic stimulation *in vivo*, a single nerve stimulation causes nerve terminals to fire repetitively (28, 29). The repetitive firing is recorded antidromically in the nerve root. This repetitive activity originates in the nerve terminals. The longer lasting increase in potassium permeability following a NAP may cause a small overshoot in the return of the membrane potential to its resting level. This overshoot may be longer lasting in the unmyelinated nerve terminal than in the more proximal sheathed nerve. The result is that a potential difference between nerve terminal and the first node of Ranvier may follow a depolarization, and this difference may be exaggerated by prior repetitive stimulation. The potential difference generates a current sufficient to cause "spontaneous" repetitive depolarization (29). Muscle relaxants and anesthetics supress this repetitive firing in concentrations below those required for neuromuscular blockade (28). In addition, facilitory drugs such as neostigmine cause similar repetitive nerve terminal firing even without prior tetanic stimulation. Although these data demonstrate a presynaptic effect, the relation of inhibition of repetitive firing to blockade of normal neuromuscular transmission is only speculative, as is its relation to normal neuromuscular transmission. Clinical electromyography in normal man fails to routinely demonstrate repetitive compound action potentials in response to single nerve stimulation. Finally, the presynaptic effect of subparalytic drug concentrations in no way excludes a concomitant action at postsynaptic receptors. Lack of apparent paresis would result from the margin of safety of transmission.

The second line of evidence for presynaptic effects relates to the effect of relaxant drugs on acetylcholine release (30, 31). Statistical analysis of the distribution of epp size and the ratio of the epp to the mepp permits an estimate of the number of transmitter quanta released by nerve stimulation. Using such techniques curare has been reported to depress release of transmitter (quantal content), implying a presynaptic locus of action. However, these studies can be challenged on technical grounds. In these studies the muscle fibers either were cut or prestretched to block or obtund contraction and the dislodgement of microelectrodes. Furthermore, the same statistical methods failed to demonstrate that curare affects transmitter release in a study which used voltage clamping to prevent contraction (32). The conflict between these investigations has not been resolved but the experiments done under voltage clamp conditions appear to most closely reflect the normal state.

Site of Action in Man

Methodological problems severely hinder any investigation of the site of action of blocking drugs at the neuromuscular junction in man. Repetitive muscle depolarization does occur after single indirect stimulation in approximately one-third of all anesthetized men (33). The increase in contraction is generally small although occasionally may be double the normal evoked tension. Most anesthesiologists overlook this phenomenon because they use tension measurements rather than electromyography. Repetitive firing complicates the interpretation of the results of earlier evoked tension studies since changes in tension may have resulted from changes in repetitive depolarization rather than neuromuscular blockade. This form of repetitive depolarization differs from that described as originating in the nerve terminal in animal preparations. Deep anesthesia and subparalytic doses of curare fail to depress it while tetanic stimulation abolishes it. In this regard it resembles direct electrical (ephaptic) re-excitation of the nerve from the muscle action potential and therefore would involve postjunctional rather than presynaptic structures (34). Studies in man are required to characterize the type of block produced by a drug, its time course and its interaction with other relaxants, anesthetics and antagonists. They have been of little use in revealing the details of their mode of action.

QUESTIONS

1. Under what conditions does quantal content increase? Decrease?
2. Distinguish between quantal content and size. What might decrease quantal size?
3. Distinguish between the mepp, epp and action potential. What effect would you expect curare to have on the mepp?
4. What factors cause muscle relaxation during clinical anesthesia?
5. What is the evidence for and against the thesis that curare competes with acetylcholine?
6. What effect might (extracellular) hypokalemia be expected to have on the membrane potential? What effect might this have on muscle strength and the action of curare?
7. How can curare-like and succinylcholine-like drugs be distinguished experimentally? How can they be distinguished clinically?
8. In myasthenia gravis there is tetanic fade and a long lasting decrease in

twitch tension after tetanus. Contrast this with a curare block. What drug produces an effect similar to that found in the myasthenic state? Propose a mechanism of myasthenia gravis based on this similarity.

9. What is the meaning of "desensitization?" What might be its mechanism?
10. How does one determine whether a patient can breath adequately after he has been given curare?

REFERENCES

1. Paton, W. D. M., and Waud, D. R.: The margin of safety of neuromuscular transmission. J. Physiol. 191: 59–90, 1967.
2. Katz, R. L., and Katz, G. J.: Clinical use of muscle relaxants. In *Advances in Anesthesiology*, Ch. 6, p. 69. Harper and Row, New York, 1967.
3. Gissen, A. J., Karis, J. H., and Nastuk, W. L.: Effect of Halothane on neuromuscular transmission. J. A. M. A. 197: 770–774, 1966.
4. Elmquist, D., and Quastrell, D. M. J.: Presynaptic action of hemicholinium at the neuromuscular junction. J. Physiol. 177: 463–482, 1965.
5. Karis, J. H.: Myasthenia gravis: anesthesia for thymectomy and postoperative care. In *Highlights of Clinical Anesthesiology*, edited by L. C. Mark and S. H. Ngai, pp. 94–100. Harper and Row, New York, 1971.
6. Desmedt, J. E.: Neuromuscular defect in myasthenia gravis: electrophysiological and histopathological evidence. In *Myasthenia Gravis*, edited by H. R. Viets, pp. 150–178. Charles C Thomas Co., Springfield, Ill., 1961.
7. Katz, R. L.: Clinical neuromuscular pharmacology of pancuronium. Anesthesiology 34: 550–556, 1971.
8. Ngai, S. H., Hanks, E. C., and Farhie, S. E.: Effects of anesthetics on neuromuscular transmission and somatic reflexes. Anesthesiology 26: 162–167, 1965.
9. De Jong, R. H., Hershey, W. N., and Wagman, I. H.: Measurement of a spinal reflex response (H reflex) during general anesthesia: association between reflex depression and muscular relaxation. Anesthesiology 28: 382–389, 1967.
10. Katz, R. L.: Neuromuscular effects of diethyl ether and its interaction with succinylcholine and d-tubocurarine. Anesthesiology 27: 52–63, 1966.
11. Katz, R. L., and Gissen, A. J.: Neuromuscular and electromyographic effects of halothane and its interaction with d-tubocurarine in man. Anesthesiology 28: 564–567, 1967.
12. Dale, H. H., Feldberg, W., and Vogt, M.: Release of acetylcholine at voluntary motor nerve endings. J. Physiol. 86: 353–380, 1936.
13. Karczmar, A. G.: Neuromuscular pharmacology. Ann. Rev. Pharmacol. 7: 241–276, 1967.
14. Waser, P. G.: Receptor localization by autoradiographic techniques. Ann. N. Y. Acad. Sci. 144: 737, 1967.
15. Waser, P. G.: On receptors in the postsynaptic membrane of the motor end plate. In *Ciba Foundation Symposium on Molecular Properties of Drug Receptors*, edited by R. Porter and M. O'Connor, pp. 59–79. J. and A. Churchill, London, 1970.
16. Gissen, A. J., and Nastuk, W. L.: The mechanism underlying neuromuscular block following prolonged exposure to depolarizing agents. Ann. N. Y. Acad. Sci. 135: 143, 1966.
17. Jenerick, H. P., and Gerard, R. W.: Membrane potential and threshold of single muscle fibers. J. Cell Comp. Physiol. 42: 79–102, 1953.
18. Katz, B., and Thesleff, S.: A study of the "desensitization" produced by acetylcholine at the motor end plate. J. Physiol. 138: 6380, 1957.

19. Nastuk, W. L., and Parson, R. L.: Factors in the inactivation of postjunctional membrane receptors of frog skeletal muscle. J. Gen. Physiol. 56: 218–249, 1970.
20. Feldman, S. A., and Tyrell, M. F.: A new theory of the termination of action of the muscle relaxants. Proc. Roy. Soc. Med. 63: 692–695, 1970.
21. Epstein, R. A., and Epstein, R. M.: The electromyogram and mechanical response of indirectly stimulated muscle in anesthetized man following curarization. Anesthesiology 38: 212–223, 1973.
22. Waud, B. E., and Waud, D. R.: The relation between tetanic fade and receptor occlusion in the presence of competitive neuromuscular block. Anesthesiology 35: 456–464, 1971.
23. De Jong, R., Freund, F. G.: Characteristics of the neuromuscular block with succinylcholine and decamethonium in man. Anesthesiology 28: 583–591, 1967.
24. Miller, R. D., Eger, E. I., II, Way, W. L., Stevens, W. C., and Dolan, W. M.: Comparative neuromuscular effects of forane and halothane alone and in combination with d-tubocurarine in man. Anesthesiology 35: 38–42, 1971.
25. Heisterkamp, D. V., Skovsted, P., and Cohen, P. J.: The effects of small incremental doses of d-tubocurarine on neuromuscular transmission in anesthetized man. Anesthesiology 30: 500–505, 1969.
26. Barnett, R. I.: The fine structural localization of acetylcholinesterase at the myoneural junction. J. Cell Biol. 12: 247–262, 1962.
27. Okamoto, M., Longnecker, H. E., Jr., and Riker, W. F.: Destruction of mammalian motor nerve terminals by black widw spider venom. Science 172: 733–736, 1971.
28. Riker, W. F., and Okamoto, M.: Pharmacology of the motor nerve terminals. Ann. Rev. Pharmacol. 9: 173–176, 1969.
29. Standard, F. G.: Post-tetanic activity in the cat soleus nerve: its origin, course, and mechanism of generation. J. Gen. Physiol 47: 53–70, 1965.
30. Hubbard, J. I., Wilson, D. F., and Miyamoto, M.: Reduction of transmitter release by d-tubocurarine. Nature 223: 531–533, 1969.
31. Galindo, A.: Prejunctional effect of curare: its relative importance. J. Neurophysiol. 34: 289–301, 1971.
32. Auerbach, A., and Betz, W.: Does curare effect transmitter release? J. Physiol. 213: 691–705, 1971.
33. Epstein, R. A., and Jackson, S. H.: Repetitive muscle depolarization from single indirect stimulation in anesthetized man. J. Appl. Physiol. 28: 407–410, 1970.
34. Lloyd, D. P. C.: Stimulation of peripheral nerve terminations by active muscle. J. Neurophysiol. 5: 153–165, 1942.

Chapter 19

Muscle Relaxant Uptake and Elimination

The intravenous injection of a muscle relaxant rapidly decreases the muscular contraction that results from indirect (i.e., nerve) stimulation. A maximum depression occurs in 1 to 5 minutes and returns to normal in the ensuing 10 to 40 minutes. The course of this waxing and waning largely depends on the factors which determine the distribution and elimination of the muscle relaxant.

The Fall in Plasma Levels of Relaxant following Intravenous Injection

The rate of disappearance of relaxant from blood (1–4) superficially is similar to that seen for barbiturates (5) (fig. 19, 1). There is a rapid initial disappearance which is followed by a slower decay. For either a barbiturate or a muscle relaxant, distribution to tissues is the major cause of the initial decrease, whereas the later decay is due to redistribution and elimination (elimination here means both excretion of the unchanged molecule and/or its metabolism).

Despite these superficial similarities, the time courses of the uptake and distribution of relaxants and barbiturates differ enormously. Unlike barbiturates, the distribution and redistribution of muscle relaxants are essentially complete in 5 to 15 minutes. After 15 minutes, the decline in blood drug concentration is entirely due to elimination.

The same blood flows and tissues receive barbiturates and relaxants; what then accounts for the far more rapid progression of events with relaxants? The answer lies in the difference in the volumes into which these agents distribute. The relaxants are confined to a much smaller volume (6).

The muscle relaxants differ from the other drugs described in this book in that they are almost completely ionized (6, 7). As such, they cannot cross cell membranes or do so only very slowly or under special circumstances. They can cross the blood capillary wall where holes between the capillary cells permit the passage of molecules with molecular weights of up to 40,000. But having reached the extracellular space, the relaxant molecule usually can go no further. Contrast this with a barbiturate or local anesthetic or inhaled anesthetic molecule which readily traverses cell membranes and therefore has a much larger volume of distribution. Volume of distribution here describes the apparent volume which dilutes the concentration of agent in blood. For example, suppose the initial concentration of relaxant in blood (prior to any loss to tissue) were 100 units/liter and that with equilibration this fell to 20 units/liter. The volume of distribution then must be 4 times the blood volume. Usually we want to know what the tissue volume of distribution

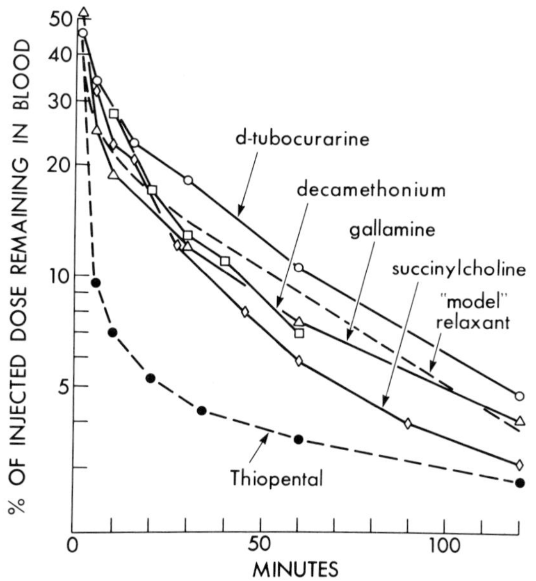

FIG. 19, 1. When compared to thipental, a greater fraction of the intravenously injected dose of relaxant remains in blood at any given time following injection. Data for curare (1) are from human studies; those for decamethonium (2) are from cats; while the data for gallamine (4) and thiopental (5) were from studies in dogs. The data for succinylcholine were obtained from dogs (3) treated with hexafluorenium to prevent hydrolysis by pseudocholinesterase. The computer simulation of a "typical" relaxant blood decay assumed a five compartment model. Lung tissue was assumed to equal 0.4 liters and possess a tissue/blood partition coefficient of 3. Vessel rich group, muscle group and vessel poor group-skin-fat made up the next 3 groups: they equalled 3, 25 and 30 liters, respectively, and received 1.4, 1.2 and 0.4 liters/minute of blood flow, respectively; all possessed tissue/blood partition coefficients of 0.2. Liver and kidney were separated from the vessel rich group and made up the fifth compartment. The liver-kidney volume equalled 3 liters; their blood flow equalled 2 liters/minute; and they possessed a tissue/blood partition coefficient of 1. In addition, it was assumed that 15 percent/minute of relaxant in or delivered to the kidney-liver group was destroyed or eliminated.

is in the absence of elimination. Since elimination contributes to even the earliest fall in blood relaxant levels, we cannot estimate the tissue volume of distribution from the blood relaxant concentration at say 20 or 30 minutes. However, in the case of muscle relaxants, we can obtain a reasonable estimate by extrapolating the "tail" of the blood disappearance curves back to zero time (i.e., the time of injection). For the relaxants in figure 19, 1 this extrapolation crosses the *Y* coordinate at 15 to 25 percent of injected dose remaining in the blood. This would indicate respective tissue volumes of distribution of $5\frac{2}{3}$ (i.e., $\frac{85}{15}$) to 3 (i.e., $\frac{75}{25}$) times the blood volume.

The tissue volume of distribution greatly influences the rate of onset, the potency and the duration of action of muscle relaxants. A limited volume of distribution is analogous to a low solubility or capacity to hold agent. This is, it indicates a low tissue/blood partition coefficient. As a result, the tissue time constants for relaxants (time constant equals tissue capacity/blood flow) are all far smaller than those for anesthetic agents. This, in large part, explains the rapid onset of relaxant effect despite a limited blood flow to the affected (muscle) site. The smaller volume of distribution also affects the *in vivo* potency of relaxants by limiting the dilution of drug. Finally, since the smaller volume of distribution confines more relaxant to blood, the kidney and liver have access to a larger fraction of the total relaxant in the body. Thus, the smaller the volume of distribution, the more rapid the rate of elimination. Each of these effects will be discussed subsequently.

Uptake and Distribution of a "Typical" Muscle Relaxant

Following an intravenous injection, relaxant travels to lung where a minor fraction is temporarily held by lung tissue (fig. 19, 2). Despite its small size, the lung may hold appreciable amounts of relaxant. A portion of the relaxant that enters lung tissue must lie within the extracellular space. However, Cohen *et al.* (8) have shown that the concentration of curare in lung exceeds that in blood (fig. 19, 3), thereby implying that curare distributes itself to a space with a capacity greater than interstitial lung water alone. This suggests that curare binds to the lung cell, perhaps to the surface of the cell membrane. A similar, but less dramatic picture is seen for gallamine and decamethonium (8). The binding of relaxant does not imply an irreversible fixation. The curare attached to the surface membrane is in equilibrium with that in interstitial fluid. Binding simply enlarges the capacity to hold relaxant. That is, a tissue which binds a greater amount of relaxant has a greater tissue/blood partition coefficient.

From lung the relaxant is delivered to the tissues of the body in proportion to the fraction of the cardiac output accorded each tissue. In

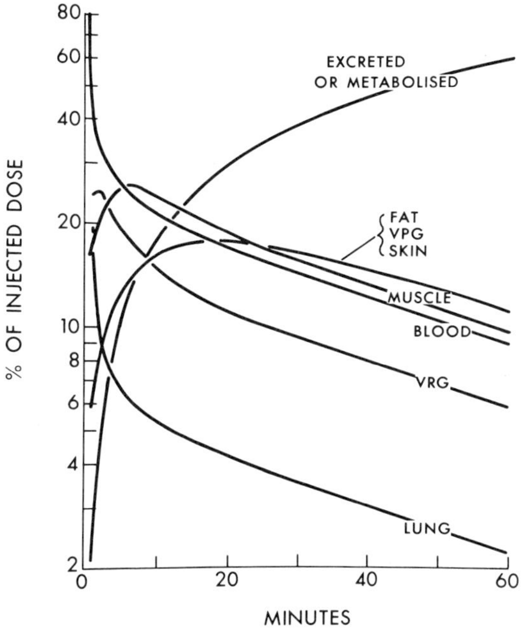

FIG. 19, 2. An intravenous dose of a "typical" relaxant initially equilibrates with lung where 20 percent of the injected dose transiently may be sequestered. From lung the relaxant is distributed to the tissues in proportion to the fraction of cardiac output given to each tissue. Thus, the largest amount of relaxant first goes to the vessel rich group (VRG) which at 1 to 2 minutes contains a peak level of 25 percent of the injected dose. The VRG thereafter returns relaxant to blood for redistribution. Muscle "peaks" at 5 to 6 minutes and also contains 25 percent of the injected dose at this time. Skin, fat and the vessel poor group (VPG) are the last to equilibrate with blood. Throughout and beyond this period, kidney and liver are eliminating relaxant. During the second hour following administration, the rate of elimination is sufficient to produce a 60 percent decrease in blood relaxant level. The assumptions used in this simulation of a "typical' relaxant are given in the legend to figure 19, 1.

this respect the distribution of relaxants is identical to the distribution of barbiturates (or any drug). Thus, peak tissue levels are first attained in the vessel rich group, next in the muscle group and last in the vessel poor group, fat and skin (fig. 19, 2). The difference between relaxants and barbiturates lies in the far greater speed with which relaxant peak levels are reached. Compare figure 19, 2 with figure 17, 4. The relaxant peak is reached in muscle in 5 minutes but peak muscle barbiturate levels are not attained for 20 minutes. The disparity is still greater for fat. As noted above, these differences result from the low tissue/blood partition coefficients and hence shorter time constants for relaxants (see fig. 19, 3). For example, muscle has a coefficient of about 0.2 for relaxants which, with a 3 ml of blood flow/100 ml of tissue, gives a time constant of 7

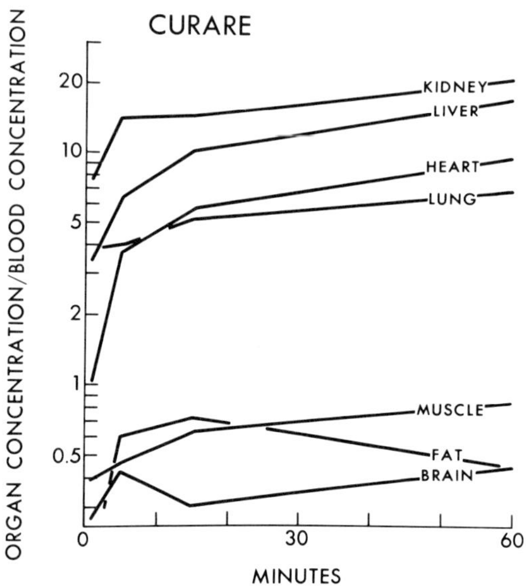

FIG. 19, 3. These tissue/blood concentration ratios give a relative and very approximate estimate of the tissue/blood partition coefficients for curare. Note that the organ concentration also includes curare in the blood perfusing the organ and hence the "organ"/blood concentration ratio depicted is higher than the true ratio. The bulk of the body tissues (muscle, tendons (not shown), cartilage (not shown), fat and brain) have partition coefficients of less than 1. A small fraction of the body tissues (kidney, liver, spleen, heart and lung) have partition coefficients in excess of 5. (Adapted from Cohen, E. N., Hood, N., Golling, R.: Use of whole-body autoradiography for determination of uptake and distribution of labeled muscle relaxants in the rat. Anesthesiology 29: 987–993, 1968.)

minutes as compared with a time constant for barbiturates of over a half hour.

As with barbiturates, the sequential nature of the peak tissue concentrations indicates an initial distribution of relaxant which is followed by redistribution. Immediately following injection, drug enters all tissues and the blood level falls (fig. 19, 2). The relaxant partial pressure (i.e., activity) in the vessel rich group soon reaches that in blood. As the blood relaxant partial pressure falls further, drug re-enters blood from the vessel rich group and is redistributed to muscle and other tissues. Within 5 to 6 minutes, the relaxant partial pressure in blood also falls below that in muscle and redistribution from muscle occurs. Finally, the blood level falls sufficiently to allow relaxant to re-enter blood from fat, skin and the vessel poor group.

Throughout and beyond this early period, the kidney (and for some relaxants the liver) removes and eliminates relaxant. The removal is sufficient to rapidly decrease the blood levels. Recall that for barbiturates the late fall in blood level occurred at a rate of 10 to 20 percent/hour. In contrast, the relaxant decay rate is almost 60 percent/hour.

How accurate is the above description of the uptake and distribution of a "typical" relaxant? At the onset it must be admitted that no single simulation can apply exactly to all relaxants. However, the closeness with which the simulated blood levels follow those found *in vivo* (see fig. 19, 1) indicates the reasonableness of the simulation. Several facts support the general validity of the approach. The fall in blood level after 15 to 30 minutes is primarily the result of removal by kidney and liver. Redistribution cannot explain this "tail" of the curve since tissue drug levels (with the possible exception of cartilage and tendons (2)) are falling after 15 to 30 minutes (8). That is, no tissue takes up more relaxant with time and thus the decay in the blood levels must result from elimination. This is what the model would predict.

The "tails" of the *in vivo* curves have a time constant of about 65 minutes (the time for a 63 percent decrease in blood levels). This time constant may be used to estimate the volume of distribution of the relaxant. If renal and hepatic mechanisms remove 15 percent of drug brought to them in their 2 liter total perfusion, then a total volume of distribution can be estimated as:

$$65 \cdot 0.15 \cdot 2 \text{ liters} = 19.5 \text{ liters}$$

Five of the 19.5 liters are blood. The remaining 14.5 liters are about 20 percent of a 70 kg man or roughly the volume of the extracellular, extravascular fluid space.

The model also accounts for the rapid onset of relaxant action. We know that maximum paralysis from curare, gallamine, pancuronium or decamethonium administration appears in 3 to 6 minutes and it is likely that this coincides with peak drug levels in muscle. Given that muscle blood flow is about 1 liter/minute, this rapid attainment of peak drug levels can only be achieved if the volume of distribution is limited to the extracellular space. When we altered our simulation by doubling the volume of distribution in muscle, the peak concentration of relaxant in muscle was reached 10 minutes after injection—a time which does not correspond to data from clinical experience or animal investigations.

Although the general validity of the model is easily defended, specific points may be questioned. The assumed tissue/blood partition coefficients must vary between relaxants and for any one relaxant may vary with concentration or pH. Total blood flow and flow distribution may be altered by anesthetics or by relaxants themselves. Renal and hepatic elimination may differ between relaxants and some relaxants may not undergo hepatic elimination at all. It should be noted that the metabolism of succinylcholine by plasma pseudocholinesterase is not covered by the model. These and other points will be discussed in succeeding sections.

Renal and Hepatic Elimination of Relaxant

Feldman *et al.* (4) demonstrated the importance of excretion to the blood relaxant level. They found that the blood gallamine level of normal dogs decreased more rapidly than that of anephric dogs (fig. 19, 4). A striking difference was apparent as early as 1 minute following injection where the level in normal dogs was 90 percent of that in the anephric animals. By 30 minutes the level was 69 percent and by an hour was 43 percent. Cohen *et al.* (9) found similar but less dramatic differences between normal and anephric dogs given curare. The smaller difference in the latter study is attributable to the compensatory increase in excretion of curare by the liver in the anephric dogs.

There are two reasons why the renal excretion of relaxants efficiently and rapidly reduces the blood levels. First, the relaxants are limited in their distribution and therefore, in contrast to the case with barbiturates, the kidney has access to a sizeable fraction of the total relaxant residing in the body. If the volume of distribution of muscle relaxants were equal to that for barbiturates, the time constant for elimination would be

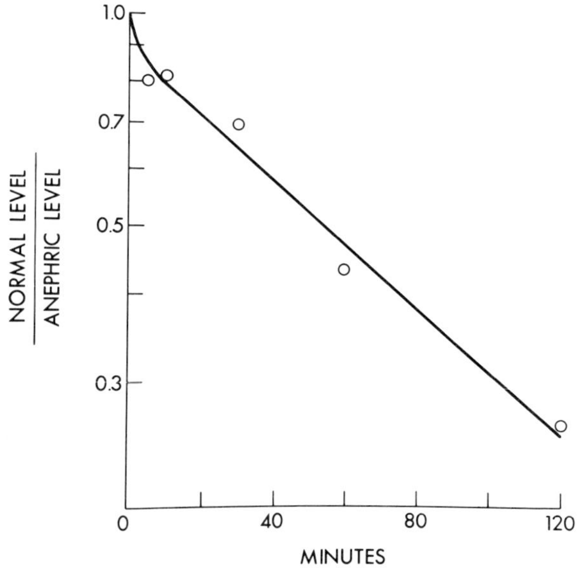

FIG. 19, 4. Plasma gallamine concentrations were obtained from normal and from anephric dogs following the injection of 2 mg/kg in each (4). The ratio of these concentrations is given here and demonstrates the importance of renal excretion to the elimination of gallamine paralysis.

increased many fold. Since the effect of the relaxant then would outlast the effect of antagonists such as prostigmine, the problem of recurarization would exist for every patient.

The second reason for the efficient renal elimination of relaxants is that the ionization of relaxant prevents the tubular reabsorption of the relaxant after it is filtered in the glomerulus (7, 10). That is, all the relaxant contained in the glomerular filtrate is excreted. Thus, the quantity excreted equals the volume of plasma filtered times the concentration in the filtrate. Now the concentration in the filtrate itself is a function of two factors: 1) the plasma concentration; and 2) the extent of binding to plasma proteins. The impact of binding is illustrated in figure 19, 5. When binding is high (fig. 19, 5*A*), most of the relaxant molecules are attached to proteins (80 percent in this example). Since the proteins are not filtered, there is little relaxant in the filtrate; most of the relaxant is concentrated in the remaining plasma (19, 5*B*). Reabsorption of water in the renal tubules (19, 5*C*) returns the concentration to nearly the same level as that which entered the kidney (19, 5*A*).

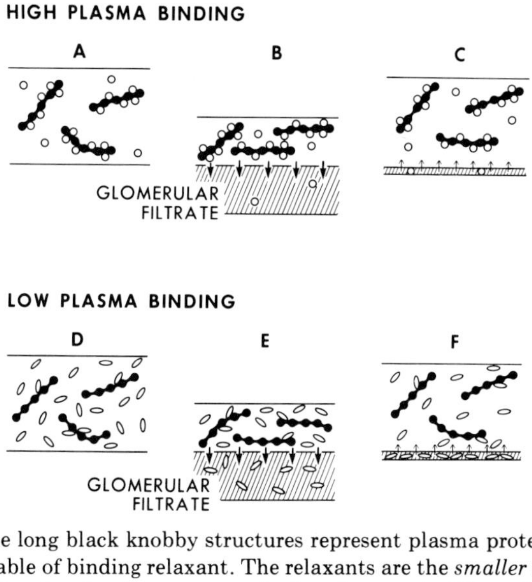

FIG. 19, 5. The long black knobby structures represent plasma proteins, each having 8 concave sites capable of binding relaxant. The relaxants are the *smaller circles* (*A*, *B*, *C*) or *ovals* (*D*, *E*, *F*) either free in plasma or attached to the protein. When the relaxant affinity for the protein is high, most of the relaxant clings to the protein (*A*); when the affinity is low, most is found free (*D*). For purposes of illustration we have assumed that half the plasma water is filtered at the glomerulus (*B* and *E*). The concentration of relaxant in the filtrate equals that free in the plasma; the bound relaxant is held back since the proteins cannot pass through the pores in the glomerular wall. Water, but not the highly ionized relaxant, is absorbed in the tubules (*C* and *F*). The final plasma concentration is only slightly changed with the highly bound relaxant (*C*) but considerably decreased with the poorly bound agent (*F*).

When binding is low, only a small fraction of relaxant molecules are attached to proteins (19, 5*D*); most are free to pass with the plasma filtrate (19, 5*E*). Reabsorption of water significantly dilutes the plasma relaxant concentration (19, 5*F*). Four times as much of the poorly bound relaxant was excreted (compare fig. 19, 6 *C* and *F*) and conversely the final plasma concentration of the highly bound agent was reduced 10 percent while that of the poorly bound agent was reduced 40 percent.

Binding of relaxant to blood proteins has a 2 fold conflicting effect on the rate of whole body clearance of relaxant. As noted above, an increase in binding decreases renal clearance and hence should delay recovery. However, an increase in binding decreases the tissue/blood partition coefficient and the resultant reduction in the tissue volume of distribution acts to *increase* the rate of whole body elimination. That is, when binding is great the kidney clears a smaller fraction of blood but the blood contains more relaxant. The balance between these two factors still favors a slower rate of whole body elimination with greater binding, but the effect is not as great as might have been anticipated from the effect on renal blood clearance alone. Parenthetically, it should be noted that binding also affects potency by limiting the amount of relaxant which is free to diffuse to the neuromuscular junction. An increase in binding decreases the blockade produced by a given dose of relaxant (11).

The volume of filtrate was exaggerated in figure 19, 5 to illustrate the importance of binding. Normal plasma filtration is about 125 ml/minute or about 20 percent of the renal plasma flow. Similarly, figure 19, 5 used extreme examples of binding to plasma proteins: 80 percent in the case of high binding and 20 percent in the case of low binding. Cohen *et al.* (12) found that slightly more than 30 percent of curare is bound. In line with this relatively low binding, Cohen (9) determined that the kidney clears approximately 20 percent of the curare delivered in the renal plasma flow.

An adequate renal blood flow and glomerular filtration are important to the relatively rapid fall in relaxant concentration and thus to recovery from paralysis. Impaired renal function may limit relaxant removal and thereby extend the relaxant effect (fig. 19, 4). Impairment of function can pre-exist or can be imposed by the stress of surgery and/or anesthesia. Conversely, several factors may act to augment elimination. The administration of large fluid volumes both may increase glomerular filtration and may dilute the plasma proteins which bind relaxant. Similarly, plasma hypoproteinemia may allow a greater clearance of relaxant. Finally, binding may be altered by changes in pH. A decrease in pH decreases the binding of curare and thereby should increase the free (active) curare which in turn should increase renal clearance (1). In accord with this, Hughes (13) found that a decrease in pH increased the activity of curare as evidenced by a greater blockade from a given dose. An opposite effect was seen with gallamine suggesting a reduced binding with an increase in pH.

The impact of renal excretion must be greatest during the moments immediately following injection of relaxant. During the first minute after injection, each passage of blood through the kidney delivers a greater fraction of the dose within the body than 15 minutes later when the relaxant has been dispersed to a larger volume. An example may serve to illustrate this point. Assume that 25 percent of the cardiac output goes to the kidney. Thus, in the first circulation following injection, 25 percent of the injected dose is subject to renal extraction. If the clearance is 20 percent, then 0.2 times 25 or 5 percent of the injected dose is removed. However, after distribution of relaxant, only about 20 percent of the agent remaining within the body is contained in blood. With a 20 percent clearance, only 0.2 times 0.2 times 25 equals 1 percent of the remaining dose is removed per minute. A second factor may further augment the early elimination of relaxant. The higher concentrations that exist immediately following injection may saturate the plasma protein binding sites. This would decrease the fraction of relaxant bound (i.e., increase the fraction free in plasma water) and thereby increase renal clearance.

The greater impact of excretion immediately following injection is similar to that seen for hepatic extraction of thiopental. However, the magnitude of the effect of time is far greater for barbiturates than for relaxants. This follows from the greater volume of distribution of barbiturates. Immediately following injection, both barbiturates and relaxants are confined to blood (i.e., their volumes of distribution are identical) and the kidney (or liver) has equal access to both drugs. But when barbiturates are distributed throughout the body, less than 1 percent of the residual barbiturate in the body remains in blood. In contrast, at the same time, blood contains 20 percent of the residual relaxant. Thus, long after injection, the kidney (or liver) still has access to only a small fraction of remaining barbiturate.

The liver also participates in the excretion of curare (7, 9) and pancuronium (14), but not gallamine (7) or decamethonium (15). The potential importance of biliary excretion is that the excretory function of the liver can substitute for the excretory function of the kidney. The process of biliary excretion partially depends on the lipid solubility of the relaxant: curare is slightly lipid soluble (as indicated by its extractability into octanol) (7) whereas other muscle relaxants are not. The lipid solubility is pH dependent: it decreases as pH falls (7). Biliary excretion of curare also depends on some unknown active transport system. The importance of such a system is indicated by the inhibition of excretion consequent to the administration of k-strophantoside (16). These studies were conducted *in vitro*. We do not know if patients receiving digitalis preparations similarly would have a reduced rate of curare excretion.

Binding of Relaxants to the Motor End-Plate

Relaxants reaching muscle not only are found in extracellular fluid, but also bind to the neuromuscular end-plate (fig. 19, 6) (2, 17–21). The affinity of the end-plates for relaxants is indicated by the very low "apparent" dissociation constants for the receptor site of acetylcholine. This dissociation constant may be obtained from the equation

$$R + S \overset{K}{\rightleftharpoons} RS \tag{1}$$

where R is the relaxant, S is the binding site and RS is the relaxant-site combination. Then,

$$K = [R][S]/[RS] \tag{2}$$

where K is the dissociation constant. For curare, K is 1.6×10^{-7} M; for gallamine it is 3.0×10^{-7} M; and for decamethonium it is 12×10^{-7} M (17). It is apparent that the relaxants have a great affinity for receptor.

Both figure 19, 6 and the affinity constants noted above suggest a difference between the nondepolarizers like curare, and the depolarizers such as decamethonium. The distribution of curare is sharply localized to the end-plate (fig. 19, 6*B*), whereas there is a diffuse distribution of decamethonium about the end-plate sites (fig. 19, 6*C*). This accords with Waser's theory that curare-like compounds are affixed to and block the

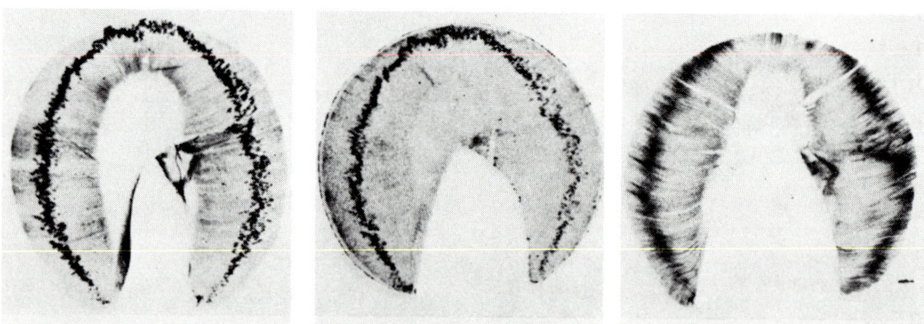

a b c

FIG. 19, 6. Acetylcholinesterase sites and hence the end-plate regions in a mouse diaphragm are identifiable as the *blackened area* in *a*. Autoradiographies of mouse diaphragms 2 minutes after intravenous injection of lethal dose of ^{14}C-toxiferine (*b*) and ^{14}C-decamethonium (*c*) both show a concentration of radioactivity in the end-plate region. Like toxiferine, curare (not shown) is distributed only to the end-plates whereas decamethonium also is distributed around the end-plates and along the muscle fiber. (Reproduced with permission from Waser, P. G.: Eine Molekulare Therorie zur Wirkungsweise curarisierender Stoffe. Der Anaesthesist 20: 23–29, 1971.)

pores whose opening permits the depolarization of the end-plate (see Chapter 18). In contrast, decamethonium occupies sites peripheral to these pores, sites which are sensitive to the direct effects of acetylcholine. These sites are diffusely located within and about the end-plate region (fig. 19, 6*C*). A second reason also may explain the diffuse decamethonium spread about the end-plate: some of this relaxant moves through the end-plate and into the muscle cell itself. The pharmacological effect within the cell is negligible except that it must serve as a reservoir of agent which may subsequently act on the end-plate (22).

Equilibrium between Muscle and Blood: Implications of Motor End-Plate Binding

The great affinity of muscle relaxants (particularly the nondepolarizing relaxants) for the motor end-plate suggests that during recovery from paralysis, the relaxant at the neuromuscular junction may not be in equilibrium with the relaxant in the plasma perfusing the area. That is, muscle relaxant molecules are concentrated at the receptor sites on the end-plate with only a small fraction of these free at any one time to diffuse through the extracellular fluid to the capillaries. Even though the process of diffusion for any one molecule may be rapid, the limited number of molecules free to traverse this path at any one time may hinder depletion of the end-plate stores.

An ingenious experiment by Feldman and Tyrrell (23) demonstrated the lack of equilibrium that may exist between the relaxant in muscle and that in blood. In anesthetized patients they injected 3 mg of curare or 8 mg of gallamine into an arm whose circulation was arrested by a tourniquet. Paralysis developed in the arm within 3 minutes, after which the tourniquet was released. As might be expected, the release of the tourniquet did not produce paralysis in the rest of the body. Somewhat more surprising was the finding that contractility in the injected arm did not rapidly return to normal. In fact, the duration of paralysis was only modestly shorter than that which resulted from the injection of a full paralyzing dose to the whole body. These results suggest that an activity gradient for relaxant may exist between the end-plate and plasma.

Feldman and Tyrrell performed two other related experiments which indirectly examined the effect of binding at the end-plate. In one experiment they injected a paralytic dose of curare intravenously and measured the contractile (twitch) response to faradic nerve stimulation in both arms. They superimposed intermittent tetanic nerve stimulation to one arm and found an accelerated recovery of the twitch response in that arm. They suggested that the acetylcholine release by a tetanic stimulus displaced curare from the end-plate (i.e., reduced the binding and thereby increased the number of free curare molecules). This curare diffused way from the end-plate. The resultant decreased occupancy of the end-plates allowed a greater subsequent twitch response. The action of neostigmine would be similar to that of a tetanic stimulus. The increased acetylcholine at the neuromuscular junction would displace curare and thereby both decrease receptor occupancy and increase the rate of loss from the end-plate. Against this hypothesis is the fact that although a single tetanic stimulus undoubtedly releases acetylcholine and displaces curare, the subsequent increase in twitch height is not sustained if the tetanus is not repeated. It may be that repeated tetany (as in the Feldman-Tyrrell experiment) simply increases the amount of readily releasable transmitter.

Finally, Feldman and Tyrrell found that the injection of a small dose of decamethonium (0.5 mg) into the arm isolated by a tourniquet produced paralysis just as had small doses of gallamine or curare. However, unlike the results with gallamine and curare, when the tourniquet was released, recovery from decamethonium occurred within a few minutes. This accords with the difference in the affinity constants noted earlier (17, 18): decamethonium has the smallest affinity for acetylcholine receptors. Feldman and Tyrrell suggested that succinylcholine would have an affinity similar to that of decamethonium. It also might be noted that recovery from gallamine, though slow, was far more rapid than curare. The affinity of gallamine for the acetylcholine receptor is less than the affinity of curare.

A Summary of the Distribution, Redistribution and Excretion of Nondepolarizing Relaxants

The almost complete ionization of muscle relaxants plays a primary role in their uptake, distribution and excretion by limiting their tissue solubility. Thus, although the order of time to peak tissue concentration (first lung, then VRG, then muscle and finally fat and VPG) is the same as for other drugs, the peak levels are reached far more rapidly with relaxants. Renal and hepatic eliminations are aided by the access to a larger fraction of drug (less is "hidden" in peripheral tissue depots). Ionization also prevents the reabsorption of excreted drug.

Some tissue binding of relaxant occurs. This appears to be of minimal importance to the volume of distribution. However, binding to the neuromuscular junction may be of considerable importance to the duration of relaxants action. Elimination of relaxant from the motor end-plate may require dislodgement by acetylcholine as well as removal by perfusion with relaxant-free blood.

Succinylcholine

In the absence of plasma pseudocholinesterase the distribution and excretion of succinylcholine follows the pattern of other muscle relaxants (fig. 19, 1). The volume of distribution is similar as is the excretion rate via the urine. In dogs pretreated with hexafluorenium to prevent plasma hydrolysis of the succinylcholine, 60 percent of the relaxant is eliminated in the urine in 1 hour (3)—a figure which agrees closely with the elimination predicted in figure 19, 2. The relatively rapid excretion may partially relate to the minimal plasma binding of succinylcholine (but not succinylmonocholine) (3).

The above description disregards the impact of succinylcholine hydrolysis by plasma pseudocholinesterase. This destruction of succinylcholine markedly shortens the duration of paralysis. Unfortunately, no *in vivo* data in man or a comparable animal directly demonstrated the rate of fall of plasma succinylcholine in the presence of normal pseudocholinesterase. We only know that the fall must be very rapid.

The rate of fall of plasma succinylcholine and the shape of the plasma decay curve depend on the kinetics of succinylcholine hydrolysis. *In vitro* studies suggest that the hydrolysis rate is very high and follows zero order kinetics (6, 24, 25). Zero order kinetics mean that the absolute rate of destruction is constant regardless of concentration and implies that the enzyme responsible for hydrolysis is saturated with substrate. The absolute rate of destruction may be calculated from the data of Schmidinger *et al.* (24) or Hobbiger and Pick (25) who, respectively, obtained values of 35 or 27 mg hydrolyzed/liter of normal plasma per minute. These results suggest that if 100 mg of succinylcholine were placed in a liter of plasma, 27 to 35 mg would be hydrolyzed in the first minute. In the second minute, an additional 27 to 35 mg would be hydrolyzed and after the third or fourth minute no succinylcholine would remain intact. If these *in vitro* data applied *in vivo*, they would have considerable implications to the clinical use as well as to the uptake and distribution of succinylcholine.

Recent studies we have conducted indicate that the above *in vitro* data do not apply to anesthetized man. (Eger, E. I., and Miller, R. D.; unpublished observations). Our *in vivo* results suggest that the rate of destruction is far less than implied by the *in vitro* data and that hydrolysis follows first order kinetics. In first order kinetics, the rate of destruction is proportional to the amount of substrate present. Thus, if 50 mg of a 100 mg dose were destroyed in the first minute, 25 mg would be destroyed in the second minute and 12.5 mg in the third minute, etc.

We found that a 4 mg/minute constant infusion provided a 90 percent reduction in twitch height. If we assume that 1) the infusion is diluted by the total plasma in the cardiac output (3 liters/minute); 2) that the transit time from right atrium to muscle is at least one-fifth of a minute; and 3) that no succinylcholine recirculates, then we may calculate a maximum rate of hydrolysis of $6\frac{2}{3}$ (i.e., $4/(3 \times 0.2)$) mg/liter of plasma per minute. This likely overestimates the hydrolysis rate since a 0.2

minute circulation time is probably an underestimate and since there likely is recirculation of succinylcholine. In any case, it is far less than the 27 to 35 mg/liter of plasma per minute found *in vitro*.

Evidence for *in vivo* first order kinetics came from a second study in which we produced a sustained 90 percent or greater paralysis by giving succinylcholine as repeated intermittent, bolus injections of either 2, 4, 8, 16 or 32 mg of succinylcholine/square meter of body surface (only one size bolus was given to any one patient). The cumulative dose for the initial half hour of injections was never less for the bolus mode of administration than for the continuous infusion mode (which produced the same minimum relaxation). This is contrary to what would be predicted from zero order kinetics. That is, with zero order kinetics the amount of succinylcholine destroyed in the time between injection and arrival at the muscle directly depends on the plasma volume into which the succinylcholine is distributed. Distribution to a larger volume exposes the succinylcholine to a greater number of enzyme molecules and hence would increase the hydrolysis rate. A continuous infusion provides a greater plasma volume of distribution than does a bolus injection and therefore should require a higher rate of administration—if zero order kinetics apply. In contrast, enzyme saturation is not present with first order kinetics and the hydrolysis rate is proportional to the amount of substrate (i.e., the volume of distribution is irrelevant). First order kinetics thus would explain our finding of no difference between the cumulative dose produced with a continuous infusion or with small intermittent bolus' when both were given so as to produce the same degree of paralysis.

A Composite Picture of Succinylcholine Uptake, Distribution and Elimination

Insufficient data are available to give a certain picture of succinylcholine pharmacokinetics, and thus the following represents a mixture of speculation and fact. A bolus of succinylcholine initially is distributed to tissues in proportion to the fraction of the cardiac output accorded each tissue. Since considerably less succinylcholine returns to muscle in succeeding circulations, the initial distribution of blood is of much greater importance than the later recirculation from other tissues. This property is one of the principal differences between uptake and distribution of succinylcholine and the uptake and distribution of other relaxants. A change in the muscle fraction of cardiac output will cause a proportional change in the delivery of succinylcholine to the myoneural junction. Shock preferentially reduces muscle flow and therefore should decrease the effect of a given succinylcholine dose. By markedly increasing muscle flow (26) isoflurane may enhance the effect of succinylcholine (27). The patient can augment muscle flow by muscle activity. This explains why the diaphragm usually is paralyzed first and most profoundly. Similarly, the anesthetist can augment paralysis of specific muscles immediately prior to injection of succinylcholine. For example, we have asked patients to chew before a "crash" induction where we wanted rapid and complete jaw relaxation.

Hydrolysis

Throughout and beyond the period of initial relaxant distribution, pseudocholinesterase hydrolyzes the succinylcholine in proportion to the amount administered. Note that this means that if a larger dose is administered, more is metabolized per minute. Similarly, anything which prolongs the succinylcholine sojourn in plasma prior to its arrival at muscle will cause less relaxant to reach the myoneural junction. Thus, a factor which lengthens the time between injection of relaxant and its arrival at muscle will decrease the effect of a given succinylcholine dose between subsequent recirculations.

Halothane (28) or methoxyflurane (29) can decrease cardiac output and thereby may antagonize the effect of succinylcholine. Similarly, shock may reduce recirculation of relaxant. On the other hand, by increasing cardiac output, ether or fluroxene may do the reverse (28). An increase in cardiac output from surgical stimulus or an increased $PaCO_2$ might increase the effect of succinylcholine regardless of the anesthetic.

Variations in the pseudocholinesterase level may also significantly influence the dose recirculated. Thus, more recirculation may occur in a patient who is heterozygous for atypical pseudocholinesterase, and a great deal of recirculation must occur in the homozygous atypical patient (6). Liver disease may reduce the quantity of pseudocholinesterase and this will proportionately reduce hydrolysis (25).

Some factors may reduce the effectiveness of pseudocholinesterase without altering the number of enzyme molecules. Organophosphates ranging from insecticides to cancer chemotherapy agents may inhibit pseudocholinesterase (30, 31). Local anesthetics such as procaine may compete with succinylcholine for substrate sites (32). Finally, pseudocholinesterase activity may be cut in half by a reduction in body temperature from 37° to 26° C (24).

Recirculation

As noted above, 4 mg/minute of intravenous succinylcholine will produce a 90 percent reduction in twitch height. Larger doses used clinically increase both the magnitude and duration of blockade. However, since *in vivo* hydrolysis increases in proportion to the amount present (first order kinetics), the greater duration is related to the square root of the increase in dose rather than to the increase in dose itself. This implies that recirculation of succinylcholine cannot occur many times. The evanescent effect of succinylcholine also supports this notion.

Recovery

Further support for a very limited recirculation of succinylcholine comes from a study by Walts and Dillon (33). They measured the time to 10 percent (T_{10}), 50 percent (T_{50}) and 90 percent (T_{90}) recovery of muscle twitch following the intravenous injection of 0.5, 1.0, 2.0 or 4.0 mg/kg of succinylcholine in man (fig. 19, 7). On a logarithmic dose scale an increase in the time to recovery occurs which is directly proportional to dose. If at a given level of recovery the same concentration of relaxant exists at the site of action and if the initial concentration imposed on the site of action is proportional to the administered dose, then we can calculate a time constant for the disappearance of succinylcholine from that site (the time it takes to reduce the concentration by 63 percent). For example, at a dose of 4 mg/kg, T_{50} is reached in 16.7 minutes. A 63 percent reduction of 4 mg/kg leaves 1.48 mg/kg. This dose results in a T_{50} of 11.6 minutes. Thus, the time constant is 16.7 minus 11.6 or 5.1 minutes. Similar values may be obtained from the T_{10} and T_{90} curves.

I have implied that the results illustrated in figure 19, 7 are explained by the plasma decay rate. Two additional explanations suggest themselves. First, recovery is determined by the rate of diffusion of succinyl-

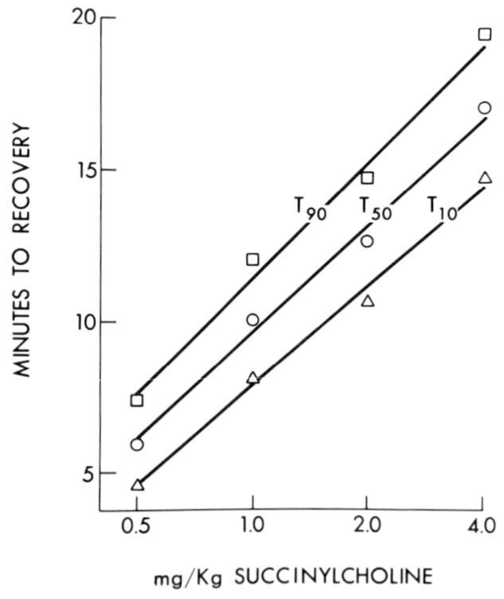

FIG. 19, 7. The time to recovery from succinylcholine paralysis is proportional to the dose administered (33). T_{90}, T_{50} and T_{10}, respectively, indicate 90, 50 and 10 percent recovery of twitch height.

choline away from the myoneural junction to the zero concentration in the plasma perfusing the junction (34). Second, recovery is determined by the perfusion characteristics of the junction. This latter explanation is appealing, since it fits the time constant of 5.1 minutes from the Walts and Dillon studies (33). That is, normal muscle perfusion is about 3 ml/100 ml/minute, but the volume of succinylcholine distribution in muscle may be only 15 percent of the muscle volume (extracellular water). Therefore, the effective flow is 3 ml/15 ml/minute, giving a time constant of 15/3 or 5 minutes. Against the thought that recovery is perfusion limited is the experiment by Argent *et al.* (34). They found that the rate of recovery from a dose of succinylcholine in cats was not altered by stopping blood flow at the time of peak paralysis. However, observations we have made in man (Dolan, W. M., Miller, R. D., and Eger, E. I., II, unpublished data) do not completely agree with the observations of Argent *et al.* We measured the rate of recovery of the thenar muscles in both hands following succinylcholine injection. At the peak of paralysis we occluded flow to one arm. The rate of recovery in that arm was significantly slowed (by roughly 50 percent) but, as in the experiment by Argent *et al.*, recovery did occur. Thus, we are left with the thought that recovery from succinylcholine is a function of 1) clearance from the active site by diffusion or by local destruction in the capillary; and 2) removal by muscle blood flow.

Summary of the Distribution and Destruction of Succinylcholine

Most of the effect of succinylcholine is achieved by the fraction of the injected dose which reaches the myoneural junction during the first few circulations to muscle. The fraction reaching the myoneural junction mainly is a function of the fraction of the cardiac output which perfuses muscle, and thus is increased by prior muscle activity, by drugs such as isoproteranol, or by an anesthetic such as isoflurane.

The fraction of the injected dose which normally recirculates quickly decreases in a logarithmic fashion. Any factor which decreases pseudocholinesterase (genetic abnormalities, liver impairment, hypothermia) and any factor which increases cardiac output (surgical stimulation, increased CO_2) will increase the amount of succinylcholine which is recirculated to muscle. A factor which reduces cardiac output (shock, anesthesia) will decrease the recirculation of succinylcholine.

The time required for the reversal of succinylcholine paralysis appears to depend on 1) the size of the dose which initially reaches the motor end-plate; 2) the rate of diffusion of succinylcholine from the end-plate or its local destruction by plasma in the muscle capillary; and 3) muscle blood flow.

QUESTIONS

1. What are the similarities and differences between the uptake and distribution of muscle relaxants and barbiturates?
2. From figure 19, 1, calculate the apparent volumes of distribution and elimination time constants for gallamine and for decamethonium.
3. Why would injection of curare into the left atrium produce a more rapid onset of action than injection into the right atrium? What additional factor would have to be considered if the drug were succinylcholine?
4. What factors increase the rate of excretion of a relaxant?
5. How may increased binding of a relaxant to blood proteins influence the distribution and elimination of that relaxant? Which effects may act in opposite ways on the rate of total relaxant excretion?
6. Why is the rate of elimination of muscle relaxant greater immediately following intravenous injection than a half hour following injection? Why is the difference less than the difference with barbiturates?
7. Cite the implications of the Feldman-Tyrrell experiments.
8. In a patient lacking plasma pseudocholinesterase, what are the factors which terminate the neuromuscular effect of succinylcholine?
9. What evidence suggests that *in vivo* succinylcholine hydrolysis follows first order kinetics?
10. A new anesthetic is said to potentiate the effect of succinylcholine. How might it do so without any direct effect on the myoneural junction?
11. What factors determine the rate of recovery from succinylcholine paralysis?

REFERENCES

1. Cohen, E. N., Corbascio, A., and Fleischli, G.: The distribution and fate of d-tubocurarine. J. Pharmacol. Exp. Ther. 147: 120–129, 1965.
2. Waser, P. G., and Luthi, U.: Distribution and metabolism of curarizing and depolarizing drugs in cats. J. Nucl. Biol. Med. 12: 4–11, 1968.
3. Dal Santo, G.: Kinetics of distribution of radioactive labelled muscle relaxants: III Investigations with ^{14}C-succinyldicholine and ^{14}C-succinylmonocholine during controlled conditions. Anesthesiology 29: 435–443, 1968.
4. Feldman, S. A., Cohen, E. N., and Golling, R. C.: The excretion of gallamine in the dog. Anesthesiology 30: 593–598, 1969.
5. Brodie, B. B., Bernstein, E., and Mark, L. C.: The role of body fat in limiting the duration of action of thiopental. J. Pharmacol. Exp. Ther. 105: 421–426, 1952.
6. Kalow, W.: The distribution, destruction and elimination of muscle relaxants. Anesthesiology 20: 505–518, 1959.
7. Meijer, D. K. F., and Weitering, J. G.: Curare-like agents: relation between lipid solubility and transport into bile in perfused rat liver. Eur. J. Pharmacol. 10: 283–289, 1970.
8. Cohen, E. N., Hood, N., and Golling, R.: Use of whole-body autoradiography for determination of uptake and distribution of labeled muscle relaxants in the rat. Anesthesiology 29: 987–993, 1968.
9. Cohen, E. N., Brewer, H. W., and Smith, P.: The metabolism and elimination of d-tubocurarine-H^3. Anesthesiology 28: 309–317, 1967.

10. Albert, A.: Ionization. In *Selective Toxicity*, p. 208. John Wiley and Sons, Inc., New York, 1965.
11. Baraka, A., and Gabali, F.: Correlation between tubocurarine requirements and plasma protein pattern. Brit. J. Anaesth. 40: 89–93, 1968.
12. Cohen, E. N.: Uptake, distribution, and elimination of the muscle relaxants. In *Scientific Foundations of Anaesthesia*, edited by C. Scurr and S. Feldman, Ch. 4, pp. 350–356. Heinemann Medical Books, Ltd., London, 1970.
13. Hughes, R.: The influence of changes in acid-base balance on neuromuscular blockage in cats. Brit. J. Anaesth. 42: 658–668, 1970.
14. Adler, L., and Pilon, R. N.: The duration of neuromuscular blockade with pancuronium in anephric cats. In *Abstracts of Scientific Papers*. American Society of Anesthesiologists' Annual Meeting, October 1972.
15. Christensen, C. B.: Distribution and biliary excretion of decamethonium in doubly nephrectomized rabbits. Acta Pharmacol. Toxicol. 23: 275–286, 1965.
16. Meyer, D. K. F., and Scaf, A. Y. J.: Inhibition of the transport of d-tubocurarine from blood to bile by k-strophantoside in the isolated perfused rat liver. Eur. J. Pharmacol. 4: 343–346, 1968.
17. Changeus, J. P., Meunier, J. C., and Hachet, M.: Studies on the cholinergic receptor protein of Electrophorus Electricus. Mol. Pharmacol. 7: 538–553, 1971.
18. Lu, T. C.: Affinity of curare-like compounds and their potency in blocking neuromuscular transmission. J. Pharmacol. Exp. Ther. 174: 560–566, 1970.
19. Waser, P. G.: Receptor localization by autoradiographic techniques. Ann. N. Y. Acad. Sci. 144: 737–755, 1967.
20. Waser, P. G.: On receptors in the postsynaptic membranes of the motor end-plate. In *Molecular Properties of Drug Receptors, Ciba Foundation Symposium*, edited by R. Porter and M. O'Connor, pp. 59–75. J & A Churchill, London, 1970.
21. Waser, P. G.: Eine Molekulare Theorie zur Wirkungweise curarisierender Stoffe. Der Anaesthetist. 20: 23–29, 1971.
22. Jenkinson, D. H.: The antagonism between tubocurarine and substances which depolarize the motor end-plate. J. Physiol. (London) 152: 309–324, 1960.
23. Feldman, S. A., and Tyrrell, M. F.: A new theory of the termination of the action of the muscle relaxants. Proc. Roy. Soc. Med. 63: 692–695, 1970.
24. Schmidinger, S., Held, K. R., and Goedde, H. W.: Hydrolysis of succinylcholine by pseudocholinesterase at low concentrations. Humangenetik 2: 221–224, 1966.
25. Hobbiger, F., Peck, A. W.: Hydrolysis of suxamethonium by different types of plasma. Brit. J. Pharmacol. 37: 258–271, 1969.
26. Stevens, W. C., Cromwell, T. H., Halsey, M. J., *et al.*: The cardiovascular effects of a new inhalation anesthetic, Forane, in human volunteers at constant arterial carbon dioxide tension. Anesthesiology 35: 8–16, 1971.
27. Miller, R. D., Way, W. L., Dolan, W. M., *et al.*: Comparative neuromuscular effects of pancuronium, gallamine, and succinylcholine during Forane and halothane anesthesia in man. Anesthesiology 35: 509–514, 1971.
28. Eger, E. I., II, Smith, N. T., Cullen, D. J., *et al.*: A comparison of the cardiovascular effects of halothane, fluroxene, ether and cyclopropane in man. Anesthesiology 34: 25–41, 1971.
29. Libonati, M., Cooperman, L. H., and Price, H. L.: Time dependent circulatory effects of methoxyflurane in man. Anesthesiology 34: 439–444, 1971.
30. Kalow, W., and Davies, R. O.: The activity of various esterase inhibitors towards atypical human serum cholinesterase. Biochem. Pharmacol. 1: 183, 1956.
31. Wang, R. I. H., and Ross, C. A.: Prolonged apnea following succinylcholine in cancer patients receiving A B-132. Anesthesiology 24: 363–367, 1963.

32. Foldes, F., McNall, P. G., Davis, L. D., *et al.*: Substrate competition between procaine and succinylcholine diiodide for plasma cholinesterase. Science 117: 383, 1958.
33. Walts, L. F., and Dillon, J. B.: Clinical studies on succinylcholine chloride. Anesthesiology 28: 372–376, 1967.
34. Argent, D. E., Dennick, P. O., and Hobbiger, F.: Prolonged apnea after suxamethonium in man. Brit. J. Anaesth. 27: 24–30, 1955.

Chapter 20

Local Anesthetic Structure, Activity and Mechanism of Action

R. H. LEVY

Structure and Activity

Unlike general anesthetics, local anesthetics form a fairly homogenous chemical and pharmacological class of drugs. Two important facts underlie many of the concepts regarding their mode of action at the macroscopic as well as the molecular level: 1) most local anesthetics are weak bases, generally tertiary or secondary amines, therefore ionizable; and 2) a typical local anesthetic molecule contains a lipophilic region separated from a hydrophilic region by an intermediate chain (fig. 20, 1). Thus, the general structure of local anesthetics is:

LIPOPHILIC GROUP—INTERMEDIATE CHAIN—HYDROPHILIC GROUP

where the lipophilic part usually consists of an aromatic or heterocyclic nucleus and the hydrophilic portion often is a tertiary or secondary amino group. The intermediate chain contains either an ester or an amide linkage (1).

This general structure suggests the orientation of local anesthetics at their site of action—the axon membrane. That the membrane is the site of action is supported by an experiment in which the axoplasm was replaced by a potassium rich-sodium poor solution. Not only did this axon act like the normal nerve in terms of propagation of a nerve impulse but local anesthetics blocked the nerve action potential both in such a "washed" axon as well as in the unaltered axon (2). Recall that, in either the classic or more recent concepts of the structure of the axon wall (Chapter 2), the outer layers are hydrophilic, while the inside layer is lipophilic. Accordingly, the local anesthetic must orient with the hydrophilic portion to the outer layers and the lipophilic portion to the inner layer.

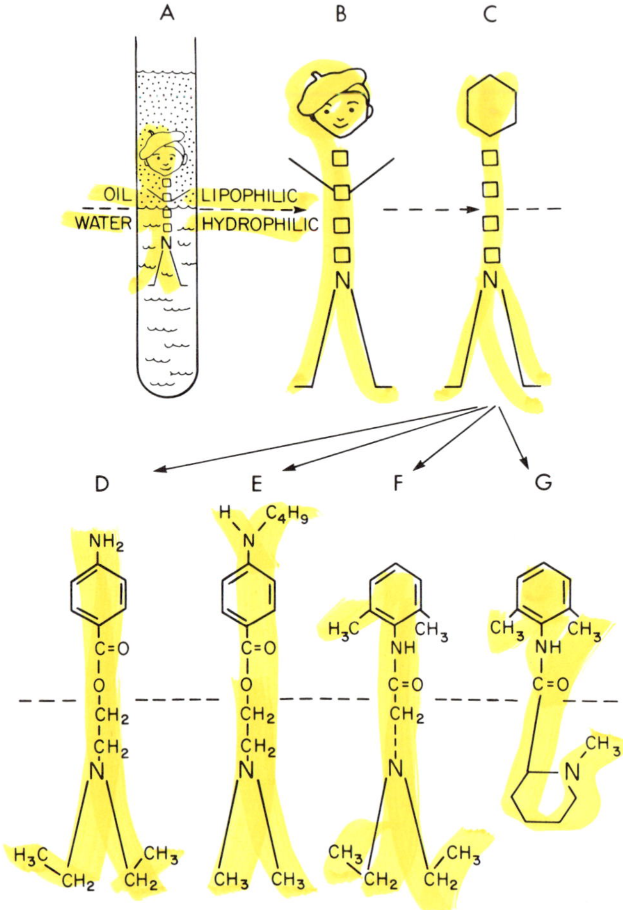

FIG. 20, 1. Structure of four representative local anesthetics illustrating the importance of a balance between the lipophilic ("head") and hydrophilic ("legs") parts of the molecule. Local anesthetic (Loan) "evolution" is described in three stages. Mr. Loan "partitioning" in an oil-water phase system is illustrated in *A*. Note: A local anesthetic molecule always "keeps its head above the water." Remember that "oil" may correspond to the hydrophobic center of the membrane and "water" to the hydrophilic surface. Mr. Loan is ready for metamorphosis (*B*) into the bare essentials (*C*) Procaine (*D*), Tetracaine (*E*), Lidocaine (*F*) and Mepivacaine (*G*) are born.

Each of the three parts of the local anesthetic contributes other properties. The aromatic moiety provides the lipid solubility which enables the drug to cross numerous cellular barriers that must be traversed to arrive at the site of action. The most remarkable feature of the intermediate chain is the highly reactive carbonyl group $-\overset{\displaystyle O}{\overset{\|}{C}}-$ of the ester or amide linkage. Local anesthetic activity is enhanced whenever the electronegativity of the oxygen atom is increased, leading to the formation of a dipole $-\underset{\delta}{\overset{\overset{O\delta^-}{|}}{C}}{}_{\mp}-$ (3). Thus, electron donating substituents in the para position of the ring allow and produce potent local anesthetics, whereas the converse is true when electron withdrawing groups are substituted in the ring.

Ionization

With few exceptions, local anesthetics are weak bases which are usually dispensed in their salt form because the base is poorly soluble in water and is unstable, whereas the salt is both stable and water soluble. The basic form is unionized whereas the salt form exists as an ion. The relationship between the two may be described by the equation,

$$B + H^+ \overset{Ka}{\leftrightarrows} BH^+ \tag{1}$$

where B represents the unionized local anesthetic base; H^+, a hydrogen ion; Ka the dissociation constant; and BH^+ the local anesthetic cation. From the law of mass action,

$$Ka = [H^+][B]/[BH^+] \tag{2}$$

where the brackets indicate concentration (more properly, activity).

The impact of acidosis or alkalosis is illustrated by rearranging equation 2:

$$[H^+]/Ka = [BH^+]/[B] \tag{3}$$

Since Ka is constant, the fraction of ionized base is directly related to the hydrogen ion concentration and conversely, the fraction unionized is inversely related. Thus, acidosis increases the local anesthetic cation at the expense of the unionized base, and alkalosis does the converse. Usually equation 2 is converted to the familiar Henderson-Hasselbach equation:

$$pKa = pH - \log [B]/[BH^+] \tag{4}$$

where pKa and pH are the negative logarithms of Ka and H^+, respectively. The exact proportions of ionized and unionized drug may be calculated if pH and pKa are known. Since the pKa values for several local anesthetics are not too far from physiological pH values, an appreciable percent of the local anesthetic exists as the unionized base (table 20, 1) (if the pKa and pH were equal then the local anesthetic would be half base and half cation). The unionized fraction is of great importance both because it is essential to the penetration of tissues and also because it may act to cause anesthesia. This last function is probably shared with the cation fraction.

TABLE 20, 1

Dissociation constants and percent unionized for several local anesthetics at various pHs (pKa values were obtained from references 4, 5, and 6)

Anesthetic	pKa	Percent of Unionized Base at			
		pH 7.4	pH 7.2	pH 7.0	pH 6.8
Benzocaine	2.8	100	100	100	100
Mepivacaine	7.6	39	28	20	14
Lidocaine	7.9	24	17	11	7.4
Prilocaine	7.9	24	17	11	7.4
Bupivacaine	8.1	17	11	7.4	4.8
Tetracaine	8.5	7.4	4.8	3.1	2.0
Dibucaine	8.5	7.4	4.8	3.1	2.0
Cocaine	8.8	3.8	2.5	1.6	1.0
Procaine	8.9	3.1	2.0	1.2	0.8

Ionization and Activity

Early studies of anesthetic action as a function of pH supported the view that the base is the active species. This was first proposed by Gros (7, 8) who demonstrated that local anesthetic solutions applied to the frog sciatic nerve yielded faster blocks when base was added. Later workers found that the minimum concentration necessary for local anesthetic block decreased with an increase in pH and also concluded that the base is responsible for the effect (9). However, from this evidence we cannot conclude that the base is the sole active species, for if the base was the only active form, its minimum effective concentration should remain constant over the pH range studied. In fact the minimum effective concentration of base increases as the pH increases (although the minimum blocking concentration of total anesthetic decreases) (10).

Most of the earlier work leading to the suggestion that the unionized species was the active form of the local anesthetic tended to ignore that two separate processes are involved in the development of anesthesia; namely, penetration of the anesthetic through the tissues and epineurium, and binding at the receptor site. While it is generally agreed that only the uncharged moiety penetrates the nerve membrane, the early work of Krahl *et al.* (11), studying the action of local anesthetics in inhibiting cell division in the sea urchin eggs, suggested that the cationic form might be active. Subsequent experiments by Ritchie *et al.* (12), in which lidocaine and the longer acting dibucaine were more effective on the nonmyelinated fibers of desheathed nerves when applied at pH 7.2 than at pH 9.6, tended to the conclusion that the cationic form may produce anesthesia (fig. 20, 2). These workers also demonstrated that a nerve, which had been completely blocked by dibucaine remained blocked (within a time span of several minutes) on exposure to an anesthetic-free solution at a pH of 7.2. As soon as the pH of the bathing medium was changed to pH 9.6, conduction was immediately restored. If the pH of the anesthetic-free bathing medium were returned to 7.2, blockade reappeared despite what must have been a lower anesthetic concentration within the nerve. Modification of membrane function as a cause of these events may be discounted since changes in nerve membrane potential and conduction velocity are virtually absent over the range of pH (pH 6 to 9.0) in which such experiments have been conducted. Only above pH 10 is membrane excitability altered and intraneural pH considerably elevated (13–15).

Unfortunately, the theory that the cation is the active species fails to explain two observations. First some potent local anesthetics are essentially unionized at physiological pH. For example, the unionized species of benzocaine, (pKa equals 2.8) is as active as lidocaine. Second, in desheathed nerves, C_m of lidocaine and dibucaine increases as the pH around the nerve is raised from neutrality to 9.2 but the opposite occurs

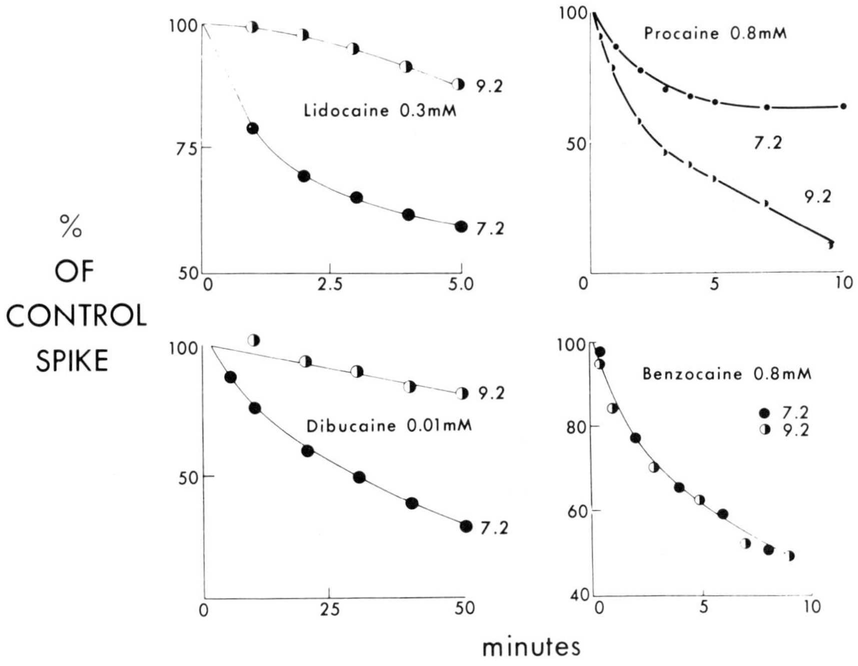

FIG. 20, 2. The effect of lidocaine (a), dibucaine (b), procaine (c) and benzocaine (d), on the size of the C elevation of the compound action potential of the nonmyelinated fibers of a rabbit desheathed cervical vagus nerve. The anesthetics were applied at pH = 7.2 (●) and 9.2 (◑). (Adapted with permission from Ritchie, J. M., and Ritchie, B. R.: Local anesthetics: effect of pH on activity. Science 162: 1394–1395, 1968. Copyright 1968 by the American Association for the Advancement of Science.)

with procaine (fig. 20, 2) (15). Thus, procaine effectiveness increases with the increase in the unionized species produced by alkalinization while the activity of the essentially unionized benzocaine is unaffected by pH. These data suggest that the uncharged molecule also must be active and perhaps, in the case of procaine, more active than the cation.

We may conclude that the unionized base is necessary to penetration of the nerve. It, therefore, is a prerequisite to *in vivo* activity. However, having crossed the barriers surrounding the nerve, we may conclude that both the base and the cation are active.

Mechanism of Action

As noted previously, local anesthetics block the nerve action potential by altering the axon membrane. Blocking concentrations prevent depolarization but do not affect the resting membrane potential. At concentrations lower than those which produce block, local anesthetics first increase the threshold for excitation, slow propagation of the impulse and reduce the rise of the nerve action potential.

Several lines of evidence suggest that local anesthetics inhibit the increased sodium conductance associated with generation of the action potential (16–22). Condouris (19), for example, reported that the conduction block caused by cocaine is similar to that produced by a low external sodium concentration and that it could be reversed if the external sodium concentration were raised. Similarly, in the presence of a reduced external sodium concentration local anesthetics become more potent (20). Experiments on bimolecular lipid membranes show that the passage of sodium ions is impaired by local anesthetics in a dose-related manner (21).

Further evidence for an effect on sodium conductance comes from studies on the interaction between calcium and local anesthetics. Recall from Chapter 2 that an increase in calcium reduces sodium conductance and that calcium may act as a "latch" which holds the sodium gate in place. Voltage clamp experiments on the lobster giant axon demonstrate that the magnitude of the reduction of maximum peak sodium conductance due to treatment with procaine is a function of the calcium concentration in the bathing medium (22). These results confirm those of several others (16, 23) which suggest that procaine may compete for nerve membrane sites normally occupied by calcium. When these sites are occupied by procaine molecules they would be less readily available than the calcium occupied sites for undergoing the reactions which permit membrane depolarization.

Finally, recall that in myelinated nerves, the sodium channels are concentrated at the nodes of Ranvier. Nerve block may be accomplished by application of local anesthetic to the node alone (24).

The fact that both the charged and uncharged species are active suggests at least two mechanisms of local anesthetic action. The uncharged base may dissolve in the hydrophobic portion of the axon membrane and thereby increase the lateral pressure within the membrane. This might compress and thereby obstruct the channels traversed by sodium. Evidence for this hypothesis is mostly circumstantial. The potency of a local anesthetic is roughly proportional to its ability to penetrate neural lipids (25, 26). Furthermore, this penetration is related to pH which also is known to affect anesthetic potency. The effect of local anesthetics on the surface pressure of a steric acid monolayer is to increase it, whereas veratrum alkaloids antagonize this effect (27). Veratrum alkaloids increase the permeability of cell membranes to sodium and potassium. This effect of veratrum could be antagonized by calcium or by lowering the pH or by the local anesthetic procaine. Finally, procaine, cocaine, tetracaine and dibucaine at minimum blocking concentrations all produce similar increases in the lateral pressure of a lipoprotein film (28).

We wonder whether the myelin sheath might be subject to a similar lateral expansion. The sheath extends for up to 2000 micra between nodes of Ranvier whereas the nodes themselves are less than 1 micron wide. The opening at the node is essential to axon function. Without the opening the extracellular sodium could not reach the sodium pores. Could local anesthetics cut off access of extracellular sodium by causing the myelin sheath to overlap the node?

The charged cation probably acts by competing with calcium to hold the sodium gate in place. The local anesthetic may combine with the polar tails of phospholipid molecules either by ion to ion or by ion induced polar bonds. This bonding may prevent the movement of lipid molecules in response to a moving electrical field (22). It may be this "swiveling" or movement of lipid molecules which opens passages for sodium transport (29). The local anesthetics in this sense are acting as a "glue." Another possibility is that the cation lodges in and directly obstructs the sodium pore.

Summary

The local anesthetic molecule consists of three parts: 1) a lipophilic hydrophobic group connected by; 2) an intermediate chain to; 3) a hydrophilic group. The lipophilic group provides the lipid solubility essential to penetrate cellular barriers. It also may be important to the mechanism of action. The carbonyl group of intermediate chain has a marked affect on anesthetic potency. The hydrophilic group shares with the lipophilic group responsibility for anesthetic effect.

The local anesthetics are weak bases and at physiological pHs exist both as the charged cation and the unionized base. The fraction of anesthetic present as the cation or base depends on the pH of the medium and the pKa of the particular anesthetic. The fraction existing as the base increases with alkalosis. The base is essential to penetration of the nerve and surrounding tissues, but once the nerve axon is reached both the base and cation may act to produce anesthesia.

Anesthesia is produced by impairment of the increase in sodium conductance required for depolarization. Solution of the unionized base in the axon membrane may obstruct sodium pores by increasing the lateral pressure within the membrane. Similarly, expansion of the myelin sheath may obstruct sodium access to the nodes of Ranvier. Finally, the cation anesthetic species may compete with calcium for a position at the gate to the sodium channel. The cation may displace the calcium and may more firmly hold the gate in place.

QUESTIONS

1. Is there a relationship between the structural characteristics of local anesthetics and those of their site of activity?
2. Lidocaine (pKa = 7.26) is introduced in a solution at pH 7.6. Determine the fraction of the total amount existing as the cation. What effect would acidosis have on this fraction?
3. Comment on the following statement: "The unionized base is the only active local anesthetic species." Illustrate your arguments pro or con by giving specific examples.
4. It has been said that "The molecular basis of the action of local anesthetics and the molecular basis of the generation and transmission of the nerve impulse are but two facets of the same problem." Explain why.

REFERENCES

1. Lofgren, N.: *Studies on Local Anesthetics. Xylocaine: A New Synthetic Drug.* Hoeggstroms, Stockholm, 1948.
2. Moore, J. W., and Narahashi, T.: Tetrodotoxin's highly selective blockage of an ionic channel. Fed. Proc. 26: 1655–1663, 1967.
3. Büchi, J., and Perlia, X.: Beziehungen Zwischen den physikalischchemischen Eigenschaffen und der Wirkung von Lokalanästhetica. Arzneimittel-Forsch. 10: 1–8, 1960.
4. de Jong, R. H.: *Physiology and Pharmacology of Local Anesthesia*, p. 75. Charles C Thomas, Springfield, Ill., 1970.
5. Parrott, E. L.: *Pharmaceutical Technology, Fundamental Pharmaceutics*, p. 219. Burgess, Minneapolis, 1970.
6. Eckenstam, B. T.: The effect of the structural variation on the local anesthetic properties on the most commonly used groups of substances. Acta Anaesth. Scand. Suppl. XXV: 10, 1966.
7. Gros, O.: Über Narkotika und Lokalanästhetika. Arch. Exp. Path. Pharmakol. 62: 380–408, 1910.
8. Gros, O.: Über die Narkotika und Lokalanästhetika. Arch. Exp. Path. Pharmakol. 63: 80–106, 1910.

9. Trevan, J. W., and Boock, E.: The relation of hydrogen ion concentration to the action of the local anesthetics. Brit. J. Exp. Path. 8: 307–315, 1927.
10. Skou, J. C.: Local anesthetics. The blocking potencies of some local anesthetics and of butyl alcohol determined on peripheral nerves. Acta Pharmacol. (Kobenhavn) 10: 281–291, 1954.
11. Krahl, M. E., Keltch, A. K., and Clowes, G. H. A.: The role of changes extracellular and intracellular hydrogen ion concentration on the action of local anesthetic bases. J. Pharmacol. Exp. Ther. 68: 330–350, 1940.
12. Ritchie, J. M., and Greengard, P.: On the active structure of local anesthetics. J. Pharmacol. Exp. Ther. 133: 241–245, 1961.
13. Ehrenberg, L.: The time-concentration curve of local anesthetics. Acta Chem. Scand. 2: 63–81, 1948.
14. Cohen, E. N., Levine, D. A., Colliss, J. E., and Gunther, R. E.: The role of pH in the development of tachyphylaxis to local anesthetic agents. Anesthesiology 29: 994–1001, 1968.
15. Ritchie, J. M., and Ritchie, B. R.: Local anesthetics: Effect of pH on activity. Science 162: 1394–1395, 1968.
16. Taylor, R. E.: Effect of procaine on electrical properties of squid axon membrane. Amer. J. Physiol. 196: 1071–1078, 1959.
17. Shanes, A. M., Freygang, W. H., Grundfesh, H., and Amatniek, E.: Anesthetic and calcium ion in the voltage clamped squid giant axon. J. Gen. Physiol. 42: 793–802, 1959.
18. Hille, B.: Common mode of action of three agents that decrease the transient change in sodium permeability in nerves. Nature 210: 1220–1222, 1966.
19. Condouris, G. A.: A study on the mechanism of action of cocaine on amphibian peripheral nerve. J. Pharmacol. Exp. Ther. 131: 243–249, 1961.
20. Condouris, G. A., and Lagomarsino, W. E.: Adrenalectomy in rats and its influence on local anesthesia of peripheral nerves. J. Pharmacol. Exp. Ther. 152: 417–424, 1966.
21. Blanstein, M. P., and Goldman, D. E.: Action of amionic and cationic nerve-blocking agents: Experiment and interpretation. Science 153: 429–432, 1966.
22. Blanstein, M. P., and Goldman, D. E.: Competitive action of calcium and procaine on lobster axon. A study of the mechanism of action of certain local anesthetics. J. Gen. Physiol. 49: 1043–1063, 1966.
23. Frankenhauser, B., and Hodgkin, A. L.: The action of calcium on the electrical properties of squid axons. J. Physiol. 137: 218–244, 1957.
24. Tasaki, I.: *Nervous Transmission.* Charles C Thomas, Springfield, 1953.
25. Skou, J. C.: Local anesthetics. V. The action of local anesthetics on monomolecular layers of stearic acid. Acta Pharmacol. (Kobenhavn) 10: 317–324, 1954.
26. Skou, J. C.: Local anesthetics. VI. Relation between blocking potency and penetration of a monomolecular layer of lipoids from nerves. Acta Pharmacol. (Kobenhavn) 10: 325–337, 1954.
27. Shanes, A. M., and Gershfeld, N. L.: Interactions of veratrum alkaloids, procaine, and calcium with monolayers of stearic acid and their implications for pharmacological action. J. Gen. Physiol. 44: 345–363, 1960.
28. Clements, J. A., and Wilson, K. M.: Interactions of narcotic agents with spread lipid and protein films. *Int. Anesth. Clin.* 1: 969–976, 1963.
29. Feinstein, M. B.: Reaction of local anesthetics with phospholipids. A possible chemical basis for anesthesia. J. Gen. Physiol. 48: 357–374, 1964.

Chapter 21

Local Anesthetic Absorption, Distribution and Elimination

M. ROWLAND

Local anesthesia is the reversible diminution of sensation in restricted areas of the body caused by blockade of axonal impulse conduction. Four variables characterize local anesthesia: 1) the time from administration of the agent to blockade of the nerve action potential (time of onset); 2) the degree of completeness of blockade; 3) the duration of blockade; and 4) recovery from blockade. In a nerve isolated *in vitro* these variables are readily assessed by changes in the amplitude of the nerve action potential. They are influenced by several factors including the dissociation constant and lipophilicity of the agent, the ionic composition (including pH) of the solution bathing the nerve and the type (myelinated versus nonmyelinated) and size of the nerve fiber. *In vivo*, where anesthesia is assessed by loss of sensation, the situation is further complicated by the anatomy and perfusion of the nerve bundle and adjacent tissue. Anesthetic which is injected near a nerve bundle must diffuse through connective tissue and cross a variety of cell membranes to reach its site(s) of action. In doing so, the injected material also passes into the numerous capillaries traversing the nerve and adjacent tissues. Together these additional factors profoundly influence the anesthetic concentration profile at the neuronal sites.

Eventually, all the agent is removed from the injection site by vascular absorption. Initially, the rate of drug absorption into the general circulation exceeds its distribution and elimination, via metabolism and excretion. The result is a rising blood concentration which may be sufficiently high to elicit systemic pharmacological effects and even toxicity. Eventually the rate of distribution and elimination exceeds systemic absorption and thereafter the anesthetic blood level declines.

This chapter will examine how each of the above factors influence the four variables that characterize local anesthesia. As with the inhaled anesthetics, we will begin with a description of a local anesthetic "MAC." Such a description is essential to an understanding of the relationship between the dose of agent injected and the effect achieved. It is also a prerequisite to any comparison of agents.

The Minimum Anesthetic Concentration

A Definition

Local anesthesia is achieved when the *minimum anesthetizing* (*blocking*) *concentration* (C_m) of local anesthetic is exceeded within an axon. C_m should be expressed as "activity" rather than concentration, but this is rarely done because of the difficulty in measuring activity (1). Activity of a local anesthetic is comparable to the partial pressure of an inhaled anesthetic. Like any other molecule, local anesthetics travel down activity rather than concentration gradients. This concept may be appreciated by considering the partition of a drug between an aqueous and lipid phase. At equilibrium, the concentration ratio (partition coefficient) between the lipid and aqueous phase may be 100. Despite this high concentration gradient, net transfer is zero because the activity of the drug in both phases is equal. Conversely, were the concentrations equal, the activity in the aqueous phase would be 100 times greater than the activity in the lipid phase and drug would move from water to lipid.

Limitations of in Vivo C_m Determination

Of necessity, C_m is assessed as the concentration of anesthetic agent in the administered solution rather than that at the neural site. Although such an assessment is clinically useful, the C_m determined in this manner is highly dependent upon the concentration gradient developed between the site of administration and the nerve, and so may be profoundly influenced by mode and site of injection, rate of injection, spreading, removal by blood and diffusion barriers created by fibrous tissue surrounding the nerve. Accordingly, in those studies where C_m is used to assess the intrinsic potency of a local anesthetic it is best determined by exposing an isolated nerve to a fixed concentration of agent under equilibrium conditions (2). However, equilibrium may take many hours by which time the preparation may no longer be viable. As a compromise, de Jong (3) has suggested a contact time of 10 minutes which should give values of C_m which are both clinically and experimentally useful.

Factors Influencing C_m

Wide variations in C_m exist among anesthetic agents. C_m decreases from procaine through lidocaine and tetracaine to dibucaine (table 21, 1). Even for a single local anesthetic, C_m varies with pH or ionic changes. For example, an increase in pH lowers C_m (Chapter 20). Hyponatremia achieved by a deficiency in the patient or by the injection of solutions lacking sodium also lowers C_m. That is, hyponatremia increases the potency of local anesthetics (5, 6) and progressive hyponatremia itself may produce a differential block (7). Higher concentrations of all local anesthetics and procaine at all concentrations are deficient in sodium (table 21, 2). This deficiency should augment the anesthetic effect of these agents. The effect of a reduced sodium concentration is to decrease the nerve action potential by decreasing the number of sodium ions available for diffusion through sodium channels. This, of course, parallels the effect of local anesthetics to reduce the number or function of available sodium channels. Similarly, an increase in calcium should augment the effect of local anesthetics, since both act to prevent the opening of the sodium channels (8).

C_m is greater in larger nerves (9, 10). This results from the constancy of the number of ions transferred per unit volume of axon during depolarization (11). Since the ratio of surface to volume is smaller in a larger

TABLE 21, 1*

Local Anesthetic	C_m	C_m
	mM/liter	% solution
Procaine	8.0	0.22
Lidocaine	2.5	0.07
Tetracaine	0.6	0.02
Dibucaine	0.2	0.01

* These are the concentrations which reduce the frog sciatic nerve action potential by 50 percent in 10 minutes (4).

TABLE 21, 2

The sodium content and pH (37°) of some commercial local anesthetic preparations

Preparation	Concentration	Sodium	pH
	%	*mEq/liter*	
Lidocaine hydrochloride (Astra)	0.5	138	6.52
	1.0	121	6.69
	2.0	103	6.73
Lidocaine hydrochloride + epinephrine (1 in 200,000) (Astra)	0.5	143	3.45
	1.0	126	3.55
	2.0	108	3.45
Prilocaine hydrochloride (Astra)	1.0	103	6.58
	2.0	103	6.59
Procaine hydrochloride (Invenex)	1.0	113	3.32
	2.0	76	3.32
Mepivacaine hydrochloride (Winthrop)	1.0	114	5.95
	1.5	97	5.94
	2.0	86	5.84
Bupivacaine hydrochloride (Winthrop)	0.25	144	5.2
Nupercaine hydrochloride (Ciba)	0.66	100	7.1

nerve, this implies a greater number of sodium channels per unit surface area in a larger nerve. To obtain a roughly constant proportion of anesthetic molecules to sodium channels thus requires an increased concentration of anesthetic. This line of reasoning also explains the greater C_m in myelinated than nonmyelinated fibers of the same size, since in myelinated nerves all the biologically active sodium channels are concentrated at the nodes of Ranvier (12). An additional reason for a difference in C_m is related to size and myelination. Larger myelinated nerves can conduct over larger distances (up to 5 mm) without regeneration of impulses because their internodal distance is greater (13, 14). This means that a longer axon segment must be anesthetized to block nerve conduction.

Since anesthetic potency is inversely related to the diameter of an axon, the concentration producing extinction of all impulse propagation in a nerve bundle must be the C_m of the largest myelinated axons. However, we may wish C_m only to be that concentration which prevents the passage of pain impulses. It would appear that pain sensation is conducted through two types of fibers. The A-delta fiber is a 3 to 4 micron diameter myelinated fiber which rapidly conducts the perception of pain. The C-fiber is a small (approximately 1 micron) unmyelinated fiber which permits a delayed perception of pain (15). Both fibers are considerably smaller than the largest (about 20 micron) A-alpha fiber which is purely motor. From the previous discussion it is obvious that the C-fiber and the A-delta fiber will be blocked at a lower concentration of anesthetic than the fiber conducting the impulses to muscle. Hence, by a judicious choice of local anesthetic concentration, it is possible to prevent pain without blocking motor function. It is noteworthy that although the above reasoning predicts a difference, in fact, A-delta and C-fibers have about the same C_m (16).

Wedensky Block

Nerve block extends the refractory period and elevates the firing threshold (10). At concentrations slightly less than C_m a single impulse may not be transmitted but may reduce the transmembrane resting potential sufficiently to allow a closely spaced successive impulse to elevate the membrane potential above the increased threshold and initiate depolarization (17). Thus, a weak stimulus (such as a pin prick) which produces only a few intermittent impulses might not be felt, whereas a strong stimulus (such as an incision) which produces many frequent impulses would be perceived—albeit as an attenuated signal. This phenomenon, known as the Wedensky block, indicates that C_m has not been exceeded.

Kinetics of Nerve Block

Induction of Block

Potential damage precludes injection of local anesthetic into a nerve bundle (18). Drug, therefore, is deposited near the nerve and moves radially into the nerve and surrounding tissue. Three elements influence the effectiveness of the local anesthetic. First, there is mass movement of the injected solution to a position around the nerve—and, of course, mass movement at the same time away from the nerve. Second, the anesthetic diffuses through the various barriers betwixt it and the axons to be blocked—diffusion away from the nerve, of course, occurs at the same time. And third, concomitant to both mass movement and diffusion, the local anesthetic is absorbed by the blood or metabolized (procaine) via local hydrolysis. The latter effect probably is of minimal importance (19).

The anesthetic must diffuse through many layers to reach its site of action. Peripheral nerves are surrounded by a sheath which apparently is penetrated easily (20). Although this sheath should not pose a significant barrier to the movement of anesthetic into the nerve, its elimination increases the potency of lidocaine (2, 21). Having crossed the nerve sheath, drug must diffuse through the epineurium, a loose areolar tissue making up about half of the cross-section of the nerve. The epineurium contains nutrient vessels and lymphatics and thus diffusion through this barrier also permits the removal of some anesthetic by uptake into the general circulation. Anesthetic passes from epineurium through the fibroelastic perineurium. The perineurium fastens anywhere from 500 to 1000 fibers into a single strand. Individual fibers within this strand in turn are surrounded by another thin membrane, the endoneurium. The inner layer of perineurium, the perilemma, may be identical with the pia-arachnoid membrane enclosing brain and spinal cord. The perineurium may be one of the main diffusion barriers through which the local anesthetic must pass (22, 23). This description of a peripheral nerve (22) does not apply to spinal nerves since these lack the perineurium and much of the fibrous support (and barrier) provided by the epineurium and nerve sheath. Edema of these structures or hemorrhage or transudation of fluid into the nerve and surrounding tissues may hinder the movement of anesthetic and thereby slow or prevent the development of anesthesia.

Since the initial local anesthetic concentration is higher outside the nerve, conduction block proceeds from mantle (outer) to core (innermost) bundles (figs. 21, 1, 21, 2). Because mantle fibers innervate more proximal regions, and core fibers more distal regions (24), it follows that block proceeds peripherally. For example, in a brachial plexus block, the

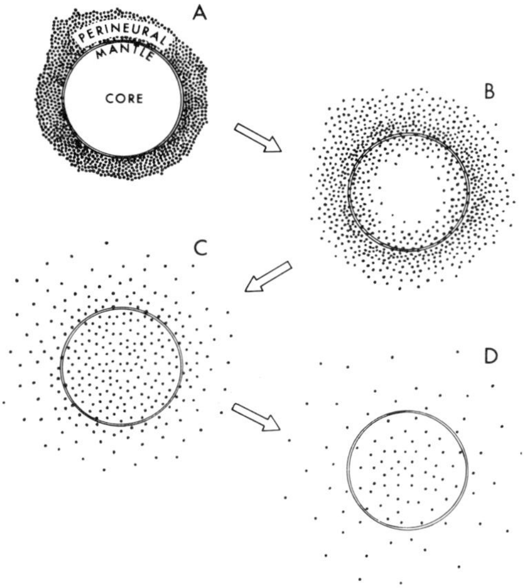

FIG. 21, 1. Immediately following perineural injection, the peripheral nerve (seen here in cross-section) is surrounded by local anesthetic (*black dots* in *A*). Agent then diffuses both inward into nerve and outward into non-neural tissue (*B*). Initially, the highest neural anesthetic concentrations are achieved in the mantle nerve fibers which are closest to the perineural space. The inward diffusion continues until the anesthetic activity in the central (core) fibers equals that in the surrounding mantle (*C*). At the same time, agent continues to diffuse away into adjacent non-neural tissue. This continuing peripheral loss reverses the activity gradient and anesthetic now diffuses from mantle fibers to the perineural space and from core to mantle fibers (*D*). Throughout this entire process, agent is removed by the perfusing blood.

upper arm becomes anesthetized prior to anesthesia of the hand and fingers. As long as the extraneural activity (recall that activity is equivalent to partial pressure) exceeds that in the encircled neural tissue, neural drug levels continue to rise.

The time from anesthetic deposition to complete conduction block is the induction or blocking time (time T_1, fig. 21, 3) and usually is much shorter than the duration of anesthesia. The induction time depends on several variables including the permeability coefficient of the undissociated local anesthetic,* the nerve size (25) (the smaller the diameter, the shorter the induction time), pH and drug concentration. Only the

---

* Permeability coefficient is a direct function of the lipid solubility and an inverse function of the size of the molecule. A smaller or lighter molecule diffuses more rapidly and therefore penetrates more readily. High lipid solubility promotes rapid penetration by facilitating passage through hydrophobic membranes. However, aqueous solubility diminishes as lipid solubility increases. If the local anesthetic molecule is too lipid soluble, the corresponding low aqueous solubility may preclude the attainment of an anesthetizing concentration of agent at the site of action.

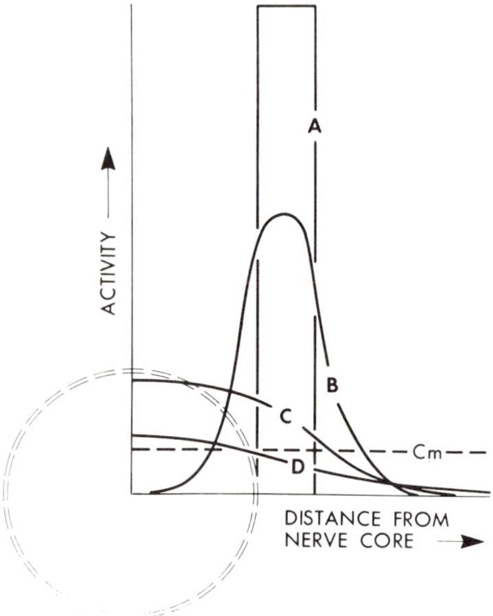

FIG. 21, 2. The activity of local anesthetic (density of black dots in fig. 21, 1) at various distances away from the nerve core after perineural injection is illustrated here as *continuous lines*. Times *A*, *B*, *C* and *D* are the same as those referred to in figure 21, 1. The activity profile becomes shallower and more diffuse with time. During uptake, C_m is exceeded and block occurs first in the mantle (curve at time "*B*") and then core fibers (curve at time "*C*"). During efflux, core fibers are the last to contain anesthetic above C_m (curve at time "*D*").

latter two can be manipulated in practice. As expected, raising the concentration decreases the induction time, and a rough inverse relationship exists between the induction time and the logarithm of the applied concentration (2, 25, 26). Since it is the undissociated base which penetrates the nerve, the induction time is diminished by increasing pH. For example, raising the pH of a lidocaine solution surrounding an intact nerve from 6 to 7.35 shortens the induction time 4 fold (2).

Onset of action usually is slower with anesthetics that are more strongly bound to (highly soluble in) neural components. Thus, using an equipotent solution, the block by the strongly bound tetracaine has a slower onset than that seen with the less extensively bound lidocaine (4, 27, 28). The reason for this difference may be that the stronger binding causes a more marked reduction in activity (i.e., leads to a larger gradient) as the drug moves into the nerve. The driving pressure therefore is more rapidly reduced with the more strongly bound compound (2, 25). This effect is analogous to the greater reduction in partial pressure between the inspired and alveolar tensions of a highly soluble versus a poorly soluble inhaled anesthetic. However, exceptions

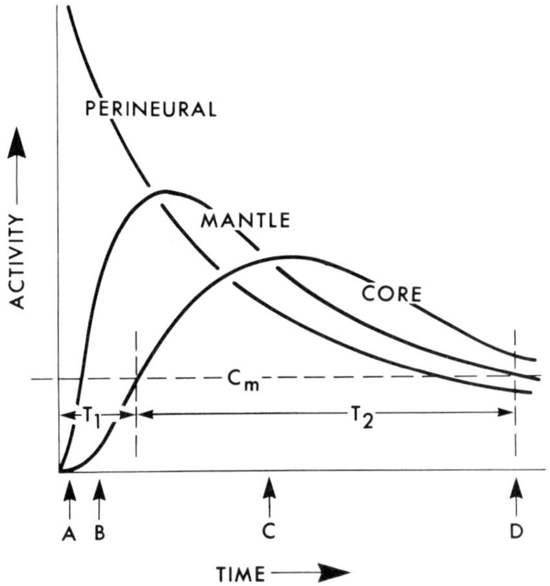

FIG. 21, 3. The events depicted at four separate points in time in figures 21, 1 and 21, 2 are illustrated here as continuous functions. Times *A*, *B*, *C* and *D* refer to the like lettered illustrations in figure 21, 1. The induction time (T_1) is the time required to raise the activity in the core fibers above C_m. The duration of action (T_2) is the time from completion of induction to the time when the activity in the mantle fibers falls below C_m.

to this rule appear to exist for local anesthetics. For example, the more highly bound bupivacaine (5 mM) has a faster onset than lidocaine (20 mM) in isolated nerves (28).

Duration of Action

The duration of action of a local anesthetic is the time from the onset of blockade to the point at which the block becomes ineffective (i.e., the local anesthetic concentration falls below C_m (fig. 21, 3)). It is roughly proportional to the logarithm of the applied concentration (fig. 21, 4). The *in vivo* evaluation of duration is complicated by the different values of C_m for nerve fibers within a nerve bundle. It thus may vary with the block desired. Since the C_m of pain conducting fibers is less than the C_m of the larger, myelinated motor fibers, duration of analgesia will exceed duration of motor paralysis.

To compare the duration of action of different anesthetics requires the use of equiactive rather than equimolar solutions (19). Equiactive concentrations are equal multiples of the C_ms. If equiactive concentrations are administered and if the rate of fall in activity is the same for two drugs, their duration of action should be the same. Differences in

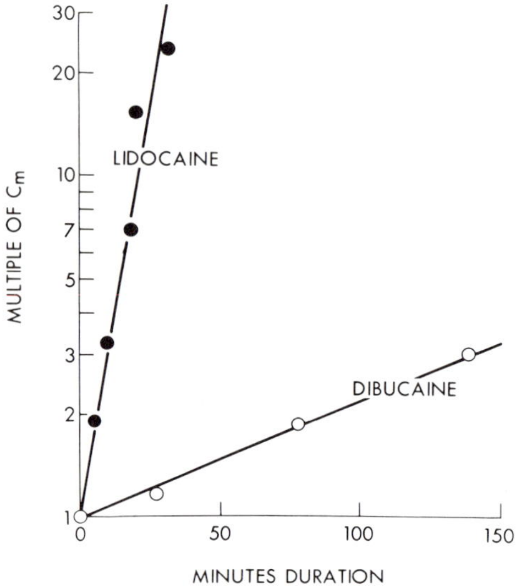

FIG. 21, 4. Duration of spinal anesthesia in the rabbit is directly proportional to the logarithm of the applied concentration, expressed in this case as multiples of C_m. At any given C_m, the duration is dependent on the affinity of the local anesthetic for nerve and adjacent tissue. A greater binding is associated with a greater duration of action, and hence dibucaine is longer acting than lidocaine. (Luduena, F. P.: Experimental spinal anesthesia. Arch. Int. Pharmacodyn. 109: 143–156, 1957.)

duration would indicate differences in the persistence of each of these anesthetics in the neural tissue. A greater persistence would result from a greater solubility of anesthetic in (binding to) neural tissue (fig. 21, 4) (30–32). The larger capacity engendered by a greater solubility would increase the time constant for removal of agent. The effect of solubility also may be thought of in terms of its effect on activity: the two are inversely related and, thus, a greater solubility diminishes the diffusion of drug out of the nerve. A greater persistence of one agent within the nerve also would result if its permeability coefficient was less than the other (2).

In an isolated nerve preparation, the major factors influencing duration of anesthesia are the specific interaction at the receptor site and nonspecific binding to neural tissue. The latter particularly diminishes the diffusional gradients and slows egress of drug from the nerve. Persistence *in vivo* also is affected by changes in local blood flow or capillary permeability induced by the agent or drugs (usually vasoconstrictors) given concomitantly (19, 33). For example, addition of the vasoconstrictor epinephrine to a local anesthetic solution usually prolongs the duration of action (19). Also, prolongation in action of (+) prilocaine, (+) mepivacaine and (−) bupivacaine over their respective optical isomers appears to be associated with an increased vasoconstrictor activity (or to differences in diffusion and binding) of the longer acting isomers rather than differences in C_m (19, 34).

Despite the importance of neural binding to the duration of local anesthesia the data on partition coefficients in nerves or nerve membranes are limited. Local anesthetics appear to be more soluble in nerves than in skin or muscle (35). We do know that the duration of action of local anesthetics correlates with their binding to plasma and erythrocyte proteins. For example, the increasing order of plasma binding of lidocaine, mepivacaine and bupivacaine (fig. 21, 4) parallels their duration of action. Similarly, the shorter acting procaine and lidocaine are less extensively bound to crude heart and brain homogenates than the longer acting dibucaine and tetracaine (4).

An additional factor which influences the duration of anesthesia *in vivo* is the rate of removal of drug from the adjacent extraneural tissue. As anesthetic diffuses into, it also diffuses away from the nerve (figs. 21, 1 to 21, 3). Eventually sufficient anesthetic is lost from perineural to adjacent tissues or is systemically absorbed that the nerve no longer receives but now releases anesthetic. Since the surrounding tissues contain anesthetic the gradient for diffusion away from the nerve is limited, and loss from nerve to other tissues must develop slowly. Diffusion away from the nerve affects the mantle bundles before the core bundles. The first return of sensation or movement, therefore, heralds the fall in local anesthetic concentration below C_m in the mantle fibers. If anesthesia is to be maintained, additional drug must be injected. Small doses rapidly restore blockade as only the outer fibers are deficient in drug and even these fibers contain some anesthetic.

Factors Modifying the Dynamics of Anesthesia

Spreading: The Roles of Mass Movement, Diffusion and Binding

The mass movement or spread of the local anesthetic probably lasts only a few seconds to a minute or two following injection of the drug. Although short-lived, spreading is an important determinant in nerve block. Mass movement is influenced by the volume of solution injected a well as by the character of the tissue at the injection site. A large volume predisposes to a greater spread and encirclement of the nerves to be blocked. Similarly, injection into a loose areolar tissue or into spinal fluid promotes the movement of local anesthetic. However, surprisingly, the extent of segmental spread of epidural analgesia depends upon the mass of lidocaine rather than on the volume of solvent (36).

Injecting a larger volume of a given dose of anesthetic (as is often done close to a peripheral nerve or into the epidural space) exposes a greater number of nerve fibers, nonspecific binding sites and blood capillaries to a more dilute solution. The concentration of anesthetic agent in this dilute solution may be barely sufficient to reach C_m in the nerve, with the result that induction of a more diffuse block is delayed and duration of action is decreased.

Like other small, lipid soluble molecules, local anesthetics probably equilibrate between tissue and blood (i.e., have the same activity in both) by the time blood leaves the tissue. At concentrations well below and well above the capacity of tissue binding sites the activity of local anesthetic in the tissue water changes proportionally with concentration, i.e., the fraction of agent not bound to tissue components remains constant and independent of concentration. Then the spread of local anesthetic would not be expected to change the overall rate of systemic absorption since any dilution is matched by a corresponding increase in the number of capillaries available for removal of agent. Supporting these considerations, 1 and 2 percent prilocaine produce the same blood levels if the same total dose is given in each case (37). Similarly, no difference in blood levels appears when the same dose of lidocaine is injected intramuscularly over a 30 fold concentration range (38).

The above conclusions do not apply when the local anesthetic concentration in the tissue is near the capacity of the tissue binding sites. Then the fraction of the molecules unbound (activity) in tissue increases disproportionally with increasing anesthetic concentration (see fig. 21, 8). Accordingly, there is a more rapid loss of agent via diffusion into blood and adjacent non-neural tissue with the more concentrated anesthetic. Perhaps this reasoning explains why the rate of absorption of mepivacaine is greater from a 2 than 1 percent solution in patients receiving the same total dose (500 mg) in each case (39). Also, since loss is less rapid with dilute solutions, a decrease in anesthetic concentration should not produce a proportional decrease in duration of anesthesia. Supporting this argument, duration of anesthesia is but slightly decreased upon going from a 2 percent to 1 percent solution of mepivacaine (39).

As with perineural anesthesia, peridural anesthesia is influenced by diffusion and spreading. Anesthesia may result from diffusion of a small (10 percent) fraction of the peridural dose across the meninges and into the subarachnoid space (40, 41). Diffusion across the entire dural membrane may occur or anesthetic may cross into the subarachnoid space through the arachnoid villi that pierce the dura in the region about the nerve roots (42). These villi are more readily traversed than the dura because they are thinner and therefore present less of a diffusion barrier (43). In addition, the villi possess pores which may allow the bulk transfer of anesthetic from the epidural to the subarachnoid space (42). Subarachnoid anesthetic concentrations equaling or exceeding C_m are achieved during peridural anesthesia (44, 45). The moderate delay (15 to

30 minutes) for complete surgical anesthesia to develop following a peridural injection (42, 46) suggests that penetration is slow since anesthetic in the sinal fluid acts on the uncovered spinal nerves almost as rapidly as on a desheathed nerve. However, diffusion into the subarachnoid space fails to explain the segmental analgesia sometimes achieved with peridural injections (44). Perhaps in addition to the passage into spinal fluid, peridural anesthetic moves via the dural sheaths and intervertebral foramina to act directly on the spinal nerves where they pierce the dura.

Subarachnoid blocks are greatly affected by spreading. The location and extent of the block can be restricted by utilizing solutions whose specific gravity differs from cerebrospinal fluid. Mixing between this fluid and the injected solution is sufficiently slow that extensive sensory blockage with lesser or no motor block in a supine patient may be achieved with a higher density (hyperbaric) solution which moves posteriorly in the lighter cerebrospinal fluid. Manipulation of the patient's position also will affect localization of the anesthetic within the subarachnoid space.

Hydrogen Ion Concentration

Any factor which diminishes systemic absorption will, by maintaining the concentration of local anesthetic at the injection site, enhance spreading and aid in a more rapid, intense and longer duration of action. Systemic absorption is most profoundly affected by pH and blood flow at the site of administration. By increasing the unionized species and hence the penetration of anesthetic, an elevation in pH of the injected solution increases the depth and rapidity of onset of local anesthesia. However, although alkalinization is desirable on pharmacological grounds, the free base often is unstable and possesses low aqueous solubility, and hence local anesthetics usually are prepared as the water soluble hydrochloride salt. Being the salt of a strong acid and weak local anesthetic base such solutions are acidic (pH 4 to 5), although the pH of many commercial preparations has been adjusted to between 6 and 7. Those solutions containing the more labile procaine and epinephrine are stabilized by adjusting the pH closer to 3 (table 21, 2).

The buffer capacity of most tissues and the blood perfusing them usually is sufficient to rapidly restore the *in vivo* pH of a local anesthetic solution to near normal (47). Since C_m increases as the pH falls, without restoration of normal pH the effectiveness of local anesthetic preparations would be compromised (see Chapter 20). Several factors may act to limit or even oppose the achievement of a normal pH in the area to be anesthetized. For example, a pH of 5 or 6 may exist in an infected area and this acidic environment may preclude any local anesthetic effect

(48). Another example is the tachyphylaxis which may follow repeated administration (49–51) particularly in the intrathecal or epidural space. Both spaces are relatively poorly perfused and lack protein buffering. Bicarbonate moves slowly from blood into the spinal fluid, thereby limiting its ability to contribute as a hydrogen ion acceptor. Tachyphylaxis may arise from the inadequately buffered reduction in pH of the acidic local anesthetic solution, with a consequent preponderance of the poorly permeable ionized species (52). Favoring this hypothesis is the observation, in the dog, that the pH of the cerebrospinal fluid fell from 7.4 to 6.8 with repeated spinal injections at 90 minute intervals of either lidocaine or procaine hydrochloride solution (fig. 21, 5). The shift in pH substantially reduces the percent of free base and consequently decreases the concentration of anesthetic at the site of action. The acidification also appears to lead to accumulation of local anesthetic with repeated injections.

Unfortunately, two observations suggest that the effects of acidosis and repeated administration are not as clear-cut as the above remarks would imply. For example, tolerance to repeated injections of mepivacaine occurs more rapidly than to repeated injections of the same concentration and volume of lidocaine. But the change in the percent of free base with a given change in pH around 7.4 should be greater for lidocaine than for mepivacaine (table 20, 1). Furthermore, one study with repeated injections of lidocaine suggests that the disappearance of lidocaine from the cerebrospinal fluid does not change with time (53).

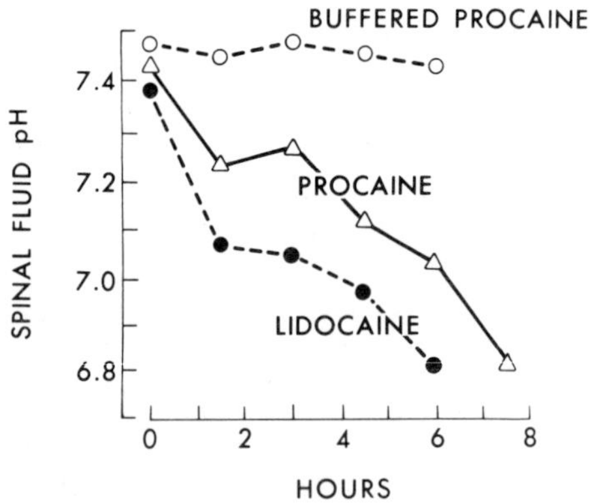

FIG. 21, 5. Intrathecal injection of 1 ml of 2.5 percent unbuffered procaine (pH 4.7) or unbuffered lidocaine (pH 4.5) every 90 minutes produces a progressive decrease in dog spinal fluid pH. This reduction in pH (from 7.4 to 6.8) would reduce the unionized fraction of lidocaine by 69 percent and of procaine by 74 percent (see table 20, 1). Injection of procaine buffered to pH 7.4 with THAM does not alter spinal fluid pH. (Adapted by permission from Cohen, E. N., Levine, D. A., Colliss, J. E., and Gunther, R. E.: The role of pH in the development of tachyphylaxis to local anesthetic agents. Anesthesiology 29: 944–1001, 1968.)

Either any change in pH did not materially alter the rate of vascular absorption, or the disappearance is related more to the capacity of the nervous tissue to absorb agent than to vascular uptake, or that clinically the pH does not change that much.

Injection of a large volume of local anesthetic may produce a dilutional acidosis which opposes the local anesthetic effect (54). Following injection, these solutions quickly equilibriate with and dilute the ambient tissue PCO_2 and also dilute the local tissue stores of bicarbonate. The carbon dioxide is replaced by metabolism. Since the solutions injected normally have little or no buffering capacity, the local increase in the CO_2/bicarbonate ratio produces an acidosis which shifts the equilibrium away from the permeable local anesthetic base.

The local pH changes may be far more complex than implied above. With the exception of the local anesthetic itself, the injected water and salts probably remain outside the cell. Carbon dioxide moves from within the cell to this carbon dioxide deficient solution. This shift would render the extracellular fluid more acidic but at the same time would cause an intracellular alkalosis. The intracellular alkalosis would be progressively reduced as metabolism replaced the transferred carbon dioxide. The above speculation implies that immediately following injection, the relative extracellular acidosis and intracellular alkalosis would limit the intracellular concentration of ionized local anesthetic. As the extracellular compartment received buffer from blood and as intracellular carbon dioxide rose, local anesthetic would move from outside the cell into the cell.

Recall also that most commercial preparations contain the hydrochloride salt of the local anesthetic base. Replacement of hydrochloric acid by carbonic acid should prevent ambient tissue carbon dioxide moving into the injected solution and thereby prevent a reduction in extracellular pH and an increase in intracellular pH. Thus, the onset would be shortened and intensity of block enhanced by administering the carbonated solution of local anesthetic (55, 56). An additional theoretical advantage of the carbonated solutions is that carbon dioxide freely permeates the neuron and can lower the intraneural pH, thereby favoring the intraneuronal formation of the active cationic form (56). This effect is likely fleeting, since the injected carbon dioxide would rapidly diffuse away. Regardless of the cause, clinical data suggest the advantage of carbonation. Carbonated lidocaine produces surgical anesthesia 30 percent faster than an equivalent lidocaine hydrochloride solution and the quality of anesthesia is more intense and reliable (55, 57). While yet to be fully evaluated, these data suggest that carbonated solutions of local anesthetics should have wide clinical application.

It has been suggested that the effect of epinephrine to prolong anesthesia may be related to its ability to reduce local blood flow, and therefore, absorption (19). The reduction in blood flow may have a second effect which is not generally appreciated: it may increase local acidosis. This increase in local acidosis would hinder the removal of anesthesia from the nerve by decreasing the nonionized species and thereby hindering the diffusion of anesthetic from the nerve. It is interesting that addition of epinephrine to a peridural solution reduces the transdural diffusion of anesthetic (40). This would support the hypothesis put forth above that epinephrine causes an acidosis which restricts diffusion. Epinephrine also may increase local cellular metabolism. This would exaggerate the acidosis and further restrict the rate of diffusion of local anesthetic to the capillary.

Solutions commonly used in topical anesthesia are 4 percent lidocaine and 1 percent tetracaine, concentrations far greater than used elsewhere. The need for higher concentrations can be partially attributed to the pH of the drug solutions (5.5 to 6.5) and the low buffering capacity of mucous membranes. These solutions lower the pH in the applied area, thereby maintaining a very low percent of unionized molecules. Of equal or greater importance is the barrier to diffusion presented by the mucous membrane and the rapid removal of agent promoted by high local blood flow (see below). Perhaps the latter factor explains why cocaine, which alone elicits sympathomimetic vasoconstriction (58), is one of the more effective topical anesthetics (59).

Blood Flow and Absorption

Vascular absorption of local anesthetics influences all aspects of the kinetics of nerve block. Induction time is shortened and intensity, duration, recovery time and degree of spreading are increased by lowering perfusion of the injection site. Also, dose requirements may be reduced and systemic effects minimized by slowing absorption. Accordingly, any factor diminishing perfusion at the site of administration is generally regarded favorably when employing local anesthetics.

Vascular absorption of local anesthetics primarily occurs at the capillary. Arteries, arterioles and venuoles also take up some anesthetic (60). Normally, blood flow rather than the capillary wall permeability is the rate limiting step in the absorption process and any increases in blood flow proportionately increase uptake. Thus, lidocaine, procaine and many other local anesthetics may facilitate their own absorption by relaxing vascular smooth muscle (58). In contrast, cocaine elicits a sympathomimetic mediated vasoconstriction.

To reduce the rate of systemic absorption and thereby prolong anesthesia, epinephrine often is added to the local anesthetic solution. Since this effect relates to the duration of action of epinephrine, which in turn relates to its metabolism and absorption, it must be proportionately greater for shorter acting anesthetics. The effect of epinephrine may be compromised by the acidosis produced by epinephrine containing solutions. Epinephrine itself does not alter the pH of the solution. However, to prevent the oxidation of epinephrine, the acidic antioxidant sodium bisulfite is added to commercial solutions which contain epinephrine. As a result, the pH of these solutions is between 3 and 4 (table 21, 2). Approximately the same concentration of sodium bisulfite (10 mEq/liter) is added to stabilize solutions of procaine without epinephrine. The ability of the tissue buffer reserve and perfusing blood to cope with this additional acid load is aggrevated by the retention of CO_2 and acid metabolites associated with the epinephrine induced localized ischemia (61–63). Thus, injection of local anesthetic solution acidified to pH 3 lowers tissue pH below 7.0 for 45 minutes, but the same solution containing epinephrine (1:40,000) may maintain this level of tissue acidosis for 150 to 250 minutes (47). As long as acidosis persists, conversion of the local anesthetic to the unionized amine is limited and anesthesia may be delayed or greater doses of agent may be required to obtain a clinically useful block. The anesthetist can help the body buffers by avoiding the use of the acid containing premixed epinephrine solutions. The same vasoconstrictor effect may be obtained by adding concentrated epinephrine to normal commercial anesthetic preparations just prior to administration. The amount of concentrated epinephrine added contains negligible amounts of sodium bisulfite (63).

The rate of local anesthetic absorption is a function of both route and site of administration. Intravenous injection produces the highest but most rapidly falling blood levels. The injection into muscle produces a lower, and subcutaneous injection the lowest blood levels (64). Absorption from topical sites varies with the site, being rapid from the trachea and slow from the oropharynx (65), probably because much of a dose applied topically to the oropharynx is swallowed.

Despite the penetration of local anesthetics into the spinal cord, apparently little local anesthetic is picked up per unit time from the subarachnoid space. Perineural injection apparently results in absorption as rapid as that from an intramuscular injection (64). Similarly, intercostal and periplexus absorption is rapid (65). Absorption from the peridural space appears to be biphasic: a fast phase followed by a slow phase. The contribution of the fast phase to the overall absorption process is greater with shorter acting agents. Early absorption of prilocaine is greater than lidocaine; lidocaine absorption is greater than mepivacaine; and mepivacaine greater than bupivacaine (Tucker, G., personal communication). This effect probably applies to perineural as well as to peridural uptake.

Absorption from the subarachnoid or peridural spaces is of particular importance, since they are frequent sites of anesthetic injection. Both blood flow and anatomic channels produced by the paravertebral foraminae constitute the main exit from these spaces. Limitation in blood flow either induced with epinephrine or by anatomic changes such as those brought about by disease or aging markedly delay absorption (44, 66). Thus, in the young the peridural cavity is richly perfused and the paravertebral foraminae are patent, thereby allowing rapid egress of anesthetic. Accordingly, infants and teenagers usually require higher doses per unit body weight to achieve the same degree of block as in more elderly patients (it is not known whether C_m itself is altered by age). The decreased vascular perfusion and closure of the foraminae in the elderly also probably accounts for a portion of the increased duration and greater spread of peridural anesthesia in the aged (46, 66, 67). Similarly, a diminished perfusion may explain the increased duration of anesthesia in shock (68, 69) and the exaggerated extradural spread of local anesthesia exhibited by arteriosclerotic patients (70). The peridural space is contracted by the presence of enlarged blood vessels in the pregnant patient at term and such patients usually require a smaller peridural dose and the degree of spreading is greater. However, the increased perfusion of the peridural space ensures a more rapid absorption than in the nonpregnant patient (71).

Local anesthesia and epinephrine may indirectly affect the duration of anesthesia by influencing tissue perfusion pressures. If the anesthetic causes loss of local control of blood flow, then tissue perfusion (removal of drug) is directly related to blood pressure. Epidural or spinal anesthesia blockade may reduce arterial pressure (72, 73), particularly in the elderly or hypovolemic (74) patient, and thereby prolong anesthesia. These hemodynamic changes appear to be primarily related to sympathetic blockade (73). However, assuming they cause equal drops in blood pressure, spinal block lasts some 2 to 3 times longer than peridural block, suggesting that other factors enter into the picture. Systemically absorbed epinephrine (or vasopressors) increase arterial pressure (75) and potentially could thereby shorten anesthesia. Instead, anesthesia is prolonged, demonstrating that the systemic effect is overridden by the local effects of epinephrine.

Systemic Considerations

Distribution

Removal of local anesthetic from the body depends upon its absorption into the bloodstream and the subsequent transport to the organs of elimination, primarily the liver. In this discussion of the disposition of local anesthetics we will use lidocaine (76–78) as representative of local anesthetics in general. Data on other drugs will be compared and contrasted where available. Figure 21, 6 gives the predicted fraction of lidocaine in various tissues with time in normal man, following an intravenous injection. The predictions assume that equilibrium partition coefficients (table 21, 3) obtained from tissue and blood analyses in the rhesus monkey following long-term lidocaine infusions are independent of concentration and apply equally to man. They also presume a

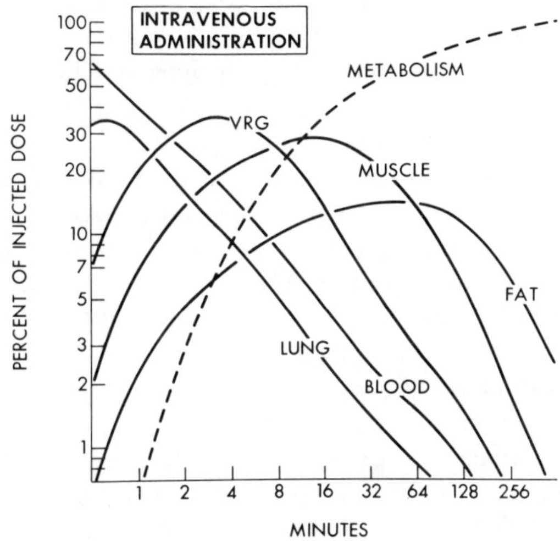

FIG. 21, 6. An appreciable fraction of an intravenous bolus of lidocaine is temporarily sequestered in lung. After passage through the lung, agent is distributed to the tissues in proportion to each tissues' share of the cardiac output. Accordingly, the vessel rich group (VRG) equilibrates first (reaches its peak concentration earliest), muscle next and fat last. Following equilibration with any given tissue, anesthetic returns from that tissue to blood where it is redistributed to organs which have yet to reach equilibrium. Throughout and beyond the time for equilibrium with all tissues, hepatic metabolism of lidocaine results in the loss of anesthetic from the body. The rate of loss is greatest immediately after injection since at this time the apparent volume of lidocaine distribution is least and the liver has access to a greater fraction of the anesthetic remaining within the body.

TABLE 21, 3

Lidocaine partition coefficients in the rhesus monkey

Tissue	Partition Coefficient
Blood	1
Lung	5.4
Liver	2.9
Brain	1.7
Other VRG	2.9
Muscle	0.92
Fat	2.9
VPG	0.84

perfusion limited model without diffusion limitations. The accuracy of the model is suggested by the agreement of prediction with *in vivo* data for lidocaine following intravenous administration in man (79).

The high arterial concentration which immediately follows the rapid intravenous injection of lidocaine is limited by lung uptake. The tissue/blood partition coefficient of the lungs allows this organ to momentarily sequester a major fraction of the intravenous dose and prevents other organs, especially the brain, from receiving the higher peak mixed venous drug concentrations. Calculations suggest that approximately 30 percent of the dose lodges in the lungs in the first minute (77).

Like other amines, lidocaine partitions into the vessel rich group (brain, liver, kidney and mesentery) (table 21, 3). Within 5 minutes these organs achieve maximal concentration and together are primarily responsible for the initial rapid fall in arterial concentration. Following this time the vessel rich group returns lidocaine to the blood. After 10 minutes the concentration in these organs closely follows the fall in the arterial concentration. These events explain the early but transient central nervous effects of lidocaine following an intravenous bolus. The rapid fall in the blood concentration following intravenously administered doses of prilocaine, procaine and tetracaine also indicates a considerable early extravascular uptake of these amines.

Although the partition coefficient of lidocaine is higher in fat than muscle (table 21, 3), the difference in perfusion ensures that redistribution from the vessel rich tissues primarily results in movement into muscle. By 15 minutes, the amount in the muscle is maximum and is 2 ½ times as great as the amount in adipose tissue. Correcting for the amount of drug eliminated by 15 minutes (35 percent of the injected dose), these tissues, respectively, contain 45 and 18 percent of the drug remaining in the body. After 15 minutes, muscle releases lidocaine to blood and thence to fat and to the organs effecting elimination. After 2 hours the majority of the drug remaining in the body resides in fat. By that time, the liver has cleared 77 percent of the injected dose.

The liver removes 70 percent of the lidocaine brought to it in the hepatic blood flow (80). Clearance of this amine essentially is limited by hepatic blood flow unless the enzymes degrading lidocaine become saturated. Analogous to the situation with thiopental, *in vivo* evidence suggests that hepatic metabolism plays a significant role in the fall of blood concentrations in the first 20 minutes following intravenous injection.

Injection into the region surrounding a peripheral nerve alters the time course of the concentration changes in blood and tissues (fig. 21, 7), but the general pattern is similar to that which follows an intravenous

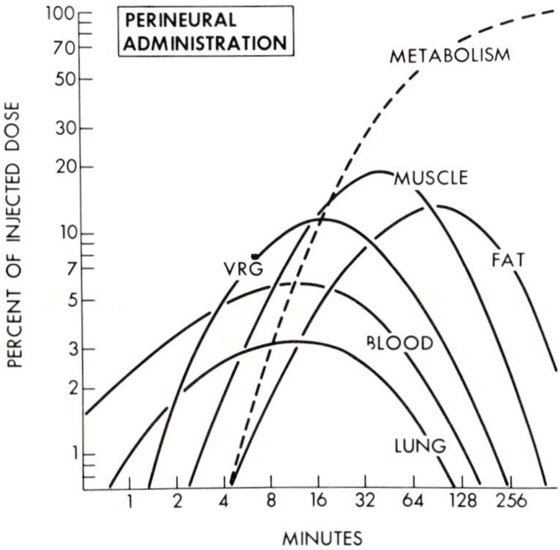

FIG. 21, 7. The uptake and distribution of lidocaine after perineural injection follows the same general pattern as uptake and distribution after an intravenous injection (fig. 21, 6). The two patterns differ in that the perineural injection delays the entry of anesthetic into the systemic circulation. As a result, the peak tissue levels are shifted to the right and are somewhat decreased. The decrease is particularly apparent for the VRG where the peak level following perineural injection is one-third the level following intravenous injection. The decrease is of considerable importance in the avoidance of toxic effects.

injection. Blood flow to the injected site is assumed to be 3 ml/100 gm of tissue/minute, and with a partition coefficient of 0.9 gives a time constant of 30 minutes. Since anesthetic is absorbed over a period of time, the peak concentration in blood, and thus in vessel rich tissues, is much lower than after intravenous injection. However, the maximum fraction of drug in the less vascular muscle and fat differ only slightly from the maximum following intravenous injection.

Lidocaine readily passes into the brain or across the placenta (81). Thus, central nervous effects appear immediately after an intravenous bolus of lidocaine, and fetal toxicity is a potential problem with peridural or pericervical anesthesia for delivery. During pericervical anesthesia the concentration of local anesthetic in umbilical vein blood may exceed that found in maternal blood (60). This apparently anomalous result stems from the injection of agent about the uterine arteries. Anesthetic agents can diffuse across arterial walls and by this route produce high concentrations in the intervillous placental space.

Protein and Tissue Binding

The relative binding by plasma versus tissue components determines the partition of local anesthetics between plasma and tissue. The tissue/plasma partition coefficient of lidocaine ranges from about 1 to 5. Bupivacaine binding to human plasma is greater than mepivacaine which in turn is greater than lidocaine (29). Despite this, the whole blood concentrations following administration of equivalent intravenous doses of mepivacaine and bupivacaine are the same as those following lidocaine, suggesting that although the tissue binding of these first two local anesthetics is greater than lidocaine the partition coefficients of all three agents are approximately equal.

Albumin, which binds many acidic drugs may be partially responsible for the binding of local anesthetics in plasma (82). Another plasma binding factor may be lipoproteins such as those present in membranes. The order of binding of lidocaine, mepivacaine and bupivacaine to plasma is similar to erythrocytic components (28) and it is interesting to speculate that the same order of binding exists at the site of action. Certainly, duration of action of these local anesthetics is in the order of their binding.

The fraction of unbound local anesthetic in plasma increases over the range (1 to 20 mcg/ml) of clinically achieved plasma concentrations (fig. 21, 8). That is, plasma binding sites may approach saturation. This is of moment since the unbound concentration is probably related to activity and therefore is more likely to be closely linked to the development of toxic effects. Plasma lidocaine concentrations normally seen in clinical practice lie between 1 and 4 mcg/ml where approximately 30 percent is free drug. Toxicity appears at levels exceeding 6 to 10 mcg/ml where the free fraction approaches 40 percent.

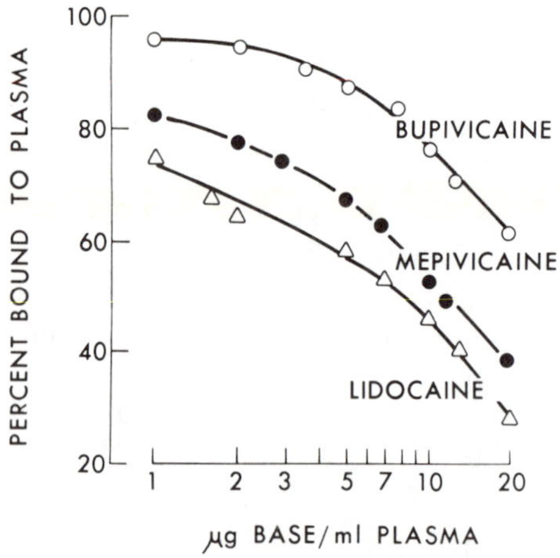

FIG. 21, 8. The fraction of anesthetic bound to plasma protein decreases as concentration increases. (Adapted with permission from Tucker, G. T., Boyes, R. N., Bridenbaugh, P. O., and Moore, D. C.: Binding of anilide-type local anesthetics in human plasma. Anesthesiology 33: 287–303, 1970.)

Elimination

All commonly used local anesthetics are rapidly cleared from the blood by biotransformation (38, 83–85). Renal excretion of unchanged local anesthetics is minor. The older local anesthetics (procaine, tetracaine) are esters which are hydrolyzed enzymatically to the acid and amino alcohol in liver and other tissues. The enzyme responsible for plasma hydrolysis of procaine appears to be pseudocholinesterase (86, 87). While some hydrolysis of procaine or the newer, more rapidly hydrolyzed, 2-chloroprocaine occurs at the site of injection, this property does not significantly affect duration of action. Thus, addition of epinephrine to 2-chloroprocaine increases the duration of intradermal anesthesia, suggesting the greater importance of systemic absorption to the termination of the anesthetic effect (19).

Anilide types which include lidocaine and the more long-acting mepivacaine and bupivacaine drugs are metabolized by the liver. With none of these drugs is metabolism of importance to the duration of nerve blockage. Although the two orthosubstituted methyl groups sterically hinder and stabilize the lidocaine amide bond against hydrolysis by either strong acid or strong base *in vitro*, lidocaine is rapidly cleared by the liver *in vivo* (76, 80). Dissociation of the drug-plasma complex is extremely rapid and does not limit metabolism. The hepatic extraction of lidocaine is so high (0.7) (80) that only between 25 to 50 percent of an orally administered dose enters the systemic circulation intact, despite rapid and complete absorption from the gastrointestinal tract (78). Thus, an oral dose of 500 mg produces plasma levels of less than 1 mcg/ml. In contrast, these levels are seen for over 30 minutes when only 100 mg are administered as an intravenous bolus (76).

If the activity of the injected lidocaine were the same in all body tissues, for each 100 mg in the body the concentration of lidocaine in blood would increase by 1 mcg/ml (76). Together with a knowledge of the elimination half-life (90 to 120 minutes (76–78)), this information allows us to assess the likelihood of reaching a certain concentration in blood in healthy patients following a given schedule of lidocaine. Thus, despite the peridural administration of 120 mg of lidocaine every 30 minutes, the concentration in blood would never exceed 5 mcg/ml, i.e., 500 mg in the body. Systemic toxicity is unlikely at this concentration (88).

Systemic toxic responses may result from "usual" doses in patients with hemodynamic dysfunction (88). Poor peripheral perfusion limits redistribution to muscle and fat, and therefore restricts a greater fraction of the dose to the vessel rich group, including the heart and brain. Furthermore, hepatic blood flow may be seriously compromised in this group and hepatic removal of lidocaine accordingly reduced. These factors would allow plasma and hence heart and brain levels to rise considerably higher during continuous or repeated injection of local anesthetic. This may explain in part the poor tolerance of patients with myocardial disease, especially those in congestive heart failure, to local anesthetic administered intravenously (88).

Despite its extensive use, the metabolism of lidocaine and the contribution of its metabolites to its systemic effects is incompletely understood. The dizziness associated with large (500 mg) oral doses cannot be caused by the low lidocaine plasma concentrations. This symptom may result from the high circulating concentrations of metabolites which must follow absorption of the oral dose (89). The metabolism of other amide linked local anesthetics also is not clearly defined, but in some instances may be of clinical importance. For example, information from prilocaine of the phenolic metabolite parahydroxyorthotoluidine formed by rearrangement of a primary metabolite, N-hydroxy O-toluidine, could cause the methemoglobinemia associated with large doses of prilocaine (90). This metabolite is readily oxidized to the quinone. The redox system between the oxidized and reduced form of the quinone can oxidize hemoglobin to methemoglobin and thereby prevents its association with oxygen. This effect is easily reversed with methylene blue which reduces methemoglobin back to hemoglobin (91).

Summary

Local anesthesia is achieved when the minimum anesthetic concentration (C_m) required to block the nerve action potential (NAP) is exceeded within an axon. Since C_m is higher in larger axons, the C_m for a whole nerve is the C_m for the largest (motor) axons. A sensory but not motor block can be produced by administering an anesthetic concentration which just exceeds the C_m for sensory fibers. At C_m, the second of two closely spaced NAPs still may be transmitted (Wedensky block).

Local anesthesia is characterized by the time of onset, intensity and duration of block. These variables are influenced by mass movement of local anesthetic, its diffusion into and away from the nerve bundle and vascular absorption. Bulk spreading (i.e., mass movement) of local anesthetics, aided by dilution, insures a more diffuse and shallower blockade. The perineurium, especially the innermost perilemma, is the major barrier to diffusion of materials into the nerve bundle. Block proceeds from the outer mantle (proximally innervating) to core (distally innervating) nerve fibers. Time of onset of blockade is much shorter than duration. Increasing the applied concentration of anesthetic agent shortens the time of onset and prolongs the duration. Associated with a much shallower activity gradient, both onset and duration of block are longer for more highly bound local anesthetics.

Changes in blood flow and pH alter the persistence of drug at the nerve and thereby influence the dynamics of nerve block. Elevating the pH increases the fraction of the more permeable unionized base, and so hastens onset of anesthesia. Most commercial solutions contain the hydrochloride salt of the anesthetic amine, and are acidic. Normally the tissue buffers plus buffers contained in the blood rapidly neutralize these solutions. Return of tissue (and solution) pH to normal after injection is slower with solutions containing epinephrine especially if rendered acidic with the antioxidant sodium bisulfite. Neutralization may also be diminished upon repeated injections of the anesthetic solution especially into the intrathecal and epidural space where the buffer reserve is low. Tachyphylaxis may be explained partially by this generation of a more acidic solution with repeated injections. Similarly, the diminished effectiveness of repeated injections of a large volume of anesthetic solution may be caused by dilutional extracellular acidosis and intercellular alkalosis. Shorter acting carbonated solutions overcome these effects.

The dynamics of local anesthesia vary markedly with the site of injection, primarily due to differences in vascular perfusion. Perfusion decreases with age and dose requirements vary with age and in altered hemodynamic states. Epinephrine, through vasoconstriction and perhaps by promoting metabolic acidosis, prolongs local anesthesia. The high anesthetic concentrations required for topical anesthesia probably result both from high vascularity, from the presence of a significant diffusional barrier and poor local buffering.

Once systemically absorbed, distribution of local anesthetic into various tissues is governed by tissue perfusion, organ size and solubility between tissue and blood. Local anesthetic amines favorably partition in lungs, kidneys and other vascular rich organs and partition moderately into adipose tissue. Initially, most of the local anesthetic resides in vascular rich organs, but the drug soon moves to muscle and fat. Elimination occurs primarily by hepatic metabolism. Elimination is sufficiently rapid that achievement of systemic toxic concentrations is unlikely with the usual anesthetic doses in normal patients.

QUESTIONS

1. What is the influence of epinephrine on the time for onset of local anesthesia?
2. Should the time between return of peripheral distal recovery to full recovery be different for the short- and long-acting local anesthetics?
3. Why is procaine a moderately good local anesthetic despite a pKa of 8.9?
4. What would be the effect on the onset and intensity of epidural block by replacing 0.5 percent bupivacaine hydrochloride by an equimolar solution of carbonated bupivacaine?

5. Why is bupivacaine relatively short-acting in the subarachnoid space, slightly longer-acting in the epidural space and very long-acting in the peripheral nerve?
6. Will lidocaine or bupivacaine have the largest drop in concentration profile as it enters the nerve?
7. Are the combined properties of a rapid onset and extremely long duration of anesthesia mutually exclusive in a single local anesthetic agent?
8. Why is the time for onset of epidural blockade shorter following an upper lumbar than either an upper thoracic or an upper sacral injection?
9. Does the absence of protein in the cerebrospinal fluid aid or hinder the kinetics of spinal nerve block?

REFERENCES

1. Shanes, A. M.: Electrochemical aspects of physiological and pharmacological action in excitable cells. Pharmacol. Rev. 10: 59–266, 1958.
2. Rud, J.: Local anesthetics: An electrophysiological investigation of local anesthesia of peripheral nerves, with special reference to lidocaine. Acta Physiol. Scand. 51: Suppl. 178: 7–171, 1961.
3. de Jong, R. H.: *Physiology and Pharmacology of Local Anesthesia*, p. 92. Charles C Thomas, Springfield, Ill., 1970.
4. Truant, A. P., and Takman, B.: Differential physical-chemical and neuropharmacologic properties of local anesthetic agents. Anesth. Analg. 38: 478–484, 1959.
5. Lorente de No, R.: On the effect of cocaine upon sodium-deficient frog nerve. J. Gen. Physiol. 35: 203–225, 1951.
6. Condouris, G. A., and Lagomarsino, W. E.: Adrenalectomy in rats and its influence on local anesthesia of peripheral nerves. J. Pharmacol. Exp. Ther. 152: 417–424, 1966.
7. Nathan, P. W., and Sears, T. A.: Differential nerve block by sodium free and sodium deficient solutions. J. Physiol. 164: 375–394, 1962.
8. Goldman, D. E., and Blaustein, M. P.: Ions, drugs and the axon membrane. Ann. N. Y. Acad. Sci. 137: 967–981, 1966.
9. de Jong, R. H., and Wagman, I. H.: Physiological mechanisms of peripheral nerve block by local anesthetics. Anesthesiology 24: 684–727, 1963.
10. Matthews, P. B. C., and Rushworth, G.: The relative sensitivity of muscle nerve fibres to procaine. J. Physiol. 135: 263–269, 1957.
11. Toman, J. E. P.: Neuropharmacology of peripheral nerve. Pharmacol. Rev. 4: 168–216, 1952.
12. Hodgkin, A. L.: *The Conduction of the Nervous Impulse*. Liverpool U.P., Liverpool, 1965.
13. Huruyama, M.: The dependence of the extinction-time upon the number of nodes of Ranvier in narcosis of single nerve fibers. Keio Igaku 21: 201–212, 1941.
14. Tasaki, I.: *Nervous Transmission*. Charles C Thomas, Springfield, Ill., 1953.
15. Melzack, R., and Wall, P. D.: Pain mechanisms: a new theory. Science 150: 971–978, 1965.
16. Nathan, P. W., and Sears, T. A.: Some factors concerned in differential nerve block by local anesthetics. J. Physiol. (London) 157: 565–580, 1961.
17. Pizzolato, P., and Mannheimer, W.: *Histopathologic Effects of Local Anesthetic Drugs and Related Substances*. Charles C Thomas, Springfield, Ill., 1961.
18. Moore, D. C.: *Complications of Regional Anesthesia: Etiology-Signs and Symptoms-Treatment*. Charles C Thomas, Springfield, Ill., 1955.

19. Luduena, F. P.: Duration of local anesthesia. Ann. Rev. Pharmacol. 9: 503–520, 1969.
20. Kristerson, L., Nordenram, A., and Nordqvist, P.: Penetration of radio-active local anesthetic into peripheral nerve. Arch. Int. Pharmacodyn. 157: 148–151, 1965.
21. Foussard-Blanpin, O., and Richer-Deville, M.: Activite comparee de quelques derives de la xylidine proches de la lignocaine sur l'excitabilite du nerf isole a gaine conjonctive intacte ou fendue. Anesth. Analg. (Paris) 25: 35–43, 1968.
22. Sunderland, S.: The connective tissues of peripheral nerves. Brain 88: 841–854, 1965.
23. Shanthaveerappa, T. R., and Bourne, G. H.: Peripheral epithelium: A new concept of its role in the integrity of the peripheral nervous system. Science 154: 1464–1466, 1966.
24. Sunderland, S., and Ray, L. J.: The intraneural topography of the sciatic nerve and its popliteal divisions in man. Brain 71: 242–273, 1948.
25. Ehrenberg, L.: The time-concentration curve of local anesthetics. Acta Chem. Scand. 2: 63–81, 1948.
26. Truant, A. P., and Wiedling, S.: A contribution to the pharmacological and toxicological evaluation of a new anesthetic, d, 1-N-methylpipecolyl-2,6-xylidide. Acta Chir. scand. 116: 351–361, 1959.
27. Bennett, A. L., Wagner, J. C., and McIntyre, A. R.: The determination of local anesthetic-potency by observation of nerve action potential. J. Pharmacol. Exp. Ther. 75: 125–136, 1942.
28. Tucker, G. J., Boyes, R. N., Bridenbaugh, P. O., and Moore, D. C.: Binding of anilide-type local anesthetics in human plasma: I. Relationships between binding, physicochemical properties and anesthetic activity. Anesthesiology 33: 287–303, 1970.
29. Luduena, F. P.: Experimental spinal anesthesia. Arch. Int. Pharmacodyn. 109: 143–156, 1957.
30. Moore, D. C., Bridenbaugh, L. D., and Bridenbaugh, P. O.: Bupivacaine for peripheral nerve block: A comparison with mepivacaine, lidocaine and tetracaine. Anesthesiology 32: 460–463, 1970.
31. Albert, J., and Lofstrom, B.: Bilateral ulnar nerve blocks for the evaluation of local anesthetic agents: III. Tests with a new agent, procaine, and with lidocaine in solution with and without epinephrine. Acta Anaesth. Scand. 9: 203–211, 1965.
32. Adriani, J., Zepernick, R., Arens, J., and Authement, E.: The comparative potency and effectiveness of topical anesthetics in man. Clin. Pharmacol. Ther. 5: 49–62, 1964.
33. Ciocatto, E. M. D., Moricca, G. M. D., and Cavaliere, R. M. D.: Studies on the effect of local anesthetics on peripheral nerve and its metabolism. Proc. 3rd World Congr. Anesthesiol. 1: 241–247, 1961.
34. Akerman, B., Persson, H., and Tegner, C.: Local anesthetic properties of the optically active isomers of prilocaine (Citanest). Acta Pharmacol. Toxicol. 25: 233–41, 1967.
35. Cotev, S., and Robin, G. C.: Experimental studies on intravenous regional anaesthesia using radioactive lignocaine. Brit. J. Anaesth. 38: 936–940, 1966.
36. Bromage, P. R., Burfoot, M. F., Crowell, D. E., and Pettigrew, R. T.: Quality of epidural blockade I: Influence of physical factors. Brit. J. Anaesth. 36: 342–350, 1964.
37. Braid, D. P., and Scott, D. B.: The systemic absorption of local analgesic drugs. Brit. J. Anaesth. 37: 394–404, 1965.
38. Covino, B. G.: Local anesthesia. New Eng. J. Med. 286: 1035–1042, 1972.
39. Tucker, G. T., Moore, D. C., Bridenbaugh, P. O., Bridenbaugh, L. D., and Thompson, G. E.: Systemic absorption of mepivacaine in commonly used regional block procedures. Anesthesiology 37: 277–287, 1972.
40. Lund, P. C.: *Peridural Analgesia and Anesthesia*. Charles C Thomas, Springfield, Ill., 1966.

41. Wilkinson, G. R., and Lund, P. C.: Bupivacaine levels in plasma and cerebrospinal fluid following peridural administration. Anesthesiology 33: 482–486, 1970.
42. Shantha, T. R., and Evans, J. A.: The relationship of epidural anesthesia to neural membranes and arachnoid villi. Anesthesiology 37: 543–557, 1972.
43. Bromage, P. R., Joyal, A. C., and Binney, J. C.: Local anesthetic drugs: Penetration from the spinal extradural space into the neuraxis. Science 140: 392–394, 1963.
44. Bromage, P. R.: Physiology and pharmacology of epidural analgesia. Anesthesiology 28: 592–622, 1967.
45. de Jong, R. H.: *Physiology and Pharmacology of Local Anesthesia*, p. 192. Charles C Thomas, Springfield, Ill., 1970.
46. Usubiaga, J. E., Wikinski, J. Wikinski, R., Usubiaga, L. E., and Pontremoti, M.: Transfer of local anesthetics to the subarachnoid space and mechanisms of epidural block. Anesthesiology 25: 752–759, 1964.
47. Bjorn, H.: The neutralization of acid local anesthetic solutions in the tissues. Svendsk Tandlak. T. 40: 853–867, 1947.
48. Watson, P. J.: The mode of action of local anaesthetics. J. Pharm. Pharmacol. 12: 257–292, 1960.
49. Brown, W. E.: Single injection caudal for obstetrical analgesia and the use of pontocaine. Amer. J. Obstet. Gynec. 55: 717–723, 1948.
50. Truant, A. P.: *Drill's Pharmacology in Medicine*, p. 151. McGraw-Hill, New York, 1965.
51. Cox, J. M. R., and Spoerel, W. E.: Continuous epidural analgesia—The use of an intermittent injection device. Canad. Anaesth. Soc. J. 11: 72–82, 1964.
52. Cohen, E. N., Levine, D. A., Colliss, J. E., and Gunther, R. E.: The role of pH in the development of tachyphylaxis to local anesthetic agents. Anesthesiology 29: 994–1001, 1968.
53. Morch, E. T., Rosenberg, M. K., and Truant, A. T.: Lidocaine for spinal anesthesia: A study of the concentration in the spinal fluid. Acta Anaesth. Scand. 1: 105–115, 1957.
54. Jorgensen, N. B.: Personal communication in reference 2, 1956.
55. Bromage, P. R.: A comparison of the hydrochloride and carbon dioxide salts of lidocaine and prilocaine in epidural analgesia. Acta Anaesth. Scand. Suppl. 16: 55–69, 1965.
56. Catchlove, R. F. H.: The influence of carbon dioxide and pH on local anesthetic action. J. Pharmacol. Exp. Ther. 181: 298–309, 1972.
57. Schulte-Steinberg, O., Harthmouth, J., and Schult, L.: Carbon dioxide salts of lignocaine in brachial plexus block. Anaesthesia 25: 191–197, 1970.
58. Nishimura, N., Morioka, T., and Sato, S.: Effects of local anesthetic agents on the peripheral vascular system. Anesth. Analg. 44: 135–139, 1965.
59. Adriani, J., Zepernick, R., Arens, J., and Authement, E.: The comparative potency and effectiveness of topical anesthetics in man. Clin. Pharmacol. Ther. 5: 49–62, 1964.
60. Hyman, M. D., and Shnider, S. M.: Maternal and neonatal blood concentrations of bupivacaine associated with obstetrical conduction anesthesia. Anesthesiology 34: 81–92, 1971.
61. Trainter, M. L.: Summary of studies on the optimal composition of local anesthetic solutions. Anesthesiology 2: 489–502, 1941.
62. Holler, W.: Die Bedeutung der Wasserstoffionenkonzentration in der lokalanasthesie. Deutsch. Zahnaerztl. Z. 8: 701–706, 1953.
63. de Jong, R. H., and Cullen, S. C.: Buffer-demand and pH of local anesthetic solutions containing epinephrine. Anesthesiology 24: 801–807, 1963.
64. Bromage, P. R., and Robson, J. G.: Concentrations of lignocaine in the blood after intravenous, intramuscular, epidural and endotracheal administration. Anaesthesia 16: 461–478, 1961.

65. Campbell, D., and Adriani, J.: Absorption of local anesthetics. J.A.M.A. 168: 873–879, 1958.
66. Bromage, P. R.: Aging and epidural dose requirements. Brit. J. Anaesth. 41: 1016–1022, 1969.
67. Lund, P. N., Curk, J. C., and Vallesteros, F.: Bupivacaine, a new long-acting local anesthetic agent. A preliminary clinical and laboratory report. Anesth. Analg. 49: 103–114, 1970.
68. Quimby, C. W., Jr.: Influence of blood loss on the duration of regional anesthesia. Anesth. Analg. 44: 387-390, 1965.
69. Morikawa, K., Tucker, G. T., Murphy, T. M., and Bonica, J. J.: Effect of acute hypovolemia on lidocaine absorption and cardiovascular response following peridural block. Anesthesiology. In press.
70. Bromage, P. R.: Exaggerated spread of epidural analgesia in arteriosclerotic patients: Dosage in relation to biological and chronological aging. Brit. Med. J. 2: 1634–1638, 1962.
71. Reynolds, F., and Taylor, J.: Plasma concentrations of bupivacaine during continuous epidural analgesia in labour: The effect of adrenaline. Brit. J. Anesth. 43: 436–440, 1971.
72. Moore, D. C., Bridenbaugh, L. D., Bagdi, P. A., Bridenbaugh, P. O., and Stander, H.: The present status of spinal (subarachnoid) and epidural (peridural) block: A comparison of two techniques. Anesth. Analg. 47: 40–49, 1968.
73. Bonica, J. J., Berges, P. U., and Morikawa, K.: Circulatory effects of peridural block: I. Effects of level of analgesia and dose of lidocaine. Anesthesiology 33: 619–626, 1970.
74. Bonica, J. J., Kennedy, W. F., Akamatsu, T. J., and Gerbershagen, H. U.: Circulatory effects of peridural block: II. Effects of acute blood loss. Anesthesiology 36: 219–227, 1972.
75. Bonica, J. J., Akamatsu, T. J., Berges, P. U., Morikawa, K., and Kennedy, W. F.: Circulatory effects of peridural block. II. Effects of epinephrine. Anesthesiology 34: 514–522, 1971.
76. Rowland, M., Thomson, P. D., Guichard, A., and Melmon, K. L.: Disposition kinetics of lidocaine in normal subjects. Ann. N.Y. Acad. Sci. 179: 383–398, 1971.
77. Tucker, G. J., and Boas, R. A.: Pharmacokinetic aspects of intravenous regional anesthesia. Anesthesiology 34: 538–549, 1971.
78. Boyes, R. N., Scott, D. B., Jebson, P. J., Godman, M. J., and Julian, D. G.: Pharmacokinetics of lidocaine in man. Clin. Pharmacol. Ther. 12: 105–116, 1971.
79. Benowitz, N., Forsyth, R., Melmon, K. L., and Rowland, M.: Lidocaine disposition kinetics in monkey and man: Prediction by a perfusion model. To be submitted to Clin. Pharmacol. Ther.
80. Covino, B. S.: Comparative clinical pharmacology of local anesthetic agents. Anesthesiology 35: 158–167, 1971.
81. Stenson, R. E., Constantino, R. T., and Harrison, D. C.: Hepatic metabolism of lidocaine in man. Circulation 40: 205–211, 1969.
82. Mather, L. E., Long, G. J., and Thomas, J.: The binding of bupivacaine to maternal and foetal plasma proteins. J. Pharm. Pharmacol. 23: 359–365, 1971.
83. Geddes, I. C.: Metabolism of local anesthetic agents. Int. Anesth. Clin. 5: 525–549, 1967.
84. Akerman, B., Astrom, A., and Ross, S.: Studies on the absorption, distribution and metabolism of labelled prilocaine and lidocaine in some animal species. Acta Pharmacol. Toxicol. 24: 389–403, 1966.
85. Moore, D. C., Bridenbaugh, L. D., Bridenbaugh, P. O., Thompson, G. E., and Tucker, G. T.: Does compounding of local anesthetic agents increase their toxicity in humans? Anesth. Analg. 51: 579–585, 1972.
86. Kalow, W.: Hydrolysis of local anesthetics by human serum cholinesterase. J.

Pharmacol. Exp. Ther. 104: 122, 1952.

87. Salgado, A. S.: The distribution of procaine in human blood: Relation to potentiation of succinylcholine. Anesthesiology 29: 1040–1045, 1968.
88. Thomson, P. D., Melmon, K. L., Richardson, J. A., Cohn, K., Steinbrunn, W., Cudihee, R., and Rowland, M.: Lidocaine pharmacokinetics in advanced heart failure, liver disease and renal failure in man. Ann. Int. Med. 78: 499–508, 1973.
89. Fehmers, M. C. O., and Dunning, A. J.: Intramuscularly and orally administered lidocaine in the treatment of ventricular arrhythmias in acute myocardial infarction. Amer. J. Cardiol. 29: 514–519, 1972.
90. Kiese, M.: Relationship of drug metabolism to methemoglobin formation. Ann. N.Y. Acad. Sci. 123: 141–155, 1965.
91. Sadove, M. S., Jobgen, E. A., Heller, F. N., and Rosenberg, R.: Methemoglobinemia, an effect of a new local anesthetic L-67 (prilocaine). Acta Anaesth. Scand. 16: 175–182, 1965.

Index